The Whiplash Encyclopedia

The Facts and Myths of Whiplash

Robert Ferrari, MD, FRCPC
Consultant
Edmonton, Alberta, Canada

AN ASPEN PUBLICATION®
Aspen Publishers, Inc.
Gaithersburg, Maryland
1999

The author has made every effort to ensure the accuracy of the information herein. However, appropriate information sources should be consulted, especially for new or unfamiliar procedures. It is the responsibility of every practitioner to evaluate the apporpriateness of a particular opinion in the context of actual clinical situations and with due considerations to new developments. The author, editors, and the publisher cannot be held responsible for any typographical or other errors found in this book.

Library of Congress Cataloging-in-Publication Data
Ferrari, Robert.
The whiplash encyclopedia: the facts and myths of whiplash / Robert Ferrari.
p. cm.
ISBN 0-8342-1661-2
1. Whiplash injuries—Pathophysiology.   2. Whiplash injuries—Complications.
3. Cervical syndrome—Etiology.   I. Title.
RD533.5.F47   1999
617.1′028—dc21   99-21053
CIP

Orders: (800) 638-8437
Customer Service: (800) 234-1660

About Aspen Publishers • For more than 35 years, Aspen has been a leading professional publisher in a variety of disciplines. Aspen's vast information resources are available in both print and electronic formats. We are committed to providing the highest quality information available in the most appropriate format for our customers. Visit Aspen's Internet site for more information resources, directories, articles, and a searchable version of Aspen's full catalog, including the most recent publications: **http://www.aspenpub.com**
Aspen Publishers, Inc. • The hallmark of quality in publishing
Member of the worldwide Wolters Kluwer group.

Editorial Services: Ruth Bloom
Library of Congress Catalog Card Number: 99-21053
ISBN: 0-8342-1661-2

Printed in the United States of America
1   2   3   4   5

Dedicated to all the workhorses, pack mules,
sled dogs, slaves, and mischievous children
who suffered a whip's lash, with no chance to litigate.

And dedicated to
Dr. John S. Percy, my mentor, my friend,
and the inspiration for this book.

Table of Contents

Preface

The Whiplash Encyclopedia was born out of the realization that although the issue of whiplash is fervently debated in the courts and elsewhere, concerned parties lack a common reference source. If scientific issues are to be debated in court, then lawyers and judges should have a thorough and balanced appreciation of the conclusions reached in the scientific literature. Without having to acquire the knowledge base or experience of a physician (that is what medical expert witnesses are for), one can still attain a better understanding of the subject by reading somewhat more widely and hearing from more than just a few medical experts.

We should all have a resource that explains all the aspects of whiplash that medical experts commonly refer to and provides the basis for those references. This resource was not generally available to most—until now.

This book examines the models that may explain why some individuals report chronic symptoms following an acute injury and others do not. To this end, I have attempted to collect all of the English language scientific literature about whiplash and other relevant topics. Readers can gain insights about whiplash from all these articles, even those whose authors have different opinions than the readers hold. Trying to understand whiplash by ignoring literature that does not accord with one's point of view is not likely to be successful. Thus, I have read, considered, and given mention to each article in at least one place in the text. Some articles are discussed within the main body of the text, others in the bibliographies.

The Whiplash Encyclopedia clearly summarizes this large amount of information for lawyers, health care providers, insurance adjusters, engineers, and so forth. All who would consider whiplash are addressed here.

There are plenty of opportunities in this text (and indeed in many) to debate the suitability and accuracy of the term *whiplash*. It is fruitless to devote too much time to such semantics, since we have much to do and cannot dillydally.

Through such a train of words if I should run,

The day would sooner than the tale be done.

—Burton R. [Democritus Junior]. *The Anatomy of Melancholy.*
London: Chatto & Windus; 1898:43.

Besides, our society has too much bastardized the English language for us to attempt recompense now. Consider the word "infinite," for example. It is used to describe both that truly great distance from our point in the universe to the most distant known galaxy, and also that distance between oneself, snugly and comfortably settled into the couch for the evening, with a cup of tea and a warm blanket at hand, and the television, upon which some villain hath left the remote control.

Acknowledgments

Many thanks to those experts who offered reviews and criticisms of *The Whiplash Encyclopedia* along the way:

Murray Allen (sports and musculoskeletal medicine)
Robert Banks (engineering medicine)
Arthur J. Barsky (psychiatry)
Jeff Burgess (dentistry/oral medicine)
Charles Conquest (grammar)
Ronald Donelson (orthopaedic surgery)
George E. Ehrlich (rheumatology)
Gary Faulkner (engineering)
Charles V. Ford (psychiatry)
Jon Friel (psychology)
Jonathan Gough (engineering)
Hamilton Hall (orthopaedic surgery)
Dean Kolbinson (dentistry)
Oliver Kwan (psychology)
Myer Leonard (oral surgery)
Stephen McAliley (law)
David Mechanic (sociology)
Christopher Pike (law)
Issy Pilowsky (psychiatry)
Anthony S. Russell (rheumatology)
Harald Schrader (neurology)
Edward Shorter (medical history)
Gordon Waddell (orthopaedic surgery)
Simon Wessely (psychiatry)
Harvey West (engineering)
Frederick Wolfe (rheumatology)

I must particularly thank Dr. Oliver Kwan for his help as we successfully struggled through the language and concepts of adoption of the sick role in Chapter 10 and of malingering in Chapter 12.

Introduction

Whiplash has become a medical, legal, and social dilemma. Physicians are not sure how to treat or cure patients with whiplash. Courts are trying to be just to whiplash claimants but also must strive to find the truth. Patients, claimants, and others want answers at a time when few seem available and those that are remain controversial.

The controversy has raged in the medical literature for more than 5 decades now. One reason for this unending contention is that the arguments are being made without a common, reliable reference source. Without this grounding, people are often ill informed, and myths about whiplash pervade discussions. There is general agreement that an acute injury may indeed have occurred in most patients labeled as having whiplash. But controversy begins when accident victims seem to have chronic symptoms and these symptoms are attributed to accidents.

To consider why some individuals report chronic symptoms following an acute injury while others do not, we first address "whiplash cultures" in Chapter 1. This chapter presents a strong argument for reevaluating long-held conceptions about whiplash. If the chronic pain of whiplash is simply due to some chronic damage in the neck, for example, then why does the problem not exist in every country with cars and collisions? Part I attempts to answer that question. Those trying to understand why whiplash is such a problem in their country may actually find the answers by examining why it is not a problem in others.

To understand these cultural differences and how they arise, we will first look at historic examples that give us clues (Chapters 2 and 3). We can then appreciate the context in which the whiplash problem evolved (Chapter 4).

Chapters 5–7 address theories proposed to explain the various chronic symptoms of whiplash. There are numerous theories to explain each symptom, but a unifying theory of acute injury leading to chronic damage that continues to produce symptoms from that original acute injury has not yet emerged.

Alternatively, unifying biopsychosocial models are addressed in Chapters 8 through 10. These models try to explain why some accident victims report chronic symptoms following acute injuries. One is tempted to conclude immediately that the model that accounts for such differences is insurance fraud. Yet it is equally possible that one of two other models better accounts for these cultural differences.

Both models accept that there is an acute physical injury and that multiple physical sources for chronic symptoms interact with each other. These models speak of the inability to pigeonhole whiplash in either a pure physical injury model or a pure psychiatric model. Maintaining these latter polarized, dualistic approaches seems unfeasible and unhelpful given current knowledge. A multidimensional, biopsychosocial approach is necessary.

The first multidimensional model, which addresses primarily the psychocultural basis for reporting chronic symptoms following a minor neck injury, can explain the reporting of chronic symptoms without resorting to labeling all whiplash patients as malingering or as having psychogenic pain that is "all in their heads." The model of whiplash as a psychocultural illness is truly biopsychosocial. It includes the biological—the possibility of acute injury and genuine, chronic symptoms with various physical origins, even though these origins are not in the form of chronic damage that follows the acute injury. The model also considers the psychosocial (wherein it becomes clearer why whiplash claimants in some cultures behave so differently). More important, this first model *does not* demand the conclusion that most whiplash patients have pain because of a psychiatric disorder. Proponents of this model argue that the pain being reported by many whiplash claimants *is not* strictly psychosomatic or psychogenic and does not have the nature of a psychoneurosis. The pain is likely to have contributions from a variety of physical origins, but it is still not, for example, the result of chronic damage in the neck from the acute injury.

A second model deals with a small subgroup of patients whose behavior is quite different from most patients with whiplash but is still culturally sanctioned or determined. The psychocultural basis for their symptoms still exists, but there must be a far greater emphasis on a nonorganic (psychosocial) basis for symptom reporting and illness behavior than the biological factors, which remain diminutive. Like those patients described by model 1, these patients in model 2 may have an acute injury and physical origins for some of their symptoms, but in addition, psychological mechanisms may generate part of their pain and grossly affect their behavior.

Chapter 11 deals with causation by way of the accident through consideration of these models. Chapter 12 deals with assessment, prognosis, and treatment in the new light of these models.

In Part II of *The Whiplash Encyclopedia*, there are two bibliographies. The first is an alphabetical list of the English language scientific literature concerned with whiplash and some related topics. This bibliography has more detailed comments for the interested reader. The second bibliography lists articles of interest under specific topics for easy reference.

Part III of *The Whiplash Encyclopedia* provides additional information, including a review of the anatomy and function of the neck, a discussion of diagnostic tools used in medicine and how studies are conducted, a set of issues specifically relevant for lawyers considering cross-examination, and detailed engineering literature data and tables. A glossary follows.

The book has one central purpose: to investigate why some individuals report chronic symptoms after an acute whiplash injury and others do not.

With that purpose in mind, fasten your seat belts and adjust your head restraints. Here we go.

Whiplash Cultures

The Making of a Whiplash Culture

KEY POINTS

- Some countries have whiplash cultures, and others do not. Although acute whiplash injuries occur wherever there are automobiles and collisions, the recovery rate can vary considerably from one culture to another.
- It is not clear what conditions produce a whiplash culture. However, studying the responses to acute whiplash injuries and the social climates of countries with and without whiplash cultures can provide some clues.
- Our current understanding of what is responsible for the chronic pain following whiplash does not account for these cultural variances. New theories about whiplash must be able to explain the differences.

INTRODUCTION

The acute whiplash injury is real. It appears to exist wherever there are motor vehicle accidents. One can readily produce acute symptoms of neck pain or stiffness in human volunteers subjected to experimental collisions.

Yet, while the acute injury (or at least the acute symptoms that we link to the injury) exists in all cultures, and even in the laboratory setting, in some cultures those with the acute injury continue to report chronic pain for months or even years and also report disability for prolonged periods. There are other cultures where this prolonged pain is not reported.

Thus, in Canada, France, Italy, Japan, the Netherlands, the Republic of Ireland, Scandinavian countries, and Switzerland, for example, there are huge numbers of whiplash patients reporting chronic pain. In Germany, Greece, Lithuania, New Zealand, and Singapore, however, even though whiplash patients report acute pain, they seem to get better within weeks. Why? What do countries in the first group have in common? What do countries in the second group have in common? How do these two groups differ? Why should Lithuanians and Greeks behave similarly even though the cultures are quite different? What makes a whiplash culture? This book addresses these questions.

CULTURAL OBSERVATIONS

A model that considers that chronic symptom reporting arises from some form of chronic damage from the injury could not account for wide differences in the prevalence of such behavior among cultures. Proponents of such a model have largely ignored these cultural differences. Indeed, such cultural differences are inexplicable by such an "injury" model. R. Ferrari and A. S. Russell (1997–1999) are among the most recent to point out these cultural differences.

Switzerland

Although whiplash patients frequently report chronic pain in Switzerland, whiplash patients appear to have a better prognosis in Switzerland than in many other Western countries. In a study, albeit unitary, published in various journals between 1992 and 1996, B. P. Radanov et al examined outcomes in Swiss whiplash patients. Switzerland was considered a useful location because at the time its national insurance system gave whiplash patients full coverage for lost wages and medical expenses. Litigation was rare.

Strictly speaking, there was no direct monetary compensation for pain and suffering. Yet monetary issues were involved. A claimant could receive full pay while not working because of reported disability. (Radanov et al did not measure levels of preaccident job satisfaction.) If a patient claimed there would be future economic loss, he or she could receive a substantial monetary award. Thus, the Swiss culture lacked the whiplash-related litigation present in most North American cultures. Radanov et al demonstrated that in Swiss patients the outcome is clearly much better than in North America.

It may be that removing the litigation process affects an individual's outcome, although Radanov et al did not explore this idea fully. The other explanation, that the different outcomes reflect vastly differing therapeutic approaches, is not valid. The difference between the two outcomes may arise from the adversarial nature and psychological distress of engaging in litigation and "battling" with insurance companies. These effects are less prominent in Switzerland (although patients do have trouble with the insurance system there). The Swiss system is now changing to a tort system (personal injury litigation), and it would be interesting to later repeat the outcome studies by Radanov et al.

Compared to Germany, Greece, Lithuania, and Singapore, however, Switzerland witnesses epidemic proportions of chronic pain in whiplash patients. There is more to the issue than litigation.

Singapore versus Australia

In 1982, J. I. Balla observed that while whiplash patients in Australia commonly report chronic symptoms, patients in Singapore do not, even though the countries have similar numbers of collisions. Singapore's residents are not anatomically or physiologically different from Australians, of course.

What happens after the acute injury may lead to the outcomes in Singapore. A welfare state such as Australia has different sanctions and a different culture than Singapore. Balla explains that in Australia at that time the courts fully sanctioned litigation after injuries, and the state would help an individual to obtain legal aid, if necessary. There would be the hope of monetary compensation for wrongs done to the victim. In Singapore, there are few such avenues open. Balla saw the "late whiplash syndrome" as a culturally constructed illness behavior based on indigenous categories and social determinants.

W. B. Maguire (1993) also described the absence of whiplash patients reporting chronic symptoms in Singapore. He had practiced in Asian cities where accidents were very common, yet he reported that he never saw someone complain of chronic pain from acute neck or back strain. One wonders why patients suffering from severe and long-term symptoms, if they existed, would not present themselves for treatment, even if they were not planning litigation (the system does not encourage this).

Singapore's residents might not routinely hear reports of acute whiplash injury leading to chronic symptoms or disability. If they do not witness such behavior in others, they might not expect such outcomes. Apparently, Singaporeans do not engage in a compensation process that encourages hypervigilance about symptoms; thus, symptom amplification (to be discussed later in Chapter 9) is not as likely. They also do not engage in a process that engenders anxiety, frustration, and resentment (battling with insurance companies and proving one's pain is real). They might not change their activity in response to what they view as a minor injury, so they do not develop poor posture. They will not amplify preaccident symptoms, symptoms from poor posture, or daily life's aches and pains. They will not attribute all these different sources of symptoms to chronic damage they believe the accident caused. In short, Singapore's culture does not encourage the behavior being seen in whiplash patients elsewhere.

New Zealand versus Australia

In 1986, H. Mills and G. Horne studied the difference between whiplash claims in New Zealand and whiplash claims in Australia. There is a very low incidence of whiplash cases in New Zealand compared with the number for the State of Victoria in Australia, even accounting for the differences in number of vehicles and collisions. As the authors explain, the obvious difference between the two countries is the opportunity for litigation. They felt the expectation of financial compensation accounted for most of the difference in chronic whiplash prevalence in the two countries.

Their conclusion may not necessarily be correct. The difference may not be about only financial gain. Mills and Horne did not taken into consideration that the litigation process, and not the ultimate goal of the litigation, may be the adverse aspect for the claimant. Eliminating the process may be the reason New Zealand patients do so well. Further, in Australia and other countries with the problem of chronic whiplash, not all patients with chronic symptoms are malingering for financial gain. What explains *their* behavior? The larger spectrum of cultural factors must be taken into consideration.

Australia, Then and Now

M. S. Awerbuch (1992) and F. T. McDermott (1993) examined the effect of legislation changes on the incidence of reporting chronic symptoms from an acute whiplash injury. They contrasted Australia and Singapore as well but examined most closely the effects of changing legislation in Australia. To claim for whiplash injury in 1987, the claimant had to bear initial costs for the claim (a few hundred Australian dollars), report the accident to the police, and have at least 30% disability. With this simple change in legislation, the annual incidence of whiplash claims in the State of Victoria dropped from almost 6,000 before 1987 to 2,000 in 1989 and is even lower now.

Perhaps there was a great deal of malingering going on and for some reason those malingerers stopped malingering. But otherwise, where did all the chronic pain go? Perhaps people decided not to bother making claims under the more difficult system. Unless one believes there were thousands of malingerers and only a minority of honest claimants, one still has to explain where all the chronic pain complaints went. There should be as many Australians walking around with chronic pain—if that pain was due to some damage caused by the acute injury. That revised legislation can cause such dramatic changes in the epidemiology of chronic whiplash in Australia compels one to ask why the chronic pain exists in the first place. Clearly, a model based on "neck damage" does not explain this.

Chapter 9, which explains the psychocultural model of whiplash (model 1), discusses how removing the claims process itself may remove many factors that are contributing to chronic pain reporting.

United Kingdom—Social Copying

M. Livingston (1992) argued that if chronic whiplash symptoms were due to some chronic physical damage from the acute injury, the existence of a "chronic whiplash syndrome" should have been reported in the United Kingdom not long after it was reported in the United States, instead of 30 years later. Reports of new diseases or forms of trauma spread quickly through the world medical literature unless the conditions are unique to a particular geographical region or culture. Rear-end collisions have presumably been present in the United Kingdom for as long as they have in the United States. Yet the social problem of chronic whiplash is, at least anecdotally, a relatively recent phenomenon in the United Kingdom.

Besides all these anecdotal reports and somewhat systematic observations, there are data tracking the recovery rate of whiplash victims in Germany, Greece, and Lithuania. Even though countries with whiplash cultures use therapies that match or very much exceed those of Germany, Greece, and Lithuania, the outcomes are much worse in whiplash cultures. For example, at 6 to 12 weeks, at least 50% to 70% of whiplash patients continue to report chronic neck pain in the Republic of Ireland (M. F. Gargan and G. C. Bannister 1994), Switzerland (B. P. Radanov and M. Sturzenegger 1994), the United Kingdom (K. Mealy et al 1986), and the United States (P. Gennis et al 1996). Compare these outcomes to those in the countries below.

Greece

According to M. Partheni et al (1997, 1999), the chronic whiplash syndrome appears to be a rare event in Greece. Of 130 accident victims, all suffering acute whiplash injury (judging by their symptoms after an accident), 91% recovered in 4 weeks, and the remainder had substantial improvement to the point where their frequency of neck pain was similar to the general population's. A more recent study in Greece (M. Partheni et al, unpublished data, 1999) included an even larger group of patients. The findings are similar. They also found that at 4 weeks, about 10% of the accident victim group and 10% of a control group of healthy subjects had minor symptoms, thus suggesting that suffering whiplash injury in Greece increases one's risk for headache and neck pain only for the initial 4 weeks after the accident. Thereafter, one's health status returns to the equivalent of an uninjured, otherwise healthy, individual.

Germany

H. Giebel et al (1997) and A. Bonk et al (1999) have shown that the prognosis of acute whiplash injury is remarkably good in Germany. In a study of physiotherapy treatment of 47 patients, by 6 weeks the treatment and control (healthy) groups were equal in their symptom reporting. A second group of 50 patients treated with a collar and medications for 3 weeks had a delayed recovery, but even so, all had recovered in 12 weeks. That is, for the 97 whiplash patients in total, the acute whiplash injury, even though it does appear to generate pain for weeks, does not appear to confer a greater risk of reporting chronic symptoms than is found in the general, uninjured population.

Lithuania

In Lithuania, the acute injury occurs as it does elsewhere in the world. Whiplash injury there, however, does not lead to patients' reporting chronic symptoms. In this country, there is apparently little knowledge of the potential of a whiplash injury to lead to chronic symptoms, and involvement of insurance companies, lawyers, and even the therapeutic community is rare. In this setting, H. Schrader et al (1996) and D. Obelieniene et al (1999) found no increased prevalence of chronic neck pain after a rear-end collision, when compared to the background risk of chronic neck pain in uninjured control subjects.

In the study reported in 1996, the prevalence of any neck pain (even minor and infrequent neck pain) in accident victims was 35.1% and in the general population was approximately 33%. For more significant neck pain (occurring on one day per week or more), the percentages in each group were understandably lower but remained equal. Clearly, being involved in an accident in Lithuania makes one no more likely to report chronic neck pain than not being involved in an accident.

Obelieniene et al (1999) also found, in a prospective study, that neck pain and headaches, besides being very frequent in the general population, occur spontaneously and fluctuate over short periods of time at the same rate and pattern of the Lithuanian accident victims. Are the chronic symptoms being reported by whiplash claimants simply these very same episodes, being attributed to the accident instead? The Lithuanian data certainly bring this possibility to light.

Consider the Lithuanian involved in a collision who suffers an acute injury such as a neck sprain. This individual lives in a culture that has not heard of the possibility that the damage in a neck sprain can routinely become chronic and produce symptoms for that reason. He may view the injury as benign. He might not change his activities as a result of this injury. He might continue working much as he always has, seek little or no medical attention, and make no claim with an insurance company. He will not engage in litigation. Does this affect his outcome?

THE TASK AHEAD

These cultural observations emphasize a need to include many factors in any model of whiplash. International studies have thus given us insight into how certain cultural factors may change the behavior of some whiplash victims. Assuming the observations (from experiments or other studies) are accurate, one's model(s) must account for those observations. If it cannot, the model(s) must be modified or discarded. Thus, any model or models proposed must accomplish the following tasks:

1. Explain why chronic symptoms are not being reported by volunteers in whiplash experiments or in accident victims in, say, Lithuania, even though both groups are frequently experiencing the acute injury.
2. Explain the great variance among cultures in the phenomenon of whiplash patients reporting chronic symptoms that they attribute to the accident.
3. Account for the genuine quality of many of the symptoms being reported.
4. Explain the apparent similarity in the presentation of whiplash patients reporting chronic symptoms.
5. Explain why some patients seem to have symptoms for days, others for months, and others for years, even when these three different outcomes appear to follow the same acute injury.
6. Explain the frequent clinical observation that whiplash patients develop abnormal posture and the relevance of this observation in symptom reporting.
7. Account for the entire symptom complex, such as chronic neck and back pain, dizziness, cognitive symptoms, jaw pain, and so forth.
8. Account for the failure of researchers to identify the source of chronic injury damage after the acute whiplash injury.

The two models proposed in this book represent the beginning, not the end, of our fuller understanding of whiplash.

Before we leap into our exploration of whiplash, there is one more culture from which we can learn: the nineteenth century, when there was railway spine. Railway spine is the medicolegal predecessor of whiplash. For decades, the medical and legal communities struggled to understand railway spine, much as they struggle to understand whiplash now. Our ancestors found a solution, but it took a drastic change in the model they had been using. In Chapter 2, we begin to learn something from them.

Railway Spine

KEY POINTS

- In many ways, the nineteenth-century debate about railway spine resembles the twentieth-century debate about whiplash.
- In the case of railway spine, two opposing views (one that the patient was malingering, the other that the spine was chronically damaged) about the pain's origin eventually gave way to a third theory, that of traumatic neurosis. Might the whiplash debate follow a similar path to resolution?

INTRODUCTION

At the outset, it should be said that railway spine, a nineteenth-century malady, and whiplash are not the same. Diagnoses of railway spine and whiplash follow different types of accidents. Symptoms in the two conditions have separate origins. Yet there is much that we can learn from the history of railway spine and the medicolegal controversy about it.

Railway accidents were quite horrific events, often resulting in explosions, serious injury, and many fatalities. Some train occupants with minor injuries and members of the medical, legal, and insurance community behaved much as similar players do in whiplash-related cases today.

Just as with whiplash, there were two extreme views regarding railway spine. One (chiefly that of the railway insurance companies) was that patients were malingering. The other view was that chronic symptom reporting was due to chronic damage that continued after the acute injury. Insurance fraud could easily have existed then (indeed, some settlements in the late 1800s were equivalent to close to a million dollars today). And various serious injuries may not have been readily detected then. Yet there was also a subset of patients whose symptom reporting

10

appeared to occur when they "had not received a scratch." These patients puzzled medical science.

As a result, the two divergent views were debated in the courts for decades. While a search for the physical damage from the accident went on, only decades later was the basis for chronic symptom reporting understood.

Railway spine found its beginning in the courts. It was popularized when the orthopaedic surgeon Erichsen gave a series of lectures on the basis for chronic pain and other symptoms seen in railway accident victims who, like most whiplash victims today, had no objective and readily provable injury. When compensation for railway injuries became mandatory, railway accidents appeared to produce a peculiar group of accident victims reporting chronic and disabling symptoms, the cause of which no one could quite understand or explain. Nevertheless, the notion that the railway accident was the cause was seemingly undeniable at the time. The legal professionals needed more information from the medical community to satisfy, in part, their clients' desire to be compensated for this personal injury. The medical community was more than willing to comply. Decades of controversy and conjecture ensued. Eventually, people recognized that it was not chronic damage to the spine but a host of psychological factors that led to symptom reporting. Reviewing this history may help us understand how the whiplash controversy has evolved, what it is today, and where we need to look for a solution.

> The first duty of history [is] to ensure that merit shall not lack its record and to hold before the vicious word and deed the terrors of posterity and infamy.
>
> —Jackson J., trans. *The Annals of Tacitus.* Book III, section LXV.
> London: William Heinemann Ltd.; 1962:625.

> He who lives to see two or three generations is like a man who sits in a conjurer's booth at a fair, and witnesses the performance twice or thrice in succession. The tricks were meant to be seen only once; and when they are no longer a novelty and cease to deceive, their effect is gone.
>
> —Schopenhauer A. On the sufferings of the world. In: Saunders T. B., ed.
> *Studies in Pessimism. A Series of Essays by Arthur Schopenhauer.*
> London: Swan Sonnenschein & Co.; 1898:14.

> The novelties of one generation are only the resuscitated fashions of the generation before last.
>
> —Shaw G. B. On Diabolonian ethics. In: *Three Plays for Puritans.*
> Middlesex, England: Penguin Books Ltd.; 1976:24.

"DISCOVERY" OF RAILWAY SPINE

J. E. Erichsen, a British physician, gave a series of lectures in 1866 in which he described railway spine. In his text (1867), he states that he noticed others using the "absurd appellation" of "railway spine" to describe a specific type of injury associated with railway collisions.

He went on to say that he would "endeavor to trace the *train* of progressive symptoms and ill effects that often follow such injuries." (Did he really think he could get away with that pun?)

Patients had sustained no injuries at the actual time of the accident, with "no blow or injury upon the head or spine." Instead, according to Erichsen's theory, "the whole [nervous] system [had] received a severe shake or shock."

Individuals responded with sufficient similarity to such events that they "all present very analogous *trains* of symptoms and phenomena."

Presenting a series of cases, Erichsen characterized the various symptoms. The patients were "anxious and depressed" and "felt ill and shaken." They exhibited symptoms and signs of a "remarkable *train* of nervous phenomena," as listed in Exhibit 2–1.

The patients were not considered to have been malingering. They had grossly limited all aspects of their lives, spending most hours in bed, discontinuing their work altogether, and losing sexual drive and the desire to socialize. They seemed to be giving up their prior good health and livelihood and suffering for months or years.

THEORIES ABOUT RAILWAY SPINE

Erichsen presented two chief theories of how a physical disorder in the spinal cord came about in railway spine patients. Erichsen initially believed that "terror" had much to do with symptom production, but he believed that the terror had somehow caused physical changes in the spinal cord that then led to symptoms. He even wrote that anxiety could cause inflammation in the spinal cord. This is, of course, seemingly impossible. One must realize, however, that in 1866 psychology had not yet formally developed. Erichsen's statement that terror and anxiety had much to do with the production of physical changes to the spinal cord should not be interpreted to mean that the physical damage resulted from psychological factors. That was not likely Erichsen's intent. That is, today we realize that psychological trauma from frightening events can lead to bodily symptoms such as pain. What we would now consider to be an obvious relationship between a psychological (terror) event and a bodily symptom, however, was not an accepted concept in Erichsen's time. Thus, although he was correct about what caused the symptoms of railway spine, he was wrong about the mechanism, as obviously we know today that terror and anxiety do not cause disorder in the spinal cord. Had

Exhibit 2–1   The Symptoms of Railway Spine (as Described by Erichsen, Paraphrased with Current Medical Terminology)

Memory impairment
Poor concentration
Sleep disturbance
Anxiety
Irritability
Back stiffness and pain
Pain on movement of spine
Headache
Hearing problems
Extremity numbness
Arm and hand pain
Loss of sexual desire

Source: Data from J. E. Erichsen, *Railway and Other Injuries*, 1867, Henry C. Lea.

---

he written his text about 30 years later, when psychology was more established, he likely would have been able to understand railway spine as a psychological illness from the beginning. (Indeed, today the explanation for railway spine might be post-traumatic stress disorder or a less severe form of anxiety disorder.)

In a later publication (1886), Erichsen considered a second mechanism. He thought that railway spine might somehow be due to the "jarring back and forth" of the spine, although he could not explain what exactly happened to the spinal cord as a result. (This sounds remarkably familiar to the explanation proposed for whiplash decades later.)

Erichsen did thus provide some insight into the pathogenesis of this illness, railway spine, when he recognized that terror of the accident led to the illness. The medical community and the culture, however, did not have sufficient appreciation of psychology to understand railway spine as a psychological illness. Erichsen remained convinced, as did many, that the chronic symptoms were due to some form of physical disorder. Much of his discussion of what the spine damage was and how it came about was theoretical. Nevertheless, the medical and legal communities at the time accepted these theories as fact. As explained by M. R. Trimble (1981) in his review of the subject:

> Erichsen's work was extremely influential and attracted much attention. . . . The disorder and its accompanying pathology were seized upon by litigants and their friends. . . . Few cases it seems were taken to court without the book appearing and being quoted. The tone of litigation claims changed. In the nineteenth century and before, legal cases involved with personal injury were mainly to do with material injuries,

such as loss of a limb or an eye, where objective evidence was unmistakable and quantifiable. With the advent of "concussion of the spine" the situation changed, and the concept that the injured were victims of at best "shock" . . . became prevalent.

Again, it is probable that insurance fraud did exist in some cases. Yet many physicians at the time, even if they did not accept that symptom reporting was due to some form of chronic spine damage, agreed that there was a genuineness to many patients' complaints. Thus, a model of malingering alone was insufficient, and researchers did not verify a model of chronic spine damage despite decades of trying.

After about 40 years of controversy, a different model evolved. This one took into account the apparent genuineness of many claimants, the nature of the accidents, and the effects of societal influences (including the influences of the medical and legal communities) on the accident victim's behavior. The model explained railway spine as involving a "traumatic neurosis."

This is not to suggest that the mechanism for reporting chronic symptoms after the acute whiplash injury is a traumatic neurosis or post-traumatic stress disorder. An analogy is simply being drawn between how the railway spine controversy evolved and how the whiplash controversy is evolving. It is possible that a very different theory will replace the two divergent views (malingering versus chronic injury) about whiplash, just as it did with railway spine. Are we prepared to consider such a bold step today?

CHAPTER 3

Traumatic Neurosis

A neurosis is a secret you don't know you're keeping.
> —Tynan K. *The Life of Kenneth Tynan*. London: Widenfeld and
> Nicolson Ltd.; 1987:188.

Neurosis is the way of avoiding non-being by avoiding being.
> —Tillich P. *The Courage to Be*. London: Nisbet & Co. Ltd.; 1955:62.

KEY POINTS

- Traumatic neurosis, the concept that solved the railway spine dilemma, accepted that patients had genuine symptoms (including pain) but not that chronic damage was the cause of their symptoms.
- A third, previously unknown theory ended the railway spine controversy. Therefore, those involved in the whiplash debate should stay open to theories other than those around which the debate now centers.

A THIRD POSSIBILITY

The solution to the nineteenth-century medicolegal controversy about railway spine involved an ability and willingness to look at other possibilities. Initially, there were two chief models used to explain chronic symptoms in railway spine patients. One was that everyone was malingering, a view that remained largely unverifiable and seemingly unconscionable to the medical community and others. The second possibility was that the symptoms arose from some chronic damage in the spine that could not be identified but was responsible for not only chronic pain but a host of other chronic symptoms.

15

Erichsen's theory was, of course, that there was a form of chronic damage. Many physicians, including H. Page, who published his book in 1883, challenged this model. M. R. Trimble (1981) quotes Page's thoughts on railway spine (1883), especially after minor collisions (and there was indeed an alarming increase in the number of claims even after minor railway collisions): "Small wonder when a man gets a slight sprain of his vertebral column in the most trifling collision on a railway that, labouring under the belief he has received a 'concussion of the spine,' his anxiety should be needlessly great and prolonged."

As Trimble further explains, "Page . . . introduced into his argument the concept of nervous shock, which was essentially psychological in origin." Page was clear to point out that most patients were not malingering and noted that "they are examples free . . . from the taint of conscious exaggeration."

In 1888, A. Strümpell (A. M. Stalker 1894) also felt that patients with traumatic neurosis were not "shamming" or "intentionally exaggerating their complaints." From observations of patients at various stages, he was able to elucidate the series of psychological events that produced the patient's illness. Thus, Strümpell opened the way for discussion of concepts not fully appreciated by many members of the medical community just decades earlier. From the early 1900s to the 1930s, there was greater realization in the medical literature, the courts, and society that reporting of chronic symptoms in the railway spine victim was not a result of ongoing, chronic physical damage. Instead, there may have been no or a minor physical injury. Symptoms evolved partly through a psychological injury, with genuine symptoms (albeit modified by circumstances such as feelings of victimization, preaccident psychosocial factors), and partly through the influences of the medical, legal, and insurance communities.

SUMMARY

Railway spine came to be viewed as a complex illness evolving from specific psychological events related to the accident, and as such it remained a "personal injury." This phenomenon—then labeled "traumatic neurosis"—provided a new explanation of railway spine. This made it unnecessary to consider all railway spine patients malingering, or to insist on some unidentified physical damage as the explanation for chronic symptom reporting. Traumatic neurosis produced genuine symptoms mediated by psychological mechanisms.

Again, traumatic neurosis does not explain why whiplash victims report chronic symptoms. The lesson that the railway spine debate has for the whiplash debate is the importance of considering other theories. With these thoughts, the discussion turns to whiplash.

The Medical History of Whiplash

In 1928 as a young man in orthopedic surgery I presented eight cases of neck injury to a medical meeting in San Francisco simply to ask the members of the audience to tell me what on earth had happened to these injured persons. . . . I have regretted the coinage ever since because the coinage proved to be counterfeit. . . . I never published the term "whiplash injury" but it spread across the country, got into published literature and became a household word which is used thoughtlessly by the layman, the attorney and the physician.

—H. E. Crowe (1958)

KEY POINTS

- Whiplash was originally defined as a mechanism of injury.
- Early theories were produced and propagated in the media and the courts as if they were factual.

INTRODUCTION

When H. E. Crowe coined the term *whiplash injury* in 1928, he could hardly have imagined the medicolegal and social controversy that was to unfold. Whiplash was to become a complex topic inciting frequent contention in both medical and legal circles.

Physicians did not introduce "whiplash" into the medical literature until 1945. Recall that by 1945 the medical and legal professions should have been aware of the illness of traumatic neurosis. Further, there was ongoing discussion about compensation for traumatic neurosis. When physicians introduced the proposed physical mechanism of whiplash, the focus interestingly shifted from traumatic neurosis to physical injury of a chronic nature, and, in the courts, to compensation for that physical injury.

THEORIES

Whiplash has had many definitions since 1928. Originally, some used it to explain how a rear-end collision would cause the subject's neck to bend backward (extend) because the collision moved the body forward. The head, which did not experience the same sudden acceleration of the body (not being rigidly aligned to the rest of the body), "fell behind." The result was neck extension (or hyperextension if the degree of extension was extreme). As the subject's vehicle slowed down, the head would begin to move forward. When the car and the subject's body stopped altogether, the head would still continue to move forward for a short time on its inertia, with the chin moving toward the chest. The result here was neck flexion (or hyperflexion if the degree of flexion was extreme). Whiplash seemed appropriate to describe this movement. Presumably, in frontal collision, there would be a reversal of these head movements. If there was a component of impact from the side (lateral), then the head would tilt to one side during this whiplash motion. Thus, researchers first based theories of whiplash on these concepts.

In 1945, A. G. Davis opened the discussion: "Starting with the fact that the great majority of injuries of the cervical spine are in the nature of a 'whip lash,' and accepting the meaning of the term 'whip lash' as a *hyperflexion* [emphasis added] followed by spontaneous extensor recoil, the nature of a great variety of injuries of this section of the spinal column becomes understandable." He argued that "automobile head-on collision is the most prolific cause. The extreme mobility of the cervical section of the spine permits the weight of the head to continue its forward momentum after the moment of impact."

As we shall see, the dogma of whiplash would evolve so that hyperextension, not hyperflexion, was the mechanism of injury. Whatever the mechanism, the concept of injury in patients suffering chronic pain from automobile accidents was now being firmly established in the medical literature.

In 1953, J. R. Gay and K. H. Abbott began the characterization of symptoms, and with this and Davis's theories, the term *whiplash* was used to indicate a physical injury producing certain symptoms.

> Most of the accidents that involved a whiplash injury were caused by a collision in which one vehicle was rammed from behind by another vehicle. . . . The mechanics of the injury were interpreted as a sudden and forceful flexion of the neck, followed, in some instances, by several other less violent oscillations of the neck in alternating flexion and extension. The basic pathological change was mechanical trauma of the supporting ligaments of the cervical spine.

> Symptoms consisted of pain in the lower cervical spine, limitation of motion of the neck, and spasm and tenderness of the cervical spinal musculature. Tenderness and spasm were often present in adjacent

musculature, including the muscles of the upper thoracic spine and shoulder girdle. . . . Cervical radiculitis . . . [led to] . . . intense pain in the posterior cervical region, with radiation of pain into the occipital region of the skull, lower jaw, shoulder girdle, upper anterior chest, or upper extremities.

Other symptoms included "neuromuscular tension, restlessness, irritability, subjective vertigo, poor concentration, insomnia . . . vasomotor instability, recurrent headaches, mood changes, and general nervousness." (See Exhibit 4–1.)

If there was "a profound emotional reaction due to the circumstances of the accident, or a predisposition for a psychoneurotic reaction to develop, it was usual for the nervous symptoms to return, recur, and persist for many months."

Gay and Abbott (1953) also noted other psychological aspects.

The accident involved a sudden, violent, and unexpected jolt that was a disturbing experience. Since the victim was seldom incapacitated immediately after the accident, there was opportunity for development of considerable hostility toward the offending motorist. A tedious investigation usually followed the accident at a time when the patient was bewildered, emotionally disturbed, and uncomfortable. . . . [The] next day frightening symptoms began, such as pain in the neck and head, radiating pain and paresthesias in the limbs, or aching in the lower back. Most of these sensations had never been experienced before. Lacking

Exhibit 4–1 The Symptoms of Whiplash (as Described by J. R. Gay and K. H. Abbott, Paraphrased with Current Medical Terminology)

Memory impairment
Poor concentration
Sleep disturbance
Anxiety
Irritability
Back stiffness and pain
Pain on movement of spine
Headache
Extremity numbness
Arm and hand pain
Flushing

Source: Data from J. R. Gay and K. H. Abbott, Common Whiplash Injuries of the Neck, *Journal of the American Medical Association*, Vol. 152, No. 18, pp. 1698–1704, © 1953, American Medical Association.

understanding on the variety, extent, and nature of their injuries and ill-prepared to alleviate their discomfort, these patients were prone to the development of apprehension, anxiety, and neuromuscular tension.

The development of psychoneurosis was the most important factor in delaying recovery. In some patients, the aggravation of legal action was considered important, but even after settlement, these patients were often partially disabled by recurrent nervous symptoms.

Sound familiar? What followed was an attempt to identify the physical tissue damage that was responsible for not only the initial neck pain but also chronic neck pain. For certain complications of automobile accidents, such as fractures or spinal cord damage with neurologic signs, the site of damage was not difficult to identify. In the much larger group of patients who did not have fractures or spinal cord injury, however, no one had firsthand knowledge of the actual site that was supposedly chronically damaged. Instead, physicians made "educated guesses." Theories abounded. The task for researchers was difficult. It was not simply a matter of defining the damage that occurred with the acute injury but showing that the damage persisted in actively producing chronic symptoms.

The scientific literature reveals that for 5 decades researchers have been able to provide only theories of this chronic damage that continues to cause symptoms. The theories sound very plausible and logical, but they remain unverified theories. Unfortunately, these theories have been passed down as fact through much of this controversy, because they seem so scientifically valid.

> For men's opinions are accepted in the trains of ancient beliefs, by authority and on credit, as if they were religion and law. They accept by rote what is commonly held about it. They accept this truth, with all its structure of apparatus and arguments and proofs, as a firm and solid body, no longer shakable, no longer to be judged. On the contrary, everyone competes in plastering up and confirming this accepted belief with all the power of their reason, which is a supple tool, pliable, and adaptable to any form. Thus the world is soaked with twaddle and lies.
>
> —Frame D. M., trans. Apology for Raymond Sebond. In: *The Complete Works of Montaigne.* Stanford, CA: Stanford University Press; 1957:403.

It will become apparent that many researchers were prepared to accept the theories as facts before the proof was available. Researchers were perhaps hopeful that their beliefs would soon prove themselves true through science and, in the meantime, would satisfy the hasty appetite for quick solutions to the whiplash controversy.

My observation is made from the hill of song, and not from that of science, and will, I trust, be found sufficiently accurate for the present purpose.

—Longfellow H. W. The occultation of Orion. In: *The Poetical Works of Henry W. Longfellow.* London: Ward, Lock, Bowden and Co.; 1860:488.

SUMMARY

The following chapters discuss some of the theories proposed to explain how an accident injury could cause some form of damage that in turn could be the basis of chronic symptoms, chiefly neck pain, but also many other symptoms. In each chapter, the flaws of each theory are discussed. Not every relevant medical article is mentioned, but they are all listed in Part II, Literature Review.

Before considering in detail the models that can explain the cultural differences in the problem of chronic whiplash, however, it is necessary first to ask a question: On what basis do specialists presume that the chronic symptoms arise from some form of chronic damage caused by the acute injury? To date, researchers have not been able to find the mysterious origin of the chronic damage. (If they had, whiplash would not be a controversy.) The following chapters discuss the arduous attempts researchers have made over the years to find the physical damage that causes all these chronic symptoms.

To appreciate the search for theories and models, one needs at least a rudimentary understanding of the anatomy of the neck, the diagnostic tools researchers use, and the principles they consider when conducting studies. Readers unfamiliar with these important concepts are referred to Chapter 15, Anatomy and Function of the Neck, and Chapter 16, Diagnostic Tests.

Chronic Neck Pain

KEY POINTS

- Most whiplash patients have either a Grade 1 or a Grade 2 whiplash-associated disorder as defined by the Quebec Task Force on Whiplash-Associated Disorders (1995). This ultimately means that they do not have any injury that can be objectively proven. They report pain, tenderness, and other symptoms that are very subjective (difficult to refute or prove).
- There are many theories attempting to explain chronic neck pain as a consequence of physical damage from the acute injury. Researchers have employed various diagnostic tools to find a site of chronic damage and explain the chronic pain.
- Engineering analysis is very important in low-velocity collisions. Engineering concepts such as striking velocity, change in velocity (ΔV), and head acceleration are used to indicate the risk of injury from a given collision.
- Experiments using human volunteers have not shown that collisions lead to the type of chronic neck pain reported by many whiplash patients. Human volunteers in experiments have behaved much like Lithuanian accident victims.

INTRODUCTION

Most research has been directed toward understanding why some who suffer an acute injury go on to report chronic neck pain. Back pain is also frequently reported in a chronic fashion, but the discussions here, because many of them apply to back pain in any case, will focus on neck pain, where the research has also focused.

NECK PAIN AND WHIPLASH

The Quebec Task Force (QTF) on Whiplash-Associated Disorders classification (see W. O. Spitzer et al 1995) grades whiplash-associated disorders from 1 to 4. Grade 1 is characterized by a complaint of neck stiffness only, with no abnormalities reportedly found on examination. Grade 2 is characterized by reporting of neck pain and sites of tenderness, and a reduced range of spine motion. Within this grade, patients may be reporting other symptoms including back pain, jaw pain, dizziness, and so forth. Grades 3 and 4 are distinguished by the requirement of clearly objective findings (ie, findings that do not rely on patient input for positive identification of the sign). These include loss or diminishment of deep tendon reflexes, objective muscle weakness, and sensory deficits in a specific dermatomal pattern reflecting nerve injury (Grade 3) or where X-ray findings include fracture or vertebral dislocation (Grade 4). These latter two grades apply to few "whiplash" injury claims. In contrast, Grades 1 and 2, which account for most claims of whiplash injury, are diagnosed largely by symptom reporting. There are no truly objective findings (ie, findings that are independent of the patien's input). One cannot, by physical examination, truly prove or disprove the injury.

This is not only true of the whiplash claimant reporting neck or back pain. It may seem surprising, but the precise anatomical structure responsible for spontaneous episodes of acute neck or back pain in the general population remains unclear in all but a few patients. Not surprisingly, in most whiplash patients, one cannot readily determine whether pain reporting stems from lesions of facet joints, discs, muscles, ligaments, or all or none of the above. The importance of this is that it may be entirely possible that the chronic symptoms being reported by whiplash patients may arise from a number of sources. These other sources may have nothing to do with the acute injury.

Again, many are prepared to accept that individuals who have mild and short-lived symptoms have suffered a neck muscle sprain (microscopic tears in muscle and surrounding tissue have occurred). Efficient and ready healing is the expected and observed outcome of muscle sprains elsewhere in the body. Many are not prepared to accept, therefore, that a muscle sprain will produce a form of damage that remains chronically active in producing symptoms. That is why, after almost 5 decades of discussion in the medical literature, L. Barnsley et al (1994) stated openly that no studies have identified a chronic, painful muscle pathology following trauma in whiplash patients. The traditional expectation is that muscle sprains will heal in weeks, forming a scar within the muscle as in other parts of the body and producing no residual pain.

The general assumption is that Grade 1 or Grade 2 whiplash-associated disorders represent a sprain. This assumption may find support in certain experimental observations. First, volunteers in whiplash experiments and German, Greek, and Lithuanian accident victims behave as if they have had a minor sprain, with symptom reporting resolving after days to weeks (see later in this chapter under "Whiplash Experiments"). Second, Kallieris et al (1991) demonstrated the point (in terms of collision severity) at which human volunteers report acute symptoms. The simultaneous subjection of cadavers to these symptom-producing collisions shows the cadavers to have sustained microscopic tears in the muscles or ligaments of the neck. Third, bone scans and magnetic resonance imaging (MRI) scans are capable of detecting more serious and significant muscle or ligament tears (ie, more than microscopic bleeding, which is what occurs with minor sprain), disc rupture, spinal joint disruption, or nervous system injury. Yet studies have failed to detect these in the vast majority of whiplash patients (see "Radiology of Whiplash" below). There is thus no evidence that in most patients the injury is anything more than a minor sprain.

Similar muscle or ligament tears occur in ankle sprains. In some severe cases, ankle sprains may represent a complete tear of a muscle or ligament, but these are readily detectable by tests such as MRI scans (C. De Simoni 1996). For these more severe sprains, there appears to be a correlation between outward and objective, clinical signs of injury and the MRI findings. As such, in Grade 1 or 2 whiplash-associated disorder (that is, most whiplash patients), one expects the sprain to be minor (microscopic tears) because MRI findings reveal no evidence of more severe damage.

Nevertheless, many have argued that ongoing, chronic muscle or other damage does exist and persist and that the initial physical injury thereby explains both the initial pain and the chronic pain as well. Theories became more fanciful with time.

In 1953, for example, H. E. Billig Jr argued that "narrowing of one or more of the cervical dorsal intervertebral discs, by compression, as revealed by roentgenographic studies" was the source of chronic neck pain.

To this, J. R. Gay and K. H. Abbott (1953) added a separate theory: "There is trauma of the spinal ligaments because of the characteristic symptoms of a sprain of the neck. . . . It is likely that there is hemorrhage and edema in the region of the damaged ligaments that may be a source of nerve irritation. Later on, fibrosis and cicatricial changes may be a chronic source of irritation of the nerve roots."

Billig (1953), M. M. Braaf and S. Rosner (1958), A. Fields (1956), O. L. Huddleston (1958), and E. Seletz (1958) all attempted to explain a source of chronic "damage." They believed this came from the initial injury and that the chronic damage caused ongoing pain complaints. They each selected a specific anatomical site in the neck and theorized on how acute injury there could cause neck pain. They then theorized how that injury would manifest chronic damage in the neck that would then cause chronic neck pain. They offered no objective study or evidence, merely conjecture. (See Chapter 13 for comments on these articles.)

Eventually, articles appeared to remind others not only that they were dealing with theories but that some theories did not even seem sensible. T. A. R. Dinning

(1993), for instance, questioned whether the acute tissue trauma was responsible for chronic symptoms in whiplash patients: "In the course of some hundreds of operations on the cervical spine performed by both posterior or anterior approaches, during which severe surgical trauma is inflicted on muscles, fascia, ligaments, periosteum, bone, and joints, I can recall only two patients who complained of persistent pain and tenderness in the neck and shoulder girdle after the expected two to three months postoperative convalescence. Tissue injuries do heal."

Long before this, J. F. R. Fleming (1973) had already noted that "in major neck surgery, muscles are pulled, contused, and detached, yet these patients do not have prolonged neck and head pains."

Indeed, it is difficult to conceive of a form of acute muscle or other "soft tissue" damage responsible for chronic pain and other symptoms, that a surgeon cannot induce in an obviously traumatic event. Nevertheless, researchers have dutifully searched for evidence of both the acute injury and the chronic damage it is supposed to have caused. Radiologic tools have helped with this search.

RADIOLOGY OF WHIPLASH

It seems reasonable to assume that one could demonstrate that an acute whiplash injury causes a chronic form of damage in, say, the neck, by finding radiologic abnormalities in those reporting chronic symptoms. One would still need to demonstrate that the cause of the abnormality is the accident and that the abnormality is causing the symptom, but to find this abnormality would be a start. That is what researchers have been attempting for a number of decades now. While using each new diagnostic technique to try to capture an objective sign of the chronic damage, researchers have generated a great deal of data. There have often been, however, flaws in the research, leaps in logic, and misconceptions. The discussion below deals with examples of this phenomenon (Chapters 13 and 14 list additional articles and details about them). As it turns out, all such attempts have so far been unsuccessful. Here is an exploration of the reasons why and an opportunity to address the many myths that persist about the radiology of whiplash patients.

In 1945, A. G. Davis concluded, without any proof, that an X-ray finding of "elimination of the normal forward convexity of the cervical spine indicates mechanical derangement of the posterior intervertebral joints."

He had no way of proving this because he could not dissect the necks of his patients and study their joints. Nevertheless, many said that the straightening of the normal curve in the cervical spine (the cervical lordosis) clearly indicated some form of significant (and chronic) damage to some structure in the neck. Many ignored the need to have control populations in their studies. They allowed false conclusions to perpetuate themselves in the literature and in the courts. Researchers could have avoided years of misconception and controversy if studies had control groups (a group of asymptomatic people who have X-rays taken of their necks). Many of the scientific studies on whiplash patients lacked control groups. This phenomenon warrants closer examination, as it simultaneously reveals the success (or failure) of the search for the chronic neck damage the acute injury is reported to have caused.

Whiplash and the Straight Spine

In 1944, L. A. Hadley reasoned that:

> Arthritis or trauma interferes with the demonstrable movement between the various cervical segments so that either from spasm or fixation the flexion-extension studies may reveal a lack of movement between various segments either at one level or involving the whole cervical spine. . . . Upon subsequent examination it will be found that, in some cases, complete recovery of normal movement has taken place while in others the fixation seems to be permanent. By this method it is possible to furnish roentgen evidence of injury and of progress in recovery even when the roentgenogram does not show evidence of bone or joint injury.

Hadley did not study the issue systematically with patients. He did not attempt to find asymptomatic people or individuals who had no trauma (a control population). It is thus difficult to draw any meaningful conclusions from his study's information.

In time, researchers would combat the many falsehoods resulting from poor research. In 1958, H. E. Crowe started this movement. Crowe referred to A. G. Davis's statement in 1945 that "elimination of the normal forward convexity of the cervical spine indicates mechanical derangement of the posterior intervertebral joints" in relating his concerns. Note how deeply entrenched this misconception was in day-to-day court activities and that it had been in place for at least 11 years.

> This change in posture is something with which all of you who do trial work are familiar, viz., that the curve which is normally forward in the region of the neck, as seen in an x-ray taken from the lateral view, will be straightened or even reversed as a result of the type of [whiplash injury]. Here at last it appeared to us that as medical men we now had an objective sign to tell whether or not the accident in which the patient had been involved had actually produced physical injury or had produced only the tension, which leads to neck symptoms in the absence of any physical injury. With this positive finding now clearly visible to physicians, patients,

attorneys, and jurors it seemed as though this complicated problem would now be readily solved so that we could settle definitely and objectively on the amount of injury, the persistence of injury, and the recovery from injury. This, however, did not prove to be the case.

It was not many years until it was possible to show that in the excitement of fear, anger, and tense emotional stress the flattening of the cervical lordosis was a normal physiologic reaction in many animals including man. One of the first and most notable cases reported of this kind was that of the woman who was at home in a chair when her daughter was involved in an automobile accident. As a result of the daughter's accident the mother developed neck symptoms. Her x-rays showed the characteristic flattening of the cervical lordosis which we had thought objective evidence of physical injury. The woman herself was involved only in the excitement of having heard by telephone from the police that her daughter was in an automobile accident.

D. Munro (1960) also cautioned against the study done by Hadley years earlier with cadavers. He noted that "the ability, inherent in the ligament, to stretch and contract is a characteristic of normal live tissue. For this reason experiments on the cadaver cannot be significant, nor can this condition be expected to develop as the result of an injury to an otherwise normal spine."

Studies Remove the Misconception

The proper, controlled studies began to appear thereafter. In 1960, for example, H. R. Zatzkin and F. W. Kveton compared 50 whiplash patients to 35 normal adults. Their findings revealed that "it is apparent that the presence of a slight degree of straightening of the usual lordotic cervical curve cannot be used as a criterion for the diagnosis of a whiplash injury. . . . Segmental straightening was observed with greater frequency in the *normal* group. Slight limitation of flexion of the neck would also appear not to be a significant finding upon which to base a diagnosis of a whiplash injury."

At the same time, J. O. Lottes et al (1959) added that mild abnormalities on X-rays were being labeled as traumatic. The abnormalities exist in individuals with no symptoms or history of trauma: "If one flexes the neck forward of a normal uninjured person and then makes a lateral x-ray examination, many times one will see the vertebral segments glide forward a few millimeters upon each other. . . . If this patient has [whiplash] and one takes a similar film, one can see the same findings. In the minds of some authorities that constitutes a minor degree of subluxation. They are probably labeling a normal variation [as] a minor degree of dislocation."

In addition, J. H. Juhl et al (1962), after studying 116 volunteers ranging from 10 to 60 years of age with no known injury of the neck, found that:

> In 22 [patients] the cervical curve was straight, which we considered to be normal. Sixteen had reversal of the curve and 8 had angulation in addition to reversal. These patients were asymptomatic, with no known history of trauma. It is therefore evident that, contrary to reports in the literature, such findings are not necessarily indicative of a symptom-producing abnormality of the cervical spine. The slight variations observed following whiplash injuries do not necessarily indicate injury to ligamentous supporting structures or intervertebral disks. The significance of such alterations in the cervical spine when noted in a patient who has had an injury, is therefore open to question. Voluntary contraction of neck muscles produced alterations in the curve in most of the patients who had a normal lordosis in the neutral position.

> Albers, who studied 1,100 subjects found a straight cervical spine in nearly one-half of [normal subjects] and therefore considered that this was often entirely within normal limits and did not imply injury.

More studies of asymptomatic individuals would continue to show just how abnormal the healthy general population was. A. G. B. Borden et al (1960) studied the cervical spines of 180 individuals who had no complaints referable to the neck and no history of injury. They ranged in age from 20 to 80 years. The researchers discovered that "the cervical curve may . . . be completely flattened or even reversed in the absence of symptoms. Its loss was noted mainly after the age of fifty and was usually proportionate to the degree of hypertrophic degenerative change."

In 1986, while studying 200 asymptomatic individuals, D. R. Gore et al extended even further the concept of what was "normal" for a patient's age:

> Because the normal cervical lordosis is thought to result from the wedge shape of intervertebral discs, it is not surprising to find that decreased cervical lordosis was associated with disc space narrowing in older subjects.

> Because none of our subjects had present or past symptoms referable to their neck, it appears that loss of lordosis or actual kyphotic deformities are probably normal variations. Thus, great care must be exercised in establishing a prognosis for a symptomatic patient based on this roentgenographic finding.

> It is important to realize that although roentgenographic abnormalities represent structural changes in the spine, they do not necessarily cause symptoms.

Finally, in 1994, P. S. Helliwell et al considered whether even the argument that the cervical lordosis straightens due to muscle spasm is correct. If so, one would expect to find this more often in whiplash patients than in people without neck pain. In a study of 83 whiplash patients, and comparison to controls, they demonstrated that it is completely "normal" to find a straight cervical spine in many individuals in the general population.

Summary

It is therefore incorrect to conclude that a straight cervical spine on X-ray is necessarily a sign of physical injury in whiplash patients. Found so frequently in the general population, it may be of no significance. That is not to say that an acute injury does not occur, merely that this is not a reliable sign of such an injury.

Another consideration researchers addressed was determining whether patients involved in rear-end and other collisions develop damage to or degeneration of the cervical discs. If they did, this would at least verify the site of injury.

WHIPLASH AND DISC DEGENERATION

There are numerous signs of disc degeneration on an X-ray, including disc space narrowing, osteophytes, and changes in vertebral alignment with respect to one another. It is also possible to note abnormalities in the appearance of the facet (zygapophysial) joints. As such, in looking for evidence of chronic damage following the acute whiplash injury, researchers have considered whether whiplash victims reporting chronic symptoms developed degenerative changes sooner than healthy subjects. Researchers have thoroughly examined this possibility over the years. Along the way, many misconceptions accompanied the discussions.

There are several questions regarding the significance of X-ray findings of disc degeneration.

- Do these abnormalities on X-ray predict symptoms? Is there a correlation between the severity of changes on X-ray and the severity of symptoms?
- Do whiplash patients who begin with a normal X-ray at the time of the accident develop these changes on X-ray earlier than the general population?
- Do individuals who have preexisting X-ray abnormalities develop an acceleration of these changes after a collision, or a worse outcome?

The answer to the two questions listed in the first item above is that no, X-rays do not predict symptoms, and there is a lack of a correlation between X-ray changes and symptoms. One can have severe neck pain with a normal X-ray or have a severely abnormal X-ray with no neck pain. ("Intervertebral Discs" in Chapter 15 deals with this in more detail.) "Degenerative disc disease" is a misnomer. Disc degeneration is not a disease but rather a natural consequence of aging. As such, it does not signify disease or injury. Despite the theoretical consideration of increased vulnerability to injury, most people will develop disc degeneration as they age and yet will not have any symptoms. Everyone develops disc degeneration, and eventually everyone develops abnormal radiologic findings associated with disc degeneration. Unfortunately, the misnomer has persisted, even though many would prefer to use the phrase *disc degeneration*, with no implication that this is a disease. The message here is simply that it is incorrect to blame neck pain on the X-ray findings of disc degeneration. (Chapter 15 offers a detailed discussion of the reasons for this.)

The questions listed beside the second and third bullets above, however, deal with the possibility that acute whiplash injury might cause or accelerate disc degeneration. To date, there remains no evidence of any significant effect of trauma disc degeneration.

Misconceptions

One of the earliest articles about injury and disc degeneration reveals the faulty reasoning that may occur. In 1953, A. Myers stated that "careful questioning of the past medical history of patients with degenerative lesions of the cervical spine reveals that many of them have sustained a whip-lash injury in the recent or distant past. After an asymptomatic interval of several months to several years these patients then developed degenerative lesions of the spine."

Careful questioning of patients with degenerative lesions of the cervical spine may also reveal that many of them have not been to church in the recent past. Should that lead one to infer that failure to attend church was the reason they developed degenerative lesions of the cervical spine?

> Thus saith the Lord of hosts, the God of Israel; Behold, I will bring upon this city and upon all her towns all the evil that I have pronounced against it, because they have hardened their necks, that they might not hear my words.
>
> —Jeremiah 19:15

Obviously, many people would not accept a theory that an abnormal neck X-ray was linked to failure to attend church because it seems less plausible than the notion that a collision, producing injury, caused the X-ray changes. Plausibility and truth, however, are not the same. That injury is a more plausible cause of neck X-ray changes does not necessarily make such a conclusion correct.

To demonstrate a relationship (failure to attend church or prior neck injury as a cause of X-ray changes), one needs a control group. One compares, for example, how often degenerative lesions of the cervical spine occur in people who have regularly attended church and those who have not regularly attended church. If degenerative changes occur just as often in each group, there is no association between failure to attend church and an increased risk for disc degeneration. Myers erred in conducting a study without an appropriate control population.

Acute Whiplash Injury Does Not Accelerate Disc Degeneration

Addressing this issue in 1960, Munro noted that:

> Except for rather halfhearted attempts to explain the original degeneration of the disk that starts the process of spondylosis, on the basis of repeated and cumulative minimal "injuries" resulting from the necessarily constant motion of the cervical spine and its joints and ligaments, I have been unable to find any significant study of the relation between a single episode and either the initiation or aggravation of spondylosis or the production of symptoms by the spondylitic process in a patient with previously asymptomatic and hence previously unsuspected spondylosis.

He therefore conducted a study looking at the relationship between symptoms and disc degeneration, and the aggravation or causation of those symptoms due to neck injury. He looked at patients who had various types of accidents, including those thought to produce a whiplash injury. As he stated:

> An acute injury of significant proportions to the cervical spine and its contents cannot be held to be the proximal or direct cause of any osseous, ligamentous, articular, or neurologic signs or symptoms resulting from spondylosis cervicalis [since the majority had symptoms prior to the accident]. There is also no tenable evidence to support the theory that injury to the cervical spine and its contents aggravates the symptoms of spondylosis [since they had not appreciably changed from the symptoms prior to the accident].

M. Hohl (1974) also revealed an interesting finding in his patients. He found that 58% of patients with radiological evidence of disc degeneration had no symptoms later, but 44% of patients who had normal X-rays continued to have symptoms. This points out that X-ray findings have little to do with outcome and little relationship to symptoms.

J. I. Balla and R. Iansek (1988), C. Hildingsson and G. Toolanen (1990), K. A. Miles (1988), H. V. Parmar and R. Raymakers (1993), and J. M. S. Pearce (1989, 1992) have all confirmed that disc degenerative changes in the neck do not develop any more rapidly in whiplash patients than they do in the general population. And acute whiplash injury does not worsen any preaccident changes.

In addition, Balla (1988), in a review of more than 5,000 cases, found a very poor correlation between neck X-ray findings and the reporting of chronic symptoms of headache, neck pain, neck stiffness, and arm pain. That is, the reporting of these symptoms in whiplash patients did not predict the finding of an abnormal X-ray. Equally important, an abnormal X-ray did not mean that these symptoms would be present, and they could be present almost as often when the patient had a normal X-ray. Balla concluded that X-rays are of no value in the assessment of why accident victims report chronic neck pain.

Studies by W. D. deGravelles and J. H. Kelley (1969) and D. R. Gore et al (1987) confirm that patients who already had abnormal changes on their X-ray do not have an acceleration of these changes.

There are some authors, however, who have reported conclusions that disagree with all the above studies. In 1991, A. Watkinson et al reported on the radiologic progression of neck X-ray abnormalities in whiplash patients. Many quote this study to suggest that whiplash causes progressive radiologic changes. The study has many potential flaws (see Chapter 13) and so does not satisfactorily counter the conclusions of the other studies above. Other studies quoted to suggest that there is such a correlation between the X-ray and outcome have many potential flaws as well. These include very low rates of follow-up (Hohl 1974), inclusion of patients with fractures (S. H. Norris and I. Watt 1983), and small patient numbers (B. P. Radanov et al 1996). C. Hildingsson et al's study (1990) lacks these flaws and biases, with larger numbers of patients, and reveals that disc degeneration, angulation, and kyphosis on X-ray at the time of the accident do not predict a worse outcome.

Summary

The literature contains a number of studies whose results demonstrate that X-ray signs of disc degeneration do not predict or correlate with symptoms. The acute injury does not appear to accelerate the development of degenerative changes in the spine.

MYELOGRAMS, BONE SCANS, AND DISCOGRAMS

The search with many other radiological tools (other than X-rays) for the chronic damage that follows the acute injury (and is then responsible for reporting of chronic whiplash symptoms) has been unsuccessful. G. L. Odom et al (1958) and W. E. Hitselberger and R. M. Witten (1968) showed why myelograms failed to demonstrate this supposed chronic damage.

S. E. Sneider et al (1963) and E. P. Holt Jr (1964) demonstrated that discography could not provide an answer to the search for the whiplash injury. Since those early studies, there have been a number of studies in nonwhiplash patients attempting to evaluate the diagnostic value of discography. The pendulum appears to swing back and forth every few years on discography, with some experts saying it cannot accomplish a great deal, and then an equal number arguing the opposite. We need more studies of discography in whiplash patients, particularly comparing findings at the same time to MRI findings.

Hildingsson and S.O. Hietala (1989) and D. Barton et al (1993), using bone scans to study whiplash patients reporting chronic symptoms, could not find evidence of chronic damage. Bone scans are very sensitive for signs of damage including damage to joints and even some ligament and muscle injuries. See comments on these articles in Chapter 13.

MRI

Before MRI, some believed that one might not detect significant neck damage (ie, damage beyond minor muscle or ligament sprains that produce mostly microscopic tears) if using only X-rays, myelograms, or computed tomography (CT) scans. J. R. Taylor and L. T. Twomey (1993) expressed this concern. Autopsy studies found significant ligament, joint, and disc damage due to acute trauma in a variety of accident victims (although the collision types were quite different from the typical collisions producing whiplash patients). Also, in 1991, however, S. J. Davis et al demonstrated that MRI readily detects these types of damage. (Their study has some flaws—see below—but it was at least able to demonstrate that MRI scans will detect this type of significant damage, if it occurs, in whiplash patients.) MRI studies have thus obviated the need for autopsy data in whiplash patients to detect such injuries: MRI misses only minor muscle or ligament injuries. MRI technology and bone scans can readily detect abnormalities of the joints and bones of the spine (C. R. Gundry and H. M. Fritts 1997). No longer can the argument that significant damage is being missed in whiplash patients be maintained by stating there is a lack of autopsy data. If damage beyond minor injury exists, an MRI scan (or the other radiological techniques previously mentioned) will find it. Yet studies of whiplash patients routinely fail to do so.

MRI Abnormalities Common in Healthy People

MRI reveals the imperfections of human anatomy. Indeed, in many parts of the spine, including the lumbar and thoracic spine, normal people frequently have abnormalities on scanning. With discography, myelography, CT, MRI, and studies comparing these techniques with each other, 15% to 50% of asymptomatic individuals can have apparent abnormalities, as shown by D. L. Kent et al (1992), H. Paajanen et al (1989), M. C. Powell et al (1986), J. W. Simmons et al (1991), T. R. Walsh et al (1990), S. W. Wiesel et al (1984), and K. B. Wood et al (1995).

In addition, studies by T. N. Bernard Jr (1990), S. D. Boden et al (1990), M. C. Jensen et al (1994), S. Kikuchi et al (1981), M. A. Linson and C. H. Crowe

(1990), and P. C. Milette et al (1990) have shown that in patients reporting pain, abnormalities may be found in regions of the spine where the patient is having no pain—that is, where the patient is asymptomatic. Moreover, many individuals have abnormalities even though they have no symptoms at all. As stated by Boden et al, "The finding that an asymptomatic individual has more than a one-in-four chance of having an abnormal magnetic resonance image emphasizes the danger of predicating a decision to operate on the basis of any diagnostic tests in isolation. . . . Images of asymptomatic subjects confirm observations that have been made with computerized tomography and myelography studies that these findings are part of a normal, or at least common, aging process." Jensen et al add, "On MRI examination of the lumbar spine, many people without back pain have disk bulges or protrusions. . . . Given the high prevalence of these findings and of back pain, the discovery by MRI of bulges or protrusions in people with low back pain may frequently be coincidental."

In 1987, L. M. Teresi et al further addressed the significance of finding abnormalities of the cervical spine with MRI. They examined 100 patients between 45 and 79 years old. They found that:

> Spinal cord involvement by degenerative disease was observed in a large percentage of patients in this study (23% of patients older than 64 years of age), and produced no symptoms.

> Cord compression also occurred in the absence of symptoms and was secondary to disk protrusion in all cases. These results in our entirely asymptomatic population are compatible with those of an earlier report by Pennin et al. in a study of symptomatic patients.

> Our findings indicate that a wide variety of abnormalities may be asymptomatic and that these are seen commonly in older patients. The radiologist and referring clinician, therefore, must be cautious with attributing clinical symptoms to structural abnormalities seen on MR images.

Conducting a similar study of MRI of the cervical spine, but including even younger patients, Boden et al (1990) found a relatively high incidence of abnormalities in healthy people under age 40, as did K. B. Wood et al (1995) in studying the thoracic spine.

MRI Studies of Whiplash Patients

In the more specific case of whiplash patients, studies have found either no abnormality or abnormalities expected in the general population, such as those due to the normal process of disc degeneration. As well, detected abnormalities do not correlate with where the patient's symptoms are or their severity. K. Petters-son et al (1994) demonstrated both aspects in whiplash patients and noted that "despite many pathologic findings on MRI, we found no relationship between these lesions and the neurological deficit in the acute phase. . . . Our results support earlier findings that hand and arm pain rarely are caused by nerve root compression in whiplash patients."

One can then understand why there are erroneous conclusions made by some from the controversial study of S. J. Davis et al in 1991. They showed that 5 out of 9 patients with whiplash had abnormalities on MRI. These abnormalities included spondylosis (which exists in asymptomatic normal controls) and disc protrusion (also shown by Teresi et al to be found in asymptomatic controls). Thus, there may be no significance to these findings. Their data also made it clear that there was no correlation between symptoms and these MRI findings, since all patients had symptoms, but only half had "abnormal" MRI findings. Further, as J. M. S. Pearce (1993) noted in his review of this work, "This small mixed series . . . includes major osseus and disc lesions which should be excluded by definition."

Indeed, when studying typical whiplash patients, Pearce (1989) had already shown the odd contradiction wherein 19 patients with moderate or severe symptoms after whiplash had normal MRIs.

Again, some argue that significant muscle or ligament tears may be responsible for reporting of chronic neck pain, as opposed to minor (microscopic) tears typical of a minor sprain. Bone scans are capable of detecting significant muscle and ligament injury and yet have not in whiplash patients. MRI is capable of detecting new and old muscle or ligament tears and many other injuries (see A. A. De Smet et al 1990 and De Smet 1993). Yet studies of whiplash patients with MRI have not found these. Studies by G. Borchgrevink, O. Smevik, I. Haave et al (1995), G. E. Borchgrevink, O. Smevik, A. Nordby et al (1995), M. Fager-lund et al (1995), M. Karlsborg et al (1997), C. Maimaris et al (1989), R. W. Par-rish et al (1991), Pettersson et al (1994), H. R. Ronnen et al (1996), and P. R. Yarnell and G. V. Rossie (1988) confirm this.

Borchgrevink, Smevik, Haave et al and Borchgrevink, Smevik, Nordby et al (43 patients in one and 52 in another) conducted their 1995 studies within 2 to 4 days of the accident. Ronnen et al (100 patients) conducted their study within 3 weeks of the accident. It is worth considering in detail the findings of Ronnen et al.

> No abnormalities directly related to trauma were seen on MR images obtained. . . . No bone abnormalities or signs of trauma in the musculature, ligaments, or other soft tissues were seen. No spinal cord abnormalities were detected.

> We did not observe signs and symptoms of acute disk herniation and avulsion in our study, and the disk herniations were considered to be

asymptomatic and already present before trauma occurred. . . . No abnormalities were detected in the cerebrum or in the brainstem.

In the literature, a kyphotic angle has been interpreted as a sign of ligamentous injury. Because of the lack of abnormalities seen at MR imaging, it appears that a kyphotic angle does not automatically imply soft-tissue injury such as that to the ligaments. The kyphotic angle could be the result of a muscular spasm.

Borchgrevink et al found the same.

Finally, H. Jónsson et al (1994) reveal the important difference between individuals involved in accidents who have objectively verifiable injuries and whiplash patients who do not. In their study of 50 patients involved in accidents, Jonsson et al found there were two groups of patients: "10 patients with not only persistent pain, but pain radiating down the arms in association with objective neurologic findings and unequivocal correlations with diagnostic scans; and 40 who did not have these objective findings or correlations between the examination and MRI scans (i.e., no identifiable injury)."

The patients with identifiable injury responsible for their arm pain had complete recovery from appropriate therapy for their type of identifiable physical injury. Of the remaining 42, the outcome was completely erratic. In 24 of the 42, there were no symptoms by 6 weeks after the accident. A remaining 18 had ongoing symptoms despite not having any identifiable injury that would distinguish them from those 24 who recovered fully. Some of the patients who remained symptomatic, and for whose symptoms the investigators could find no explanatory injury, had pain for up to 5 years later. Their symptoms did not in fact correlate with MRI findings (ie, some had completely normal scans while having the most severe pain). The investigators could find no physical explanation for why these patients had such a poor outcome. These observations reinforce the improbability that a physical damage produced the symptoms, given that the outcomes were so different. Pettersson et al (1997) found the same where the MRI findings in whiplash patients are not different from controls, unless specific objective, neurological abnormalities on examination distinguish them. Otherwise, the findings on MRI are irrelevant to symptoms or outcome. The study by Jónsson et al also confirmed the findings of earlier studies showing that whiplash does not cause an acceleration or appearance of disc degeneration. Their study demonstrated that from the initial postinjury radiograms to the 5-year follow-up radiograms, no progression of degenerative changes was seen in any of the 50 patients.

Summary

In the vast majority of whiplash patients, radiological findings from X-rays or MRI scans are not helpful in demonstrating the injury or source of symptom reporting. It is erroneous to conclude that MRI findings of disc degeneration and other common variations found in the general population are responsible for symptoms. If there are no abnormal neurological findings consistent with nerve compression, or the neurological findings do not correlate with the radiological findings, then those radiological findings are irrelevant to the patient's symptoms. The abnormalities merely represent the background incidence of such findings in the general population. Their description seems to confuse more than help the clinician. The identification of irrelevant, albeit "impressive," imaging abnormalities does more to serve the litigious purpose than the patient's health.

CHRONIC WHIPLASH—CHRONIC DAMAGE TO THE JOINTS?

In a series of elegant studies, L. Barnsley et al and S. M. Lord et al (1993–1996) demonstrate that specific joints in the cervical spine may be a source of chronic neck pain. This is an important series of studies. Although it has long been known that many structures of the neck have pain receptors and can therefore be a source of pain, it has not been known which structure causes a given individual's neck pain at a given time. There are few maneuvers a physician can do on examination to prove that the pain at that time is coming from a specific site. These authors (see their studies for the methodology) were able to show that, at least when they were being studied, some individuals had neck pain arising from the small joints in the spine (called facet or zygapophysial joints). Presumably this could be a persistent source of neck pain.

So is this the source of chronic neck pain in some whiplash patients? Yes, it may be. Is it a site damaged in the acute injury or does damage to these joints come from the acute injury in some way? It is unlikely.

First of all, if the acute whiplash injury leads either directly or indirectly to damage to these joints, and this causes chronic pain, how are German, Greek, and Lithuanian whiplash victims managing to avoid this phenomenon? Perhaps this type of injury does not happen very often. But then it is not very helpful in understanding thousands and thousands of whiplash patients reporting chronic neck pain. If it does happen, it is rare in other cultures.

Second, in the patients studied by Barnsley et al, it is difficult to know what relationship exists between the accident (the acute injury) and their neck pain. Because the patients were not a consecutive group who presented to, say, an emergency department and then were recruited into the study, they are highly select. Are they a rare collection of patients like a group of very rare Lithuanians who happen to have a poor prognosis and represent a rare phenomenon? Perhaps. Not all of the patients were involved in motor vehicle accidents, and perhaps they are not appropriate to study the question being asked. Two of the patients (in a later study) did not actually have any neck pain with their accident. They apparently developed neck pain 3 months later (ie, should not have that neck pain attributed to an accident). The major stumbling block in determining a relationship between the accident and their neck pain, however, is that the average duration from the accident to the time of the study was 4 to 5 years, with one case being 44 years after the accident! That a patient (or anyone else) attributes chronic neck pain to an accident injury does not mean that the *chronic* pain is actually due to tissue damage from the accident injury. More specifically, identifying the physical site of pain origin does not confirm that this site has chronic damage from an accident injury.

Finally, if the facet is a common site of injury in whiplash patients and both bone scans and MRI scans readily detect such injuries (Gundry and Fritts 1997), why have researchers *not* done so when studying large numbers of whiplash patients within weeks to months of the accident?

What are the other possibilities? Perhaps Barnsley et al were simply studying patients whose neck pain arises from sources other than an accident injury 44 years ago. Perhaps the patients' chronic neck pain comes from the same sources as the neck pain of people who have had no accident. After all, chronic neck pain in the general population is actually fairly common. The Lithuanian data (see H. Schrader et al) indicates that reporting of chronic neck pain is frequent in the general population. It is so common that some whiplash patients may be mistakenly attributing non–accident-related pain to an accident. The studies of Barnsley et al and Lord et al do not include a simultaneous control sample of nontraumatic, chronic neck pain patients to determine how prevalent facet (zygapophysial) joint pain is in the general population. Findings for such a control group might be the same as those for the "accident group."

Nevertheless, the elegant methodology of these studies is encouraging. If the studies were done again and involved patients with more recent accidents, then pain arising from these joints may be a consideration for the site of acute injury. Otherwise, these studies merely confirm the facet (zygapophysial) joint as a potential source of chronic neck pain but do not confirm what event caused that source of pain. Even identifying these joints as a source of pain in the whiplash patients at 3 months does not confirm that this was the acute injury.

In 1997, Y. Fredin et al encountered the same difficulties when considering whether damage to the neck joints or other neck structures might cause increased muscle tension and perhaps pain. They studied this phenomenon in a small group of whiplash patients and healthy controls. They found more muscle tension in whiplash patients, but they could not determine if this was due to neck damage, psychological factors, abnormal posture, or combinations of these. To determine this, they would need control groups composed of chronic neck pain patients who are not whiplash victims and patients with psychological distress not complaining of neck pain. They also would have to first correct abnormal posture (see below) and then conduct the study.

POSTURE AND CHRONIC NECK/BACK PAIN

This is a largely unstudied aspect of whiplash. Many of the studies on treatment of whiplash patients (see Chapter 12) include as part of the therapy instruction on correcting one's posture, both through simple measures such as sitting with a small cushion along the upper part of the low back (around the level of the L3 vertebra), and through specific exercises called neck (or chin or head) retractions and back extensions. This is often part of further instruction called "neck school," simply teaching the individual about "healthy neck postures."

The basis for using such therapies in whiplash patients is, again, not well studied. The presumption has been that following acute neck or back pain, particularly if one reduces activities, one adopts what appears to be a slouched posture. Therapists commonly note patients reporting that this posture reduces, at least temporarily, their pain.

The general belief and the apparent basis for posture correction in treatment protocols appears to be that abnormal posture eventually causes neck and back pain.

A few studies have shown that healthy subjects, when placed in "slouched postures" with the head forward and an overall "rounded back," will develop neck and/or back pain, albeit minor (see K. Harms-Ringdahl and J. Ekholm 1986, T. P. Hedman and G. R. Fernie 1997, K. S. Middaugh et al 1994, D. H. Watson and P. H. Trott 1993). What structures in the neck actually cause this pain is not yet known. Some argue it is muscular, whereas others refer to the facet joints. Using methodologies like that of Barnsley et al to study the facet joints might provide some answers in the future.

Whatever causes the pain, correcting the posture appears to improve the pain (see R. A. McKenzie 1990, K. S. Middaugh et al 1994, M. M. Williams et al 1991).

Is it possible that after the acute injury heals, new factors such as abnormal posture continue to lead to reporting chronic pain? This is again unproven, but in some whiplash patients, the behavior in response to pain (reduced activity, prolonged sitting, less time in upright postures, etc) may lead to abnormal posture of the neck and back. Although there has not been enough research on this aspect of whiplash, the frequent observation by physicians and others that whiplash patients present with abnormal posture is again compelling.

It seems unlikely that poor posture is the only cause of the neck and back pain reported by whiplash patients, since abnormal posture usually causes only minor symptoms to most individuals. Yet if one accepts that the behavior of some whiplash patients contributes to poor posture, then this contributes in part to their pain.

Summary

There remains as yet no definite evidence that whiplash patients report chronic neck or back pain because of persistent damage after the acute injury. Most whiplash patients likely have a minor sprain. Some may develop poor posture after the acute injury, and this may lead them to report chronic neck and/or back pain.

WHIPLASH EXPERIMENTS

There are several key findings of whiplash experiments.

- Animal and dummy experiments do not render an accurate assessment of the injury risk in whiplash patients. The damage identified in animal experiments is not what researchers find in whiplash patients, and the collisions experienced by most whiplash patients are physically incapable of producing these other severe injuries.
- Accelerations of 5 to 8g for less than 1 second are commonly experienced in everyday life without producing physical injury.
- The threshold for the most minor of symptoms (lasting hours to 1 day) from a collision in humans is probably at least a velocity change (ΔV) of 8 km/h for the struck vehicle in a rear-end collision. In a front or lateral collision, the threshold is a ΔV of at least 16 km/h for the struck vehicle. If an engineer cites the magnitude as being less than this, an injury explanation for the patient's symptoms is far less probable.
- The threshold for minor symptoms (lasting days at most) from a collision in humans is a head acceleration of 10g in most cases. If an engineer cites the magnitude as being less than 10g, an injury explanation for the patient's symptoms is far less probable.
- No experiment volunteer has reported chronic pain following the acute injury in 4 decades of human whiplash experiments, regardless of the experimental design.
- Studies with human cadavers (which provide an opportunity to dissect and look for tissue injury) have failed to reveal damage of any kind (not even minimal muscle damage) at head accelerations of 10g or less. They have confirmed minor muscle or ligament damage with 12 to 20g.

Introduction

If one is unable to identify, through radiology or other diagnostic techniques, the acute injury and the chronic damage that supposedly occurs, another option is simply to subject the neck to an experimental collision and study the result. One could simply ascertain if the acute injury produced chronic damage that then led to reporting of chronic symptoms by simply reproducing the acute injury experimentally. That is, one could put people in cars in a laboratory and subject them to collisions until they have neck pain. Then see what happens to them after that. Whiplash patients reporting chronic symptoms are so common that if physical damage from the acute injury in fact leads to chronic damage and symptoms, it really should not be that difficult to reproduce experimentally.

This chapter and Chapter 20 address the attempts to determine or define the whiplash injury by reproducing it in experimental collisions and to determine if acute injury will lead to chronic pain reporting. Animals, dummies, human cadavers, and living humans have all been used in more than 4 decades of research. So far, it has been impossible to produce any chronic symptoms with these experiments, even though it has been relatively easy to cause acute pain in volunteers. The volunteers just get better in days or weeks, despite a variety of impact directions, vehicles, subjects (of different ages and sexes, including non–military personnel), restraints or seats, or variations in how the experimental subject sits or has his or her head positioned.

Readers should understand a few of the engineering concepts behind collision forces and accelerations. First, the only forces of concern are the ones experienced by the vehicle occupant, not the vehicle. In other words, the force of collision of the vehicles is not the same as the forces experienced by the vehicle occupant. The collision force, depending on the exact nature of the collision, is dispersed in many ways. Some is lost to heat from friction, some to the sound of the impact, and some to deformation of the vehicle. Only a certain fraction may be remaining and experienced by the vehicle occupants. How do engineers then determine what force the whiplash victim's head and neck has undergone? Fortunately, engineers do not have to determine all the collision forces and subtract the other ways that force is dispersed to see what remains. Experiments with animals, dummies, cadavers, and living humans provide direct measurements of these forces by examining the accelerations they produce. The engineers can use data from experimental measurements to examine a "real-life" collision and use aspects of that collision to predict injury risk.

Measurements in Whiplash Experiments

ΔV

Most important, readers should understand the concept of the change in velocity (ΔV) of a collision. When two cars collide, their velocities change. How they change depends on the direction of impact, the mass of each vehicle, the velocity of each vehicle before the collision, and the damage. Imagine two cars of equal size (really, equal mass). The striking vehicle collides with the rear end of a stationary vehicle (the struck vehicle). The striking vehicle will have slowed down, and the struck vehicle will have gone from 0 speed to some velocity in a fraction of a second. The struck vehicle may have only gone from 0 to 10 km/h (6 mph) in a minor collision, but realize this occurs in a fraction of a second. The collision generally produces a faster increase in velocity (a greater acceleration) than simply putting a foot down on the accelerator. Going from 0 to 10 km/h (6 mph) may not seem like much, but in one tenth of a second, it is experienced as a sudden (and unexpected) acceleration for the unwary occupant.

The change in velocity and how fast the change occurs (acceleration) is what causes the occupant's head to accelerate. This is considered the basis of the whiplash injury: the vehicle and the occupant's body are accelerated in a certain direction, and the head lags behind for a fraction of a second until it is pulled along with the body. Presumably the muscles that attach the head to the body are sprained by this action.

One can then ask the question that engineers have been recently studying: Since most collisions occur over the same time period, if I just know what velocity the struck vehicle changed by, can I predict the likelihood of injury for the occupant inside? Yes. This is an important aspect of predicting injury risk. A number of studies have subjected volunteers to experimental collisions to see how much velocity change an individual can undergo in this fraction of a second before experiencing neck pain. Animal and cadaver experiments can push this velocity change higher and higher, detecting what type of damage occurs as the velocity change increases.

This change in velocity after a collision, often called "delta V" and symbolized as ΔV, is therefore a statement of the severity of the collision and a key predictor of probability of injury. ΔV is not the striking velocity. It is a change in velocity. Notice that vehicles going from 0 to 10 km/h (6 mph), from 10 km/h (6 mph) to 0, from 60 km/h (36 mph) to 50 km/h (30 mph), or from 50 km/h (30 mph) to 60 km/h (36 mph) all have a ΔV of 10 km/h (6 mph).

The ΔV that a vehicle undergoes is again one of the most important predictors of a neck injury, but not the only one. Engineers have found that the threshold beyond which most individuals will report acute neck pain depends partly on impact direction.

ΔV and Impact Direction

Different directions of impacts can produce the same ΔV for one's vehicle but carry a different risk (threshold) for injury. Volunteer studies show (even with other confounding factors accounted for) that the neck muscles tolerate less well the head moving backward suddenly than they tolerate the head moving forward or to the side (ear to shoulder). Imagine an occupant sitting in a parked car (velocity is 0). Another car strikes the parked car in a frontal (head-on) or side collision at 20 km/h (12 mph). Let us assume that the ΔV for the struck vehicle is 10 km/h (6 mph). No injury appears to occur in volunteers at that ΔV. Consider the same striking velocity of 20 km/h (12 mph) but in a rear-end collision. Again, assume the struck vehicle has a ΔV of 10 km/h (6 mph). Data shows the volunteer is much more likely to be injured by the collision striking in the rear than by the collision striking in the front at that same striking velocity. Impact direction alters the direction of head movements and therefore affects the injury threshold. Of course, if struck at much higher velocities than the threshold with the vehicle changing its ΔV at a much higher level, there will be an injury in any case. It is the threshold for injury that is raised or lowered by impact direction.

The minimal ΔV threshold for injury is about twice as great for frontal and side collisions as it is for rear-end collisions. This is one of the reasons why (in the lower range of collision velocities and changes) the offending driver in a rear-end collision (who is thus experiencing a frontal collision) is less likely to be injured than the one who was hit (who experiences the rear-end collision). It is not simply because the offending driver has no one to sue that he or she does not report an injury. He or she may not have an injury whereas the person hit legitimately does. Of course, at higher velocities of collision, the offending driver in a rear-end collision should also have an acute injury. There may be ways the offending driver can protect him- or herself, but one nevertheless expects the offending driver to have an injury on at least some occasions. That such individuals do not report chronic pain very often (no one has a figure on how often) can be explained by a number of factors, which by the end of this book may be clear.

The ΔV of the vehicle is useful, especially when the impact direction is known, because it indicates the threshold for injury and the probability for injury in the vehicle occupants. It does not matter what the velocity of the struck vehicle or the striking vehicle is. If either vehicle undergoes a certain velocity change (however that change was produced), a threshold can be reached for that impact direction, beyond which injury to its occupants is likely to occur.

ΔV, Vehicle Size, and Striking Velocity

The other intrinsic value to the concept of ΔV is that it works regardless of what size (mass) the vehicles are relative to each other. Whether it is a large vehicle striking a small vehicle or vice versa, if the end result is a certain ΔV, and if for that impact direction the ΔV exceeds the threshold of injury, then one can predict a high probability of injury.

The striking velocity is again not the same as the ΔV. The striking velocity is what happens at the time of the collision, and the ΔV is what happens afterward. The net or calculated striking velocity at impact is the initial difference between the two vehicle velocities. Consider a rear-end collision. If the striking vehicle is traveling at 30 km/h (18 mph) and the struck vehicle is parked (velocity is 0), the striking velocity is 30 km/h (18 mph). If the striking vehicle is traveling at 30 km/h (18 mph), and the struck vehicle is at 20 km/h (12 mph), the striking velocity is only 10 km/h (6 mph).

Although engineers use other factors in their analysis, the ΔV for the struck vehicle can be calculated if one knows the masses of the two vehicles and the striking velocity. The striking velocity alone cannot predict the ΔV. The formulas and other considerations for these calculations are not discussed here, as they become complex in some collisions. But the examples discussed below will allow readers to become familiar with which collision parameters are likely to lead to injury and which are not. Table 5–1 works through some simple collision scenarios and the likelihood of minor injury in each scenario. The struck vehicle is stationary.

Consider the simple example of a parked car. If the desired goal is to generate a ΔV of 10 km/h (6 mph), how fast must the striking vehicle be traveling? That depends on how massive each vehicle is relative to each other. If they are cars of the same mass, calculations indicate that a striking speed of about 20 km/h (12 mph) would be needed. If the striking vehicle is a bus (about 8 times more massive than the car), the striking speed would be less than 4 km/h (2.4 mph). Getting hit by a bus at what seems like a low velocity, say, 20 km/h (12 mph), can cause serious injury to a car's occupants.

In the reverse scenario, if the desired goal is to generate a ΔV of 10 km/h (6 mph) in a bus, and the striking vehicle is a car, the striking velocity would have to be about 100 km/h (60 mph). The people in the bus do well, with but a small risk of injury, while the driver of the car is in critical condition or dead.

Other scenarios are more complex, and most collisions require an engineering analysis to produce a more complete picture of injury risk. Nevertheless, certain thresholds are readily identified, even under crude analyses.

The bottom line is that whatever vehicle type, whatever striking velocity, and whatever analysis required, the end results will usually be expressed as the magnitude of ΔV, from which, knowing the impact direction, one can predict injury risk.

Head Acceleration

Although most studies now focus on ΔV as a predictor of injury risk, most of the early whiplash experiments have been built on understanding the magnitude of head acceleration that occurs in the fraction of a second following impact. By placing an instrument (an accelerometer) on the vehicle and occupant, one can reproduce many different severities of collisions under virtually any circumstance. In each case, one knows the exact accelerations undergone by, for example, the head and neck. An accelerometer thus measures acceleration, and from this one can also calculate force. Acceleration is a measure of how fast a body increases its velocity. Deceleration is a measure of how fast a body decreases its velocity. One can express the acceleration as a multiple of the acceleration due to gravity. When one drops a ball, for example, the acceleration of the ball is 1g. The force with which that ball moves (or the force a person would experience if it

Table 5–1 Injury Predictions in Low-Velocity Collisions

Impact Direction	Striking Vehicle	Struck Vehicle	Striking Velocity km/h (mph)	DV of Struck Vehicle km/h (mph)	Injury Risk for Occupants in Both Vehicles
Rear	Car, mass A	Car, mass A	10 (6)	6.5 (3.9)	Below threshold for all—like sneezing
Rear	Truck, mass 2 times > mass A	Car, mass A	10 (6)	8.7 (5.2)	Threshold just reached for a headache/neck pain for a few hours
Rear	Car, mass A	Car, mass A	15 (9)	9.8 (5.9)	Threshold for one day of headache/neck pain just reached
Rear	Bus, mass 8 times > mass A	Car, mass A	8 (4.8)	11.4 (6.8)	Threshold for one or a few days of headache/ neck pain just reached
Rear	Bus, mass 8 times > mass A	Car, mass A	20 (12)	23 (13.9)	Neck sprain for a few weeks, perhaps more serious injury
Rear	Car, mass A	Bus, mass 8 times > mass A	80 (48)	11.6 (8.7)	Threshold for one or a few days of headache/ neck pain just reached
Frontal or side	Car, mass A	Car, mass A	10 (6)	6.5 (3.9)	Below threshold for this impact direction—like sneezing

continues

Table 5–1 continued

Impact Direction	Striking Vehicle	Struck Vehicle	Striking Velocity km/h (mph)	DV of Struck Vehicle km/h (mph)	Injury Risk for Occupants in Both Vehicles
Frontal or side	Truck, mass 2 times > mass A	Car, mass A	10 (6)	8.7 (5.2)	Below threshold for this impact direction—like sneezing
Frontal or side	Car, mass A	Car, mass A	25 (15)	16.3 (9.8)	Threshold for headache/neck pain for a few hours or days just reached
Frontal or side	Car, mass A	Car, mass A	35 (21)	23. (14)	Threshold for one or a few weeks of headache/neck pain reached

dropped on his or her foot) is dependent on the mass of the ball (often expressed in kilograms). So one calculates force by multiplying the acceleration by the mass of the object being accelerated. The head acceleration for human volunteers can also be measured to see what the threshold is for injury.

For an accident victim, the mass of the head and neck will experience a certain acceleration and therefore a certain force. In many cases, it is assumed that the mass of the head and neck in most people is relatively similar (4.0 to 6.0 kg). For this reason, engineers often deal with just acceleration (in g), knowing that if one wanted a measure of the force, one would simply multiply the acceleration by the mass of the head and neck. Engineers often avoid the term "g-force" because it is confusing.

Whiplash experiments tell us how high the head acceleration must be before pain is reported. Thus, when an engineer states that the occupant's head underwent $10g$ acceleration, one can compare this to the known threshold for injury. A $10g$ acceleration seems like a high acceleration. It is, under certain circumstances. The time over which this acceleration is experienced is important. How long one experiences an acceleration determines the tolerability. People can, for example, tolerate a $1g$ acceleration (the acceleration due to gravity) for a lifetime. As the acceleration becomes higher, people tolerate it for less time, in a dramatically exponential fashion. For example, humans might be able to live on a planet with a $2g$ gravity for only a few months before the cardiovascular system and other body systems collapsed. Humans might tolerate a $3g$ gravity for only hours. Experiencing a $5g$ acceleration for a few seconds will cause a loss of consciousness in a pilot. Experiencing this acceleration for a small fraction of a second (when a person sneezes) does not cause a loss of consciousness. A $10g$ acceleration is thus not a big deal if the duration of exposure is around one tenth of a second—a minor rear-end collision.

Nothing seems simple in all this, but armed with a rudimentary understanding of what engineers mean when they quote the ΔV of the struck vehicle or the acceleration of the accident victim's head (now used less often because simply knowing the vehicle's velocity change is a good predictor of injury), readers can now understand the whiplash experiments.

Chapter 20 contains Tables 20–1 to 20–4, which review in detail the available data from whiplash experiments over 4 decades. The legend for this table provides more engineering details for the interested reader.

We will begin by considering the animal experiments. These are being discussed not because they adequately or accurately reflect the injuries in whiplash patients but because many people often quote them as if they do.

The Hare, the Monkey, and Their Dummy Friends

Dummies were used in whiplash experiments as early as 1957 (C. C. Purviance) and more recently by F. P. D. Navin et al (1989). Although dummy experiments help to define potential mechanisms of injury, they do not help to identify damage. In low-velocity collisions dummies are quite inadequate substitutes for living humans (see J. P. Gough 1996).

Many have thus conducted experiments with animals. In 1963, J. Wickstrom et al made little cars for hares and subjected them to rear-end impacts. The only way they could cause serious injury was to use greater than 500g accelerations. These produced forces 10 times (considering that the mass of a hare's head is much lower than that of a human) those seen in typical collisions experienced by whiplash patients.

The most frequently quoted work, however, is that of I. MacNab. In 1964, MacNab dropped monkeys from ranges of 2 to 40 feet on a horizontal platform. This platform would suddenly cause hyperextension of the neck when it hit bottom. MacNab stated clearly that the method does not "reproduce . . . the force applied to a human neck in a rear-end collision" and did not provide any data on accelerations or forces. He did not describe in his article exactly what forces or accelerations caused which pathology.

MacNab did ultimately demonstrate that if one dropped a monkey from a great enough height, the monkey could possibly die or suffer a severe injury. He repeated his article 2 years later and stated that whiplash "has been reproduced experimentally by subjecting animals to an acceleration-extension strain of the neck."

Of course, there are many caveats with attempting to use this data to understand what damage occurs in most whiplash patients. It is simply very uncommon to ever observe such damage as MacNab's monkeys demonstrated. This is not surprising, because most whiplash patients are not in such severe collisions.

A. M. Wiley, in 1981, commented on MacNab's work: "One must always be wary of interpreting animal experiments in the light of human anatomy. Whereas primates resemble humans in many respects, they do show differences in neck length, head weight, and skeletal anatomy, which may profoundly affect the soft-tissue neck damage."

Further study of MacNab's work reveals some other interesting aspects. He reported on the follow-up of 2 different patient groups. He reported on the first group in July 1971 (*Orthopedic Clinics of North America*). They reported chronic symptoms in the pre–head restraint era (before 1969), and in that article MacNab discusses the mechanism of whiplash injury, showing diagrams without head restraints. He argues that head restraints would negate the whiplash injury mechanism. In his second report (*Advocates' Quarterly,* 1979–1981), he reports on a group of patients in the head restraint era. Despite this, MacNab still used the identical diagrams showing no head restraints. He did not comment on why the two groups had a similar outcome if the one group used head restraints and the other did not. He does not explain how to reconcile a theory of whiplash injury with these facts. He did not discuss why whiplash was so prevalent in the head restraint era if his proposed mechanism of injury was in part the lack of head restraints. Thus, although often cited in the courts, MacNab's work has a number of potential flaws and may be internally inconsistent.

Researchers did eventually become discontent with the value of the early animal experiments, the monkey experiments in particular.

> "Where is it?" demanded Burbage, bursting into the living room. "Where's the monkey?" His short raincoat was soaking and his face was red and violent. . . .
>
> "It was an accident," said Allan.
>
> "The coroner will decide that," said the professor curtly. "I'm only interested in the monkey right now. Well, where is it?"
>
> . . . In a moment he was back with [the monkey's] decapitated body in a plastic kitchen bag. . . . His cheeks were purple with fury.
>
> "God help you bastards," he spat and stormed out of the house.
>
> —Stewart M. *Monkey Shines*. New York: Freundlich Books; 1983:251–252.

Thus, researchers pursued the whiplash injury and the cause of the chronic symptom reporting by conducting human experiments instead, as described below.

Human Whiplash Experiments

> The whole man . . . is a novel phenomenon; and all phenomena, however magnificent, are surely fair subjects for experiment.
>
> —Kingsley C. *Yeast*. London: Macmillan and Co.; 1889:35.

The experiments with humans are far more relevant to whiplash because they represent the closest approximation to the collisions whiplash patients experience. Thus, prior work with nonhumans would not in any event be able to contradict conclusions of the human experiments. Human cadaver experiments are to some degree useful because they provide an opportunity for neck dissection to look for even the most minor of injuries. This can obviously not be done in a whiplash patient. Cadaver experiments allow researchers to determine exactly what type of damage may exist in whiplash patients given similar collision parameters, although they underestimate the tolerance of the living human for a variety of reasons.

Readers should again refer to Tables 20–1 to 20–4 in Chapter 20. The discussion below deals with the pertinent studies. Chapter 22 discusses the effect head restraints and seat belts have had on claims of whiplash injury.

Injury Threshold—Head Acceleration

Since 1955, researchers have conducted hundreds of experiments using chiefly military personnel. They used a variety of vehicles, a variety of impact speeds and directions (frontal, rear, lateral, or combinations), and a variety of restraint systems (with or without head restraints) (see F. Bendjellal et al 1987, C. L. Ewing et al 1977–1979, R. C. Grunsten et al 1989, H. J. Mertz and L. M. Patrick 1967 and 1971, M. Severy et al 1955, R. Wagner 1979, J. Wismans et al 1987). Many of these collisions did produce acute symptoms such as headache, neck pain, and back pain. Sances and Weber (1981) reviewed a large number of these collisions and noted that when the acceleration was 10g or more, volunteers experienced headache and neck pain. At 16g accelerations, they experienced low back pain lasting for 1 day. In one case, symptoms lasted for 10 days. Cadaver experiments with head restraints indicated no damage using head accelerations that were less than 20g.

In 1991, D. Kallieris et al confirmed this neck injury criterion (the minimum acceleration of the head necessary to produce tissue damage) for frontal and side impacts. They used cadavers (so that they could dissect the subject to look for even minor damage). They found no damage occurred in frontal or side collisions until at least 13g accelerations were reached. At this acceleration the damage was minor muscle sprain. More significant damage would occur only above 21g acceleration. M. M. Panjabi, Cholewicki, Nibu, and Grauer (1998) showed that the damage in a rear-end collision is a minor sprain at a head acceleration of 10.5g. We thereby have a rough idea of what physical damage occurs in a cadaver at the accelerations that cause symptoms in human volunteers—a minor sprain of ligaments or muscles.

Whereas early studies focused on high-velocity impacts (ie, striking vehicle traveling at 20 to 80 km/h), recent research has instead focused on low-velocity impacts (see Table 20–4 in Chapter 20) because there appear to be a large number of accident victims reporting chronic symptoms following such impacts.

Injury Threshold—ΔV

From a review of human test data citing ΔV, what is the threshold below which physical injury is of low probability?

According to available research, the threshold for symptoms in a rear-end collision is at a ΔV for the struck vehicle of about 8 km/h (4.8 mph). This seems a very low threshold and indeed should be viewed as "rock bottom" minimum. The volunteers in these experiments often reported just 1 hour or 1 day of symptoms with these low-velocity collisions. There is obviously an attempt to give the lowest threshold for injury, but some believe the threshold should be that which causes symptoms to last for at least 1 day. This figure is closer to a ΔV of 10 km/h.

Thus, whenever an engineer states that the ΔV was less than 8 km/h (4.8 mph) or that the head acceleration was less than 10g, it is improbable that any physical injury would have occurred. G. P. Nielsen et al (1997) confirmed the fact that the injury threshold is even higher in frontal or lateral collisions. They cite a ΔV for the struck vehicle as having to be at least 16 km/h (10 mph).

It is not surprising that the threshold for injury in rear-end collision is about a peak head acceleration of around 10g, or a ΔV for the struck vehicle of 8 km/h (4.8 mph). We know that head accelerations of less than 10g occur in everyday life and do not produce symptoms. M. E. Allen et al (1994) gave us an indication of this when they measured head accelerations in everyday life events. As will be shown later, they found that sneezing may cause accelerations of around 3g. It is not very common for people to develop an injury with sneezing. "Plopping" back into a chair will cause the head to accelerate, much like it does in a rear-end collision, and this acceleration is about 8g. In a collision, if the head and neck undergo an acceleration of 5g, this does not appear to be much more than sneezing and around the same as plopping into a chair. W. Rosenbluth and L. Hicks (1994) have shown that one can repeatedly experience head accelerations of 2.0 to 3.0g while skipping rope without experiencing any symptoms or injury.

Yet whiplash claims occur following collisions where the collision parameters are below these thresholds. In his review, Gough notes:

> In impacts where the struck vehicle's speed change is less than 8 km/h, the range of cervical motion is generally confined within the normal range, regardless of the degree of support afforded by the headrest. However, it should be noted that in all of the tests which have been conducted using human subjects for speed changes up to and in some cases, significantly in excess of 8 km/h, if symptoms were experienced by the test subjects, they were minor and resolved spontaneously, without treatment, and within a short period of time (i.e., hours to days) following testing.

This raises again questions about why some report chronic symptoms following minor collisions. There appears to be no physical mechanism to explain this, and so Gough notes again:

> In the absence of some intervening factor . . . claims of injury cannot be rationalized within the available research into occupant dynamics in low-speed rear-end collisions. Medical treatment of individuals who have experienced such minor collisions is often based on an assump-

tion of hyperextension/hyperflexion injury to the cervical spine. . . .
Current research indicates that this mechanism of injury does not occur
for impacts resulting in a speed change of less than 8 km/h.

All the studies have confirmed this, regardless of the variety of different settings and subjects.

Acute neck pain reporting may occur by other mechanisms. In the studies by
Nielsen et al (1997), one of the volunteers was a physician.

> And Plato had reason to say that to be a good physician it were requi-
> site that he who should undertake that profession had passed through
> all such diseases as he will adventure to cure, and knowne and felt all
> the accidents and circumstances he is to judge of.
>
> —Florio J, trans. *The Essayes of Michael Lord of Montaigne*. Book III,
> Chapter XIII. London: George Routledge & Sons; 1885:554.

The physician relates his experience as a volunteer:

> Although I was not injured or strained in any manner by these repeated
> rear-enders, the part that startled me the most was the drama of the im-
> pact noise. Rear-end crashes sound horrible, the whole vehicle rever-
> berates with the echo of the impact. Yet upon looking at the bumpers
> afterwards, only minor dents were noted. It occurred to me that in per-
> sons who are emotionally fragile or dysfunctional, the fright from all
> this noise could be quite disturbing, and they might presume that cer-
> tainly something could have happened to them. Fear can be very con-
> vincing, and it is possible for some individuals, this in itself could lead
> to the display of injury behaviour.

Of course, one would not expect further reporting of pain when the fright of
the event (which is clearly recognizable as a minor accident) subsides. There is no
physical injury to perpetuate symptom reporting. There are other obvious causes
of reporting pain after such a minor accident. They include misattribution of coincidental symptoms occurring in the first few days after the accident (when the
symptoms may be unrelated to the accident) or the attribution of an ongoing pattern of preaccident symptoms to the accident. Insurance fraud would be another
obvious consideration. Since there is no objective way to prove or disprove most
acute whiplash injuries, one must rely on the probability of injury in such deter-
minations. This considerable body of engineering allows for an objective and accurate determination of that probability.

Moreover, one should realize that acute neck injury may indeed occur, especially when the ΔV is above 8 km/h (4.8 mph) or head accelerations are over 10g.

It is important to know, however, that experiments have not resulted in an individual reporting chronic neck pain after acute injury. Besides the injury threshold for lateral and frontal collisions, Nielsen et al (1997) also showed an increased risk of acute neck pain with the head laterally rotated. This often occurs in whiplash patients who are looking for oncoming traffic at the time of the collision. Yet even then, low-velocity collisions lead to only a few days of symptoms in volunteers.

What has to happen to generate these thresholds? Assuming ideal conditions, with the striking car hitting straight on, and no braking by the striking vehicle, when the two cars are of equal mass, the striking velocity may have to be about 15 km/h (9 mph) to change the struck vehicle's velocity from 0 to 8 km/h (4.8 mph) in a fraction of a second. It again seems remarkable that such a low striking velocity could cause injury, but recall that this may be a headache lasting for only a few hours, and that the collision circumstances must be ideal to allow this to happen. In the end, an engineer will analyze all the parameters of the "real-life" collision and state whether the injury threshold was reached. As low as this threshold seems, it is more remarkable that many claim chronic pain and disability at even lower values of ΔV.

Low-Velocity Collisions

Some further observations from the low-velocity experiments (see Chapter 20 for all of them) are worth noting.

In 1993, for example, D. H. West et al published the results of an important and illustrative study, using vehicles with velocities up to 20 km/h (12 mph) for some of the experiments. Another vehicle struck the test vehicle from behind, or the driver vehicle reversed into a wall. They removed rear-view mirrors to help keep the drivers unaware of an impending impact. (Obviously, the volunteers had to be aware of the fact that they were going to be in a collision that day.) Their findings include the following:

- A striking velocity of 12 km/h (7.2 mph) caused head acceleration of $8g$ maximum with no symptoms produced in any of the volunteers.
- In tests where a chain reaction collision took place (one car struck the vehicle ahead, which then struck the car in front), striking velocities of up to 20 km/h (12 mph) resulted in no symptoms. This is despite head accelerations of over $14g$.
- In tests in which the moving vehicle was reversed into a rigid barrier, there was reported neck pain lasting 1 to 2 days with no chronic symptoms. This is again despite head accelerations over $17g$ in some cases, and multiple exposures.

As summarized by West et al:

The forces experienced by vehicle occupants for impacts with [speeds] of less than 5 km/h (3 mph) are generally not sufficient to cause the heads of the vehicle occupants to be displaced rearward far enough to contact the head support. The maximum recorded levels of head acceleration for impacts of this magnitude were less than 3 g. Since no head contact to the head support is expected as a result of impacts of this magnitude, the presence or absence of adequate head support is of no significance. . . . A recent study by Allen et al [showed that] to "plop" into a chair . . . recorded levels . . . in excess of those which were measured with a 5 km/h impact.

Similar studies of low-velocity collisions conducted by W. E. McConnell et al in 1993 found that "test subject cervical extension and flexion angles . . . were always found to fall within the subject's voluntary physiological limits. Hyperextension or hyperflexion did not occur during any of the test runs, the maximum of about 40 to 45 degrees, even for test runs using the van, which had no headrests."

One of the subjects had mild neck pain that lasted 3 days, and none had chronic neck pain when followed for 18 months. This work then places doubt on the degree of hyperextension in low-velocity rear-end collisions. One could argue, as the authors of this article pointed out, that the subjects may have been expecting a collision and so had time to contract their neck muscles and prevent the neck from hyperextending. If this were the case, then those whiplash patients who became aware of an imminent collision should be able to protect themselves in the same way.

McConnell et al went on to explain the flaws in previous conceptions of what happens in most rear-end collisions.

In reviewing the voluminous literature on [whiplash] . . . one must be careful about making the assumption that the conclusions about human head and neck kinematics reached in these studies necessarily apply to low and very low velocity rearend collisions involving "real people." The majority of these studies have been primarily based on higher speed, 24 to 80 km/h (15 to 50 mph) or more, rearend collisions utilizing dummies, cadavers, animals, computer models and very few live volunteers.

Since exaggerated neck motion beyond tolerable human limits had been frequently observed in dummies and cadavers during high speed testing, it has been commonly assumed that cervical hyperextension and hyperflexion would also occur during low and very low velocity collisions. It has been conjectured by many that the forced movement of the neck beyond physiologic limits was the injury mechanism causing the "whiplash" syndrome, especially in thin necked, unprepared people.

Their study had shown, however, that such hyperextension does not occur with such low-velocity collisions.

Also in 1997, W. H. M. Castro et al confirmed this finding with regard to hyperextension. Their impressive study took place in Germany, and it showed results similar to those of other studies above (thus indicating that volunteers in experiments behave the same way in different cultures). They subjected 14 men and 5 women to rear-end collisions in automobiles and bumper cars. The ΔV was from 8 to 14 km/h (4.8–8.4 mph) in the automobiles. They found 5 subjects reported symptoms when the ΔV exceeded 11.4 km/h (6.8 mph). Even then, symptoms lasted a maximum of a few days. MRI scans taken before and after the collision found no abnormalities. Interestingly, none of the volunteers in bumper cars experienced symptoms even though they had more neck extension. The fact is, reporting of chronic pain or even pain lasting more than a few days after a low-velocity collision is not explained by physical injury.

Finally, there appear to be a large number of claims of whiplash injury by bus occupants, even when a vehicle of much lower mass strikes the bus. R. A. DuBois et al (1996) have shown that such claims of injury are entirely untenable. They found that when a vehicle strikes a bus in a rear-end collision, in order for the threshold for injury to be reached, the bus must undergo a ΔV of at least 8 km/h (5 mph). For a car with one eighth the mass of the bus, the car must be traveling at more than 100 km/h (60 mph) to accomplish this. Such a collision may often be fatal for the driver of the car. When the car was moving at much lower speeds, such as 10 to 20 km/h (6–12 mph), the volunteers in the bus could not even tell a collision had taken place. It may be that witnessing the collision and hearing a loud noise causes some fright in bus occupants, but claims of physical injury in bus occupants when a car strikes are contrary to known laws of physics. Interestingly, the researchers note that a lady approached one of the team's security officers after one of the experimental collisions. She tried desperately to find out exactly how many people were on that bus, but the security officer did not say, and she left in frustration.

Summary

The whiplash experiments have defined, then, that the probability of any neck injury due to acceleration is low with any of the following:

- head accelerations of less than 10g
- ΔV of less than 8 km/h (5 mph) for the struck vehicle in a rear-end collision (twice this velocity change in lateral or frontal collisions)

- a striking speed of at least 15 km/h (9 mph) in a rear-end collision, assuming the striking and struck vehicle are of similar mass

Experiments with humans indicate that symptoms occur with head accelerations between 12 and 20g (that is, with a ΔV of more than 8 km/h) [5 mph], and the symptoms correspond to minor muscle sprains.

One could try to argue that whiplash patients receive a more severe form of muscle injury than the experiment volunteers because of differences in physical features. This argument, however, fails because the more severe muscle and ligament injuries (ie, those that are not just microscopic) produce larger tears, more swelling, and more bleeding. As explained under "Radiology of Whiplash" above, MRI scans would detect these, and the MRI studies in whiplash patients have failed to do so. Besides, there is no scientific reason for a "more severe sprain" to lead to chronic pain than there is for a minor sprain to lead to chronic pain. Instead of days, it might take weeks to get better, not several months, years, or longer.

The initial acute injury of whiplash patients must necessarily be of essentially the same severity or similar outcome (concerning the physical outcome of healing) as in the volunteers who had pain. That is, sprains that generate microscopic tears and limited swelling and bleeding (limited enough that they are not noticeable on MRI scans) resolve in days to weeks.

Moreover, the most compelling confirmation of the validity of experimental results is that they agree with observation of the natural phenomenon. D. Obelieniene et al (1999) found that about 50% of accident victims involved in a rear-end collision in Lithuania report acute neck pain or headache. Remarkably, the duration of symptoms was just days in most cases, with a few having symptoms for as long as 3 weeks. After that, there was no reporting of chronic neck pain in relation to the acute injury event. Neck pain occurred in the future, but it occurred no more frequently in the accident injury group than it did in the noninjury group. What is equally remarkable is that the duration of symptoms is virtually identical to that of whiplash experiment volunteers. This is the case, even though those volunteers are in an entirely different culture, in a laboratory, and expecting a collision. Clearly, the experiment is reproducing an accurate picture of the events that follow collisions outside the laboratory. There are many other similarities between the data in the whiplash experiments and the observations made in Lithuania, which confirms even more clearly that the experimental collisions accurately reproduce the natural phenomenon. In both the experimental collisions and the collisions in Lithuania, the following was found:

- The injury symptoms appear to abate without any specific therapy.
- An impact speed of the striking vehicle that generates a ΔV of the struck vehicle of less than 8 km/h (5 mph) is much less likely to produce any injury. That is, in many of the Lithuanian accidents where the estimated striking ve-

hicle speed was less than 21 km/h (12.5 mph), there was a greatly reduced risk for acute whiplash injury.

- Gender was irrelevant to the risk of acute whiplash injury. It may be that chronic symptoms are more often reported by females, but this appears to have little to do with any gender difference in the risk of acute whiplash injury.
- The presence or vertical positioning of the head restraint does not reduce the incidence of acute pain.
- There are no significant differences in acute neck pain incidence between those with operating seat belts and those without.
- A rotated or inclined head position at the time of the impact is not found to increase the risk of acute injury significantly.

So, whatever the researchers are doing in the experimental collisions, whomever they are using as volunteers, they are clearly including all the necessary physical parameters to produce the acute whiplash injury. They produce an "experimental" accident victim who behaves just like the Lithuanian accident victim. One can imagine vast cultural and personal differences between experimental volunteers (experiments are usually done in North America) and the average Lithuanian, and yet they behave the same after an acute whiplash injury. Why?

The answer lies in not looking at their differences but at what they have in common. What they share is a lack of exposure to certain events. This book examines what those events are.

Yet we have to deal with the other chronic symptoms first.

Temporomandibular Disorders and Whiplash

KEY POINTS

- Many theories of temporomandibular joint (TMJ) injury have been produced, but there is no substantiated theory of "TMJ injury" in whiplash.
- Many TMJ imaging abnormalities some consider proof of injury are also found in asymptomatic subjects.
- Much literature indicates that psychological factors are important in the development and maintenance of jaw pain. A biopsychosocial model is needed to explain this phenomenon.

CONTROVERSY

The first description of a relationship between accelerated movements of the mandible and trauma is centuries old.

> Then Samson reached down and picked up the jawbone of an ass. . . .
>
> —Judges 15:15

Other aspects of the topic have interested researchers greatly in the past decade. The current controversy has been reviewed by R. Ferrari and M. Leonard (1998), and that work forms the basis for this chapter.

Temporomandibular disorders (TMD) are variously referred to as myofascial pain dysfunction syndrome, temporomandibular dysfunction, orofacial pain, and

Source: Ferrari R, Leonard M. Whiplash and temporomandibular disorders—a critical review. *Journal of the American Dental Association.* 1998;129: 1739–1745. ©1998 American Dental Association. Reprinted by permission of ADA Publsihing Co., Inc.

internal derangement. The basis of such disorders in nonwhiplash patients is very controversial, which further complicates the issue in whiplash patients.

Surprisingly, despite the decades during which experts have been arguing about TMD and whiplash, there is a paucity of studies about the incidence, course, management, and prognosis of claimed TMD following accidents.

D. A. Seligman and A. G. Pullinger (1996) studied the role of indirect trauma in producing these symptoms. They indicate that most of the evidence for a link between whiplash injury and TMD is anecdotal, and a direct etiologic role for indirect trauma has yet to be established. They found that non–motor vehicle accident trauma was correlated with these symptoms, but indirect trauma through motor vehicle accidents accounted for a minimal percentage of patients. They added, however, that even this association is not necessarily indicative of a causal relationship.

We are thus currently left with considering what the probability is that those whiplash patients reporting symptoms such as jaw pain, jaw clicking, "fullness" in the ears, pain in the ears, dizziness, and/or headache do so because of an injury to the temporomandibular joint (TMJ) or its supporting structures.

CULTURAL OBSERVATIONS

The first indication of the need to include psychosocial factors in understanding TMD following accidents comes from the observations of wide cultural variances in whiplash patients reporting symptoms associated with TMD. If TMD symptoms arise from acute injury to the TMJ or supporting structures along with the acute whiplash injury (where there is no direct jaw impact), one would expect to find a relatively similar incidence of TMD symptoms across cultures. The argument that TMD may be undiagnosed because symptoms are being attributed to other sources may be valid. Yet the presence of symptom reports should still be similar in different cultures, even if a different diagnostic label is attached to them. If, however, noninjury or nonphysical factors are more significant in symptom reporting, then one would indeed expect significant variances, for example, among various cultures.

Evidently, reporting TMD symptoms after an accident may be partly due to cultural factors, as whiplash patients virtually never or seldom do so in Australia (T. C. S. Probert et al 1994), Lithuania (Ferrari et al 1999), or Norway (Dr. H. Schrader, oral communication, January 1997). Lithuanian accident victims do report acute neck pain but not chronic neck pain or headache after a rear-end collision, and they do not appear to report the TMD symptoms either. As well, even in North America, medical and social fashion may be an important factor in the incidence of jaw pain in whiplash patients. Although it is common in some regions, A. P. Heise et al (1992) demonstrated, for example, that there are regions in the United States where the phenomenon of reporting TMD symptoms following accidents is virtually nonexistent.

Thus, cultural observations indicate that if the TMD following an accident is due to physical injury, whiplash victims in many other cultures are somehow managing to avoid that injury—an unlikely possibility.

THEORIES ABOUND

Theories of "mandibular whiplash" plague the controversy about TMD and whiplash. For decades, many have touted these theories without any substantial attempt to verify their validity.

The first theory began with V. H. Frankel (1965). He proposed that patients could develop whiplash of the TMJ, producing symptoms of "painful mastication, pain when opening the mouth, clicking in the temporomandibular joints, facial and aural pain, limited mouth opening."

He described his theory of the mechanism of this injury: "The mouth flies open. The stretch reflex (the jaw jerk) of the masseters is evoked, the jaw snaps shut. In the opening phase the anterior temporal attachments of the temporomandibular joint capsule and interarticular disc act as restraining ligaments that may be stretched or torn. In the closing phase, in the presence of malocclusion, the posterior mandibular and temporal attachments of the articular cartilage and disc undergo strain and these fibers may be stretched or torn."

Variations of this theory were published by E. Lader (1983) and by S. Weinberg and H. LaPointe (1987).

There has been more research undertaken to refute these theories (apparently held as fact by some) than to support them. First, researchers examined more closely how incredible the theories of mandibular whiplash had become. For instance, in 1991, R. P. Howard et al commented on Lader's theories.

> Others have suggested that injury to the temporomandibular joint associated with extension-flexion motion may be induced by myospasm. However, since extension-flexion maneuvers do not produce forces in a direction or magnitude that would have a traumatic effect on the temporomandibular joint or the masticatory muscles . . . no apparent relationship between masticatory myospasm and extension-flexion maneuvers exists that would have a greater potential to induce myospasm than would routinely experienced joint forces. However, myospasm produced by . . . stress . . . may be a major causative factor in temporomandibular joint disorder and myofascial pain syndromes.

Reviewing Weinberg's theories, they noted:

> The mechanism described by Weinberg was presumed to operate in the extension phase as follows (italics added):

The victim's body is accelerated with the car seat. The unsupported head will accelerate less quickly by virtue of its own inertia. . . . The mandible also due to its own inertia will move posteriorly less quickly than the cranium. This results in downward and forward displacement of the disc-condyle complex relative to the cranial base. . . . This leads to stretching and tearing of the posterior attachment and synovial tissues and loosening or tearing of the discal attachments to the medial and lateral condylar poles.

Analysis of the forces that would be created at the temporomandibular joint in the extension-flexion motion of the neck using a free body diagram shows the above mechanism to be invalid because the mandible does not "move posteriorly" with respect to inertial space.

Howard et al further added that "the forces experienced at the temporomandibular joint resulting from mild to moderate extension-flexion inertial motion of the neck not only act in a similar direction range as forces generated at the joint in normal chewing activity, but also are necessarily of a substantially lesser magnitude."

Also commenting on Weinberg's work, H. L. Goldberg (1990) stated that "these patient diagnoses and the general note about the symptoms . . . do not in any way support a relationship to a motor vehicle accident and whiplash."

He further added that "the patient who is involved in such an accident is typically prepared for [TMJ] treatment. Long-term appliance therapy and physiotherapy for 14 to 18 months without significant improvement is accepted as indicating the severe nature of the injury."

EXPERIMENTS

The most convincing arguments against the theories of mandibular whiplash come from human whiplash experiments. D. H. West et al (1993) and T. J. Szabo et al (1994) conducted experiments with human volunteers in rear-end collisions to determine whether mandibular whiplash was probable or not. They found that there is no opening of the jaw as a result of the impact forces, and they explain that the forces in such collisions are not capable of doing so.

But most formally, Howard et al (1995, 1998) have conducted extremely detailed analyses of the forces experienced by the TMJ under the conditions of a low-velocity rear-end collision. They proved that forces experienced by the TMJ are less than forces experienced in ordinary activities such as yawning, chewing, and so forth. The forces could not, therefore, possibly result in injury by the mechanisms others have proposed. They demonstrated that in such rear-end collisions the forces on the TMJ or supporting structures are not any higher than those experienced in normal daily use of the joint. They have combined specialized photography, dual plates attached to the upper and lower jaws (to see if they move with respect to each other), and monitoring of muscle activity (to test for relaxation or contraction before, during, and after the impact). They were able to cause acute neck injury (symptoms for a few days) and yet found that (Howard et al 1998):

> None of the test subjects experienced TMJ or related craniomandibular symptoms. Follow-up examinations revealed no delayed emergence of symptoms.

> There is no basis for TMJ ligament stretch since there is no distraction. The compressive forces, moreover, were only fractions of compressive forces imposed physiologically at the TMJ.

To the theorists, Howard et al suggested that "future proposals of injury mechanism hypotheses associated with these forces should be accompanied by satisfactory explanations as to why forces of greater magnitude and duration similarly directed on these structures, which are routinely experienced physiologically, impose no significant injury potential."

Finally, L. V. Christensen and D. C. McKay (1997) also undertook detailed electromyography studies of jaw motion (including during neck extension). They realized that theories of mandibular whiplash cannot be reconciled with any known principles in anatomy, physiology, or physics.

Despite this, others have looked for alternative ways to prove that TMD following an accident is due to an injury to the TMJ or supporting structures.

TMJ RADIOLOGY

To support the apparently insupportable notion of TMJ injury in whiplash patients, some have attempted to "demonstrate" the injury by showing that there is an association of reported TMD symptoms with imaging abnormalities. Such studies suffer from selection bias and from assumptions of accuracy of denial of preaccident symptoms (a study by P. D. Marshall et al 1995 indicated that accident victims tend to forget their preaccident neck pain). In addition, they suffer from retrospective design and from the misconception that finding an association between reporting of symptoms and abnormal imaging findings is equivalent to demonstrating a causal relationship. It is not.

There is also an apparent failure to appreciate the high prevalence of TMJ imaging abnormalities in the asymptomatic population. Regardless of which imaging modality is used—plain tomograms, arthroscopy, computed tomography, or magnetic resonance imaging (MRI)—many different types of abnormalities on TMJ imaging are seen in the asymptomatic subjects (see P. L. Westesson 1993).

Presumably, many whiplash patients were part of the asymptomatic population (they at least claim to have been) and had these imaging abnormalities before the accident. Despite this obvious point, when whiplash patients present after an accident, reporting TMD symptoms, some cite these very same imaging abnormalities as the cause of symptoms and as "proof" of injury.

Westesson et al (1989), for example, demonstrated using arthrography that "about 15% of persons with asymptomatic and clinically normal temporomandibular joints may have some form of disk displacement." In another study of theirs (1990), also using arthrograms in asymptomatic patients, they found that there was "a large variation of the dimensions of the joint compartments and also of the position of the disk in relation to the condyle."

Using tomograms, C. B. Muir and A. N. Goss (The radiologic morphology of asymptomatic temporomandibular joints, 1990) studied 200 asymptomatic women and found "an apparently high frequency of bony remodelling changes in asymptomatic TMJs." They explain that from the third decade of life onward, virtually everyone begins to have remodeling of the bony part of the TMJ. It is thus a normal finding in the population and is not necessarily a cause of pain. In asymptomatic subjects, they found numerous abnormalities, including sclerosis, osteophytes, flattening, cavities, erosions, and cysts.

The presence of TMJ abnormalities in the general population without symptoms (and presumably in whiplash patients before they are involved in an accident) has also been noted by T. Kircos et al (1987). They explain that internal derangement (abnormal placement of the disc in the joint) is often found on MRI imaging of asymptomatic subjects and question the view that internal derangement is the primary cause of TMJ dysfunction. They noted that:

> Clinical and autopsy studies show that many symptomatic TMJ dysfunction patients lack internal derangements. Moreover, autopsy studies of both young and mature adults show internal derangements in 10–32% of the general population.
>
> . . . In many instances anterior displacement of the TMJ disc which signifies internal derangement may be an anatomic variant of the normal TMJ rather than an actual derangement.

After further study, Muir and Goss (The radiologic morphology of painful temporomandibular joints, 1990) warned that "the clear implication of this study is that one should be cautious about overestimating the significance of radiologic abnormality in patients with pain in the TMJ region."

Likewise, J. E. Drace and D. R. Enzmann (1990) demonstrated that MRI of TMJs in normal (asymptomatic) subjects does indeed reveal the presence of abnormalities. They found a high prevalence of significant TMJ abnormalities in the asymptomatic population.

Thus, what is typically called a "TMJ abnormality causing pain" in a whiplash patient has a significant probability of having been present well before the accident. It is not necessarily responsible for any symptoms at all. For this reason, the one study by B. D. Pressman et al (1992), which purports that accident victims with TMD have many imaging abnormalities potentially responsible for symptoms, has many potential biases as it does not have a control group, is retrospective, and represents a selected group of patients (not a representative sample of patients). An appropriate study was done by H. Bergman et al (1998). These researchers performed MRI imaging of the TMJ on 60 consecutive accident victims (rear-end collision) reporting to an emergency department. They also did MRI imaging of 53 healthy controls. They found, 3 to 14 days after the collision, no increase in the incidence of disc displacement, joint effusion, or any other TMJ injury after whiplash trauma. This is despite the fact that 15% of the accident victim group had TMD symptoms.

Finally, B. A. Loughner et al (1996) have indicated that some TMJ abnormalities may be a *result* of altered jaw mechanics due to pain behaviors. One must consider that jaw pain is the *cause* and not the result of the abnormalities.

Although one could argue that the whiplash claimant might have had preaccident "silent" abnormalities that then became symptomatic following the accident, this claim seems untenable. Such "silent lesions" would presumably exist in whiplash patients in cultures or regions that do not appear to have the problem of TMD following whiplash. There is no reason for those patients to be at any less risk for the "activation" of a silent lesion. Moreover, the above experimental studies confirm that the forces affecting the TMJ during a whiplash injury are no more likely to activate a silent lesion than would battle with a 10-ounce New York steak—the latter not a commonly reported cause of TMD.

Thus, there is no convincing evidence of physical injury to the TMJ or supporting structures being responsible for jaw pain and other symptoms related to the jaw in whiplash patients. There are striking cultural variances, experimental evidence negates proposed mechanisms of injury, and one finds many imaging abnormalities in asymptomatic subjects. One must consider an explanation other than injury for the jaw pain and related symptoms. This does not mean there are no physical sources for these symptoms, merely that the physical sources are not injury related.

PSYCHOLOGICAL FACTORS AND SYMPTOM REPORTING

The TMD symptoms following an accident may yet be genuine and indeed may have a variety of physical (noninjurious) factors as the source, with psychosocial factors predominantly responsible for the pattern of symptom reporting in terms of severity and attribution to the accident.

Many have recognized that psychological factors influence TMD symptom reporting. D. E. Lupton (1969), reviewing the significant body of literature that had accumulated even up to just 1969, for example, identified that "there is a signifi-cant relationship of psychological factors to nonorganic TMJ dysfunction. These psychological factors are amenable to treatment, and treatment of the psycholog-ical factors results in relief of physical symptoms as well."

Regarding the specific aspect of postaccident chronic jaw pain, R. I. Brooke and P. G. Stenn (1978) considered that postaccident patients had different thera-peutic responses than other patients because of the psychological stressors such as the harbored resentment of a problem "someone else had caused" and the stress of litigation. J. A. Burgess and S. F. Dworkin (1993) demonstrated that the stress of litigation could indeed influence treatment outcomes in postaccident victims.

The possibility that stressful life events can lead to jaw pain has been explored by P. M. Moody et al (1982). They reviewed the fact that "a number of studies have identified psychologic factors in the etiology of [myofascial pain dysfunc-tion] syndrome. Furthermore, the literature suggests that anxiety and disturbing life events are associated with mandibular dysfunction problems."

In their own study, they found that "the data presented . . . suggest that patients suffering from [myofascial pain dysfunction] have higher life [changes] than pa-tients with other illnesses."

MECHANISMS

As M. F. Gargan et al (1997) recently demonstrated, whiplash patients experi-ence great distress during the first 3 months after the accident. It is well recog-nized that psychological distress has a physiological correlate and that somatic (bodily) symptoms are the accompaniment (see R. Kellner 1991). The relation-ship between distress and alterations in muscle activity about the jaw has been considered by many (F. M. Bush and M. F. Dolwick 1995, A. J. Cannistraci and G. Fritz 1989, S. Ruf et al 1997). The type of somatic symptomatology expressed with psychological distress is often culturally and socially determined (E. Shorter 1992), which may explain the wide variations in the epidemiology of many pain disorders among cultures (Shorter 1994). Shorter (1992) explains that within a given culture, a fashionable or widely publicized illness can preconsciously moti-vate the development of symptoms of that illness in certain settings (usually in the setting of somatization). The more discussion there is about the "TMJ injury" in whiplash, the more individuals appear with these symptoms. It is not necessary that the individual have a psychiatric disorder or overt evidence of a neurosis.

There is plenty of opportunity to receive such information from the media, from other patients, and from the medical and legal communities. This may ex-plain why patients develop jaw pain a few weeks after the accident, after being re-peatedly questioned or told about the "TMJ injury of whiplash." Thus, cultural ef-fects may produce jaw pain reporting in response to psychological distress. The distressed mind consciously and preconsciously recognizes this as an acceptable outlet in a given culture, just as headache is an acceptable response to stress.

Because accident victims are distressed, they may be highly suggestible to information from the medical and legal professionals, as well as the effects of the cultural sources of illness information. As explained by Kellner (1991), "a person who has experienced physical disease likely becomes more aware of bodily sensations, or has more fears of physical illness, or both."

Then, patients report the jaw pain to the medical and legal professionals they meet. If they subsequently receive a diagnosis of "TMJ injury" and are told they may need therapy for months or years, with the possibility of permanence of symptoms, symptom amplification may occur. Numerous studies indicate that anxiety is an important factor in "TMJ patients," and the information the patient receives from the medical and legal communities can potentially cause anxiety. Increased jaw pain can lead only to more psychological distress, as explained by Bush and Dolwick (1995), who reviewed the more recent studies of 1982 to 1994.

Numerous experimental studies suggest a relationship between stress-related muscular activity and [temporomandibular dysfunction] symptoms, and empirical findings support this notion.

[Electromyography] activities of the jaw muscles of symptomatic individuals show that stressful life events create muscular tension. Bruxism and levels of nocturnal muscle activity become elevated during episodes of daytime stress and anticipation of stress. Long-term study of patients diagnosed with chronic myogenous [temporomandibular dysfunction] showed that exacerbations of pain were preceded by increased [electromyography] muscular activity.

[Temporomandibular dysfunction] pain complaints have been reduced using stress management techniques designed to reduce muscular activity, including biofeedback training and relaxation therapy.

Thus, symptom expectation and the manifestation of psychological distress may both be a function of cultural and medical fashions. This may potentially explain the wide cultural and regional variations in the incidence of reporting of "TMJ complaints" by whiplash patients. This expectation will in turn lead to symptom amplification with the individual becoming hypervigilant for symptoms. Patients will also register normal bodily sensations as abnormal, reacting to bodily sensations with affect and cognitions that intensify them, making them more alarming, ominous, and disturbing (A. J. Barsky et al 1988).

Numerous factors (see Chapter 9) lead to symptom amplification and more severe or prolonged jaw pain. Finally, there may be symptom attribution just as there is with chronic neck pain. That is, headache, jaw clicking, dizziness, and auditory complaints are common in the general population. Presumably, even if the accident victim had not been an accident victim, he or she would carry some risk of developing such symptoms in the future. The patient may have even had symptoms in the past but did not have reason to recall them. As an accident victim, especially as a claimant, the patient is in circumstances that encourage detailed recording of symptoms. Symptom amplification occurs, and these previously nonintrusive symptoms (largely ignored in daily life) become far more intrusive after the accident. The patient will then regard them as new and attribute them to the accident. The behavior of others, deliberate or not, often encourages them to do so. In addition, as seen in the next chapter, symptoms such as dizziness and hearing disturbance can arise after the accident from factors such as medication use and the effects of neck pain on one's balance: again, a TMJ injury is not required to produce these symptoms. All these presumably physical (biological) sources of symptoms, even though noninjurious, may act as a substrate for the effects of psychosocial factors in generating an apparent TMD following whiplash.

SUMMARY

A biopsychosocial model is necessary to understand TMD following an accident. There is no substantiated theory of "TMJ injury" in whiplash. There is no experimental evidence of forces to cause "TMJ injury." Many of the TMJ imaging abnormalities some cite as proof of injury are found in asymptomatic subjects. Injury to the TMJ or its supporting structures must be a questionable cause of jaw pain and related symptoms in whiplash patients without blunt trauma to the jaw. There are wide cultural variations, and there is a large body of literature reflecting the psychological mechanisms of jaw pain. With all this, there is the real possibility that the jaw pain reported by a whiplash patient without blunt jaw trauma, while genuine, is not due to physical injury from the accident. Instead a biopsychosocial model is necessary to explain this phenomenon, and psychosocial factors are the most important.

Whiplash on
My Mind

KEY POINTS

- Many whiplash patients report dizziness, problems with their hearing and vision, and poor concentration and memory.
- Some researchers believe that these symptoms indicate a nervous system injury. But in the past 40 years, neurologic tests have not provided medical researchers with evidence of a site of chronic tissue damage that follows the acute injury.
- The associations between whiplash and headaches, and whiplash and the diagnosis of thoracic outlet syndrome, have also preoccupied many researchers.

INTRODUCTION

Although chronic pain is the predominant complaint of whiplash claimants, they also report dizziness, vertigo, hearing and visual disturbances, cognitive dysfunction (poor memory or concentration), headache, limb numbness, and other symptoms. Physicians often refer to these as "neurological" symptoms because the symptoms appear in a variety of diseases of the nervous system, including the brain (hence, "whiplash on my mind"). Experts have associated these symptoms with various sites of chronic damage and used different diagnostic tools to search for the sites. The researchers are looking for the damage caused by an acute injury that not only remains chronic damage but is responsible for chronic neck pain, chronic back pain, jaw pain, numbness, poor balance, poor memory, and so forth. It is no easy task to find a single site responsible for all these troubles. Not surprisingly, the search has been unsuccessful. It is worth-

Source: Adapted from R. Ferrari and A. S. Russell, Whiplash on My Mind. *Hippocrates' Lantern.* Vol. 5, No. 3, pp. 16–20. ©1998, Aspen Publishers, Inc.

while to review what other researchers have postulated are the causes of these symptoms.

DISTURBANCES OF BALANCE AND HEARING

Lack of High-Quality Research

Some whiplash patients report disturbances of balance (dizziness or vertigo) or of hearing (loss of hearing or ringing in the ears [tinnitus]) since the accident. Again, however, researchers have not identified the site of injury within the nervous system that would produce these chronic complaints in whiplash patients. In 1997, A. J. E. M. Fischer et al reviewed the studies that have been done. They found that most have significant flaws or biases. These include patient selection bias (including patients with head injury with whiplash), examining patients years after the accident (when other diseases or conditions may be acting), not accounting for medication use (which can cause many of the symptoms), and lack of control groups. Fischer et al also point out that emotional distress can lead to reporting of symptoms such as dizziness.

M. M. Braaf and S. Rosner (Meniere-like syndrome following whiplash injury of the neck, 1962) presented one of the earliest theories of the cause of vertigo (spinning sensation) in whiplash patients. Their article provides a good example of how willing the members of the medical profession are to draw a conclusion without complete evidence to support it. They wrote, for example, that:

> Cervical trauma of the whiplash-type produces primarily a mechanical overstretching of the longitudinal ligaments of the cervical spine. If the injury is severe, the intervertebral disk may also be damaged by fragmentation of the nucleus pulposus or rupture of the annulus fibrosus. The trauma causes an anatomic derangement of the cervical spine with its inherent structures, which may produce mechanical irritation of the cervical nerves or intermittent compression of the vertebral artery.

These authors neither presented experimental or objective evidence to prove their claim nor referred to other experiments to support their ideas. Other studies have had the same lack of objective proof of a site of nervous system injury responsible for these symptoms and relied on theoretical possibilities. Examples include those by S. L. Shapiro (1972) and M. Yagi (1967). Similarly, articles by J. B. Chester Jr. (1991), W. E. Compere (1968), W. J. Oosterveld et al (1991), and J. U. Toglia et al (1970) have many of the biases and flaws cited above. (See Chapter 13 for more detailed comments on these articles.) Finally, in a textbook, A. Cesarani et al (1996) discuss in detail the potential "lesions" responsible for symptoms such as dizziness, hearing loss, tinnitus, and visual disturbance. The discussion remains largely theoretical; researchers have not found a pathological lesion responsible for such symptoms in whiplash patients.

Balance Tests

Chester (1991), Oosterveld (1991), and Toglia et al (1970) used balance tests to find evidence of the chronic damage that could be responsible for symptoms of dizziness or vertigo (spinning) in whiplash patients. These studies had some flaws, but more important, the results showed that although all the patients complained of symptoms, the majority had normal findings, so that the abnormalities could not explain the reported symptoms.

Hearing Tests

It was a tiny sound, but one that he knew so well. A sound that whiplashed across his nerve endings and jerked him back.
—Smith W. *The Seventh Scroll.* London: Macmillan; 1995:130.

L. Q. Pang (1971) and Toglia et al (1969) attempted to demonstrate that there was a nervous system injury in whiplash patients that led to chronic hearing disturbances. Many researchers, including K. H. Chappa et al (1979) and M. J. Rowe (1978), found that there were differences in a normal group between the two ears of the same subject, between subjects, or between different occasions for single subjects. So one had to be very careful when using the abnormalities in these test results to indicate that something was wrong with the patient. Healthy subjects have a lot of these abnormalities too.

It is equally apparent that some people have hearing disturbances before the accident or develop them much later. In these cases, the finding of abnormal test results may be unrelated to the accident, and the symptoms are simply being attributed to the accident.

Probable Sources of These Symptoms

The probable sources of balance and hearing disturbances in whiplash patients include medication use, the presence of neck pain (in the case of balance disturbances), anxiety, and misattribution of common, minor symptoms in the general population (for which one cannot identify a cause in most cases).

The medications whiplash patients often use are known frequently to cause a wide range of adverse effects. Balance disturbances are common with antidepressants, antipsychotics, antianxiety agents, or other sedatives. Hearing disturbances are common with nonsteroidal antiinflammatory drugs (called NSAIDs), as shown in Table 7–1.

Table 7–1 The Adverse "Balance" Effects of Drug Therapy

Drug Type	Studies
Antidepressants	M. H. Lader 1996
	S. H. Preskorn 1995
	K. Wennmo and C. Wennmo 1988
Antipsychotics	P. E. Hayes and C. A. Kristoff 1986
	A. B. Whitworth and W. W. Fleischhacker 1995
Antianxiety drugs	K. Wennmo and C. Wennmo 1988
Narcotics	S. D. Jaanus 1992
NSAIDs	J. A. Brien 1993
	S. D. Jaanus 1992
	T. T. Jung et al 1993
	H. Seligmann et al 1996
	K. Wennmo and C. Wennmo 1988

More recent and more carefully conducted studies (with control groups and exclusion of patients who are on certain medications) have suggested additional causes for dizziness, vertigo, and other balance disturbances. A. Conte et al (1997), H. Heikkliä and P. G. Aström (1996), J. K. Loudon et al (1997), A. M. Rubin et al (1995), and C. Tjell and U. Rosenhall (1998) have found significant postural abnormalities in whiplash patients and argued that this may be an important factor in producing sensations of dizziness.

M. Karlberg et al (1996) studied a group with chronic, nontraumatic neck pain to eliminate any subjects involved in compensation. They found that physiotherapy reduced neck pain and dizziness and improved postural performance. This argues against a specific nervous system lesion as the cause of dizziness and is consistent with the findings of all the other researchers just mentioned. These researchers consider it more likely that dizziness is a secondary result of neck pain and the effects of neck pain and motion of the head movements. Normal movements of the head and neck are necessary for normal balance control and visual function. These same recent studies are also demonstrating that the results of many specific neurological tests are completely normal in the patients reporting these symptoms.

Anxiety is also known to be an important factor in the reporting of otherwise unexplainable chronic dizziness, vertigo, hearing loss, and tinnitus. L. S. Alvord (1991), J. M. Furman and R. G. Jacob (1997), G. H. Saunders and M. P. Haggard (1989, 1993), and R. B. Simpson et al (1988) have confirmed that anxiety generates these symptoms or that there are minor objective abnormalities of hearing, for example, that are grossly exaggerated and thus amplified by the anxious individual. S. I. Erlandsson et al (1991) and G. H. Saunders and M. P. Haggard (1989) have demonstrated that the patient's anxiety reflects not only chronic, unexplainable hearing disturbance but also a generalized anxiety state. Interestingly, D. Y. Aplin and J. M. Kane (1985) showed what effect anxiety traits have on symptom reporting in this regard. They asked two groups of normal subjects (no hearing loss) to fake hearing loss. The individuals who rated higher on certain anxiety scales faked a greater degree of hearing loss than those who did not rate high on anxiety scales. Thus, anxiety alters symptom reporting even when the symptoms are not real and the patient knows it. Compared with less anxious subjects, anxious subjects rate intense stimuli as being louder and weak stimuli as being softer.

Finally, one must also consider that many of the reported symptoms are common in the general population. The whiplash patient may simply be misattributing some of them to the accident.

Summary

There is no evidence that whiplash patients reporting chronic symptoms of dizziness, vertigo, or disturbance of vision or hearing have a specific nervous system injury. Instead, it is more probable that this symptom reporting arises from

1. medication adverse effect
2. presence of neck pain altering postural control (creating balance disturbance)
3. anxiety and other emotional distress
4. hypervigilance about symptoms that are common in the general population but misattributed to the accident and amplified

DISTURBANCE OF VISION

Some whiplash patients also complain of chronic visual difficulties such as visual blurring or eye fatigue or eye dryness when reading, and some have argued that physical damage somewhere in the nervous system is responsible for these symptoms. Only rarely (see R. S. Haslett et al 1994 and G. Liguori et al 1997) has a pathological lesion been found in the eye. Even in such cases, the lesions may have been there before the accident. These are merely case reports, not formal studies.

In 1956, H. Horwich described a theory of how whiplash might cause ocular abnormalities, but he did not add any experimental evidence and otherwise gave only anecdotal experience.

In 1958, W. N. M. Girling attempted to explain visual complaints of blurring, photophobia, and headache in whiplash patients. He studied 130 patients with previous rear-end collision and found various abnormalities on visual testing. The author does not describe the age of the patients. He also does not state whether

they had any preaccident ocular examinations to use for comparison, what medications were in use (many medications can cause visual disturbances), and with
what frequency these abnormalities are found in the healthy, general population.

Similarly, in 1962, H. Wiesinger and D. Guerry describe a small series of patients with minor ocular abnormalities after rear-end collision. These researchers
felt that the cause was whiplash. Unfortunately, they lacked the same information
as the researchers above lacked.

When trying to ascertain the damage from injury responsible for ocular symptoms occurring after whiplash, H. Horwich and D. Kasner (1962) wrote that this
was difficult since "by and large, we are at the mercy of the patient's volition and
motivation."

Even some of the objective signs observed during eye examinations are not
useful. One of these is unequal pupil size. It is sometimes a sign of disease but is
also common in the general population. As pointed out by T. L. Slamovits and J.
S. Glaser in 1988, "All pupils are not created equal. In fact, benign pupillary in-
equality exists in practically all individuals, but not necessarily all the time."

Articles often refer to convergence, a normal eye movement that allows for
near-reading without blurred vision. Some claimed any abnormalities here represent disease or injury, but this may again be a false conclusion. As noted by Slamovits and Glaser, "Converging power varies considerably and depends on the co-
operation of the patient."

It is more probable that the sources of visual disturbances in whiplash patients
include medication use, the presence of neck pain, and misattribution of common, minor symptoms in the general population (for which one cannot identify a
cause in most cases). The medications whiplash patients often use are known frequently to cause a wide range of adverse effects (see Table 7–2).

C. Hildingsson and B. I. Wenngren (1989) raised the possibility that neck pain
could alter the way the head and eyes work in unity, thus impairing ocular function. That is, normal vision requires normal head and neck movements and posture. They considered this a reasonable possibility because such postural problems would simultaneously explain disturbances of balance. R. Gimse et al
(1996) examined this posture control problem. From their studies, they conclude
that "the posture control system is affected in the [whiplash] subjects due to misleading information from the . . . cervical spine. This causes vertigo as well as
disturbed eye movements and reading problems." This was confirmed by H.
Heikkliä and B. I. Wenngren (1998).

Probable Sources of These Symptoms

The arguments for visual symptoms being caused by a nervous system injury
come from poor studies with incomplete information and numerous potential

Table 7–2   The Adverse Visual Effects of Drug Therapy

Drug type	Studies
Antidepressants	S. D. Jaanus 1992
	M. H. Lader 1996
	S. H. Preskorn 1995
Antipsychotics	A. B. Whitworth and W. W. Fleischhacker 1995
Antianxiety drugs	S. D. Jaanus 1992
Narcotics	S. D. Jaanus 1992
NSAIDs	S. D. Jaanus 1992

flaws. Researchers have not found a site of nervous system injury to explain these symptoms. Instead, it is more probable that this symptom reporting arises from

1. medication adverse effect
2. presence of neck pain altering postural (and eye) control
3. hypervigilance about symptoms that are common in the general population but misattributed to the accident and amplified

DISTURBANCE OF COGNITION

Many have postulated that brain injury is responsible for cognitive difficulties such as memory and concentration impairment. An ever-growing body of research refutes this notion. This literature considers the frequency of such complaints in control groups, radiological studies of whiplash patients, the experimental collisions defining brain injury thresholds, and studies correlating these complaints to specific noninjurious factors.

First, B. T. Olsnes (1989) and A. E. Taylor et al (1996) compared whiplash patients to chronic pain patients without injury. They found that whiplash patients with persistent symptoms are not impaired much in their performance in neuropsychological tests as compared with control patients with chronic pain that did not result from injury. Both groups displayed no selective impairment on neuropsychological tests said to be sensitive to the effects of head trauma.

Taylor et al warn that:

For those clinicians whose opinions rely heavily on patient reports of psychological and cognitive distress following whiplash, a further word of caution is warranted. Many such complaints, nonspecific in nature, are found in other medical disorders. They are also present in healthy individuals. In the latter regard, several investigators, using symptom checklists, have found little to no difference between normal subjects and [minor head injury] patients within a year of injury regarding, for example, "concentration difficulties, anxiety, depression, irritability, word finding problems."

Accordingly, subjective complaints of nonspecific symptoms cannot be uncritically accepted as substantive "proof" [of] organic (brain) pathology. To do so leads to the risk of over diagnosis of "brain damage," a permanent condition.

Second, researchers have used a variety of diagnostic tools to try to find some evidence of brain damage, and no evidence exists. Chapter 13 has more comments on the studies reviewed below.

Electroencephalograms (EEGs)

In 1960, S. K. Shapiro and F. Torres performed a much quoted experiment with 47 patients who had suffered whiplash without head injury. They obtained EEGs and felt that the results suggested the whiplash injury was within the brain. Others later showed these studies to be highly flawed. E. S. Gurdjian and L. M. Thomas (1970), D. E. Jacome and M. Risko (1984), and Jacome (1987) made it clear that EEG studies *had not* found the site of reported chronic damage produced by a whiplash injury.

Magnetic Resonance Imaging (MRI) and Other Brain Scans

MRI scans are very useful in detecting damage to many parts of the nervous system, particularly the brain and spinal cord. Yet all the researchers who have looked for brain damage in this way in whiplash patients have found none. These researchers include G. E. Borchgrevink et al (1995), H. R. Ronnen et al (1996), and P. R. Yarnell and G. V. Rossie (1988).

There is some evidence, however, that other forms of brain scan may be useful in detecting brain damage. These include single photon emission computed tomography and positron emission tomography (PET). The studies by A. Otte et al (1995–1997) are of particular interest, as they are sometimes misinterpreted. The brain scans they used detect changes in blood flow and activity in the brain. To their credit, Otte et al had 3 control groups in addition to whiplash patients in their original study. The 3 control groups were healthy subjects, subjects with nontraumatic back pain only, and subjects with nontraumatic neck pain only. Whiplash patients tended to have abnormalities in a specific part of the brain. The question was why, and the answer was provided by the findings in the control groups. They found that the healthy subjects and back pain–only subjects had normal scans (thus, being in pain itself is not responsible for these brain scan abnormalities—if it were, patients with back pain might have abnormal brain scans). The interesting finding is that patients with nontraumatic neck pain had the same frequency and location of abnormalities on these brain scans as did the whiplash patients. The authors explain that the same nerves that supply sensation to the neck also have branches on the blood vessels of the posterior part of the brain. Thus, having neck pain of any cause, for reasons that are not yet understood, alters blood flow in the brain in a specific region. Brain injury is not required. These studies emphasize the need for adequate control groups.

Otte et al extended their studies in 1998 to demonstrate also that the brain imaging abnormalities are not due to any contusion ("bruising") of the brain at the time of the initial injury. Finally, I. Bicik et al (1998) used PET scans in patients with late whiplash syndrome, finding that the abnormalities correlated best with measures of depression in the patients, as opposed to representing brain injury.

Whiplash Experiments

There have been no human whiplash experiments that attempt to consider if brain injury will occur. We do know from animal experiments, however, that to cause objective evidence of nervous system injury, the accelerations and their duration must be several orders of magnitude outside the impact experience of whiplash patients (see B. Saltzberg et al 1983, M. S. Weiss et al 1983).

Probable Causes of Cognitive Complaints

Studies indicate that these symptoms are correlated to the pain experience, other causes for psychological distress, and medications (G. Di Stefano et al 1995, B. P. Radanov and J. Dvorak 1996). The use of narcotic and other sedating medications often explains the problems in patients who describe a sensation that their "head just doesn't feel right" or that they have a "hangover" feeling. The cognitive impairment improves as the patient's pain improves.

Sources of psychological distress may also produce these symptoms. P. R. Lees-Haley and R. S. Brown (1993) studied 170 personal injury litigants. In these cases, the litigation was not related to a physical injury but to issues of sex, race, or age discrimination, verbal harassment at work, wrongful termination, and so forth. Although the patients were not filing a claim for neuropsychological impairment, they had a prevalence of cognitive and other neurological complaints similar to that of those who litigate for so-called mild traumatic brain injury. The researchers also showed that the base rates of these complaints is actually high in healthy people. In many cases, claimants are simply amplifying and misattributing their symptoms to the accident, although the symptoms relate instead to preexisting conditions, the stress of litigation, unrelated illnesses, malingering, the inspiration of hysteria by prior medical and legal evaluations, or the influence of third parties. There are as yet no controlled studies (controlled for these confounding variables) that demonstrate an injury basis for the neuropsychological impairment often claimed following whiplash.

Beyond this, an aspect of malingering cognitive dysfunction appears to be a particular problem in some countries. In the Netherlands, B. Schmand et al (1998) showed that some 25% of those patients reporting such symptoms months to years after the accident are malingering. Malingering was twice as common in litigants as it was in nonlitigants.

The arguments for cognitive symptoms being caused by a brain injury in whiplash patients are thus unsubstantiated, and all attempts to demonstrate underlying brain injury objectively have failed. Noninjurious factors explain such symptom reporting.

1. psychological distress from having pain, battling with insurance companies, and litigation
2. malingering
3. medication adverse effect
4. hypervigilance about symptoms that are common in the general population but misattributed to the accident and amplified

HEADACHE

To some patients, "headache" is simply what they call that pain at the back of the head, near the neck (ie, what others call "neck pain"). Headache in these patients can be understood, then, by investigating why patients report chronic neck pain. For others, the headache has different locations and seems distinct from their neck pain. This is one of the few symptoms of whiplash patients that the medical literature seems to agree is not likely the result of injury.

For example, O. D. Chrisman and R. F. Gervais (1962) looked at the incidence of Barre syndrome—headache plus dizziness, ear buzzing, ear ringing, or a sensation of hearing loss—in whiplash patients. They noted that the symptoms are all subjective with no objectivity to document a pathologic basis for the syndrome. They tried to document and objectify the etiology of Barre syndrome and relate it to whiplash by conducting audiology studies, but as they stated, "This attempt was unsuccessful."

Researchers have also been quite honest about the lack of any experimental or objective evidence of an injury to explain headache in whiplash patients. In 1964, for instance, A. P. Friedman and J. Ransohoff described a detailed anatomical basis for posttraumatic headache but admitted they had no evidence for that basis. They did note, as well, that there is a low incidence of chronic posttraumatic headache after recreational activities.

Then came a series of articles pointing to the psychological basis for headache in whiplash patients. Commenting on the similarities between tension headache (due to anxiety and stress) and that seen in patients with cervical spondylosis, R. Iansek et al (1986) noted that the features were "indistinguishable," suggesting that nociceptors (pain receptors) from deranged joint structures are not directly responsible for headache in cervical spondylosis.

Also, in 1993, B. P. Radanov et al (Factors influencing recovery from headache after common whiplash) examined the incidence of headache after common whiplash and found that a history of headache before the injury significantly increased the likelihood of patients presenting with trauma-related headache.

Looking more closely at the etiology of posttraumatic headache, D. C. Haas (1993) noted that:

> Chronic posttraumatic headache does not correlate with the degree of head trauma or with evidence of brain damage as noted on computed tomography (CT) and magnetic resonance imaging (MRI).

> Some authors, most notably Taylor in 1967 and then Kelly, have argued that postconcussional symptoms result, in part at least, from damage to the brainstem and white matter of the sort demonstrated in experimental animals subjected to concussions. This hypothesis is, however, inconsistent with the considerable data showing a lack of correlation between the occurrence of postconcussional symptoms, including headache, and the severity of head trauma. Kay et al. clearly showed the absence of such a correlation for the postconcussional syndrome, and others have shown the same for posttraumatic headache.

> The chronic posttraumatic headache has been related not only to coexistent mental states but also to preexistent personalities.

Haas (1996) also suggested that these headaches may really be no different than tension-type headaches in the general population. There are differences between patients reporting what they perceive to be posttraumatic headache and patients reporting nontraumatic headache, however, in that the distress in posttraumatic patients tends to be more focused or associated with their symptoms (see Wallis et al 1998). The question is why. Not surprisingly, posttraumatic patients engage in activities (litigation, battling with insurance companies, dealing with disability issues, and engaging the therapeutic community) more often than nontraumatic headache patients. These activities provide ample sources for anxiety to become associated with the headache. This may be why their anxiety tends to focus on their symptoms rather than the more generalized form of psychological distress Wallis et al found in nontraumatic headache patients, who were again far less likely to engage in these anxiety-provoking activities.

Finally, as headaches are a common experience in the general population, patients may have had them in the past or were due to have them in the future. They may be misattributing some of their symptoms to the accident. This possibility is highlighted in the study by D. Obelieniene et al (1998) in which it was found that 1 to 3 years after an accident, accident victims in Lithuania have the same prevalence and character of headache as the uninjured population.

There is simply no evidence that chronic headache in whiplash patients is due to some form of chronic physical damage from the accident injury.

LIMB PAIN AND NUMBNESS

Arm numbness (or when the patient has back pain, leg numbness) is a commonly reported symptom. Some patients may report that there is also pain in their limbs. Most of the research has focused on arm pain and numbness in whiplash patients. Because such symptoms are sometimes reported by those with specific neurological diseases, researchers have looked for chronic nerve damage in whiplash patients. Some have considered damage to nerves via the disorder known as thoracic outlet syndrome, whereas others have looked for nerve damage elsewhere.

Thoracic Outlet Syndrome

As discussed in Chapter 15, a group of nerves from the spinal cord come together and travel through the deep structures of the neck, under the collarbone (clavicle), and into the arm. The thoracic outlet is the space nerves travel through in the lower part of the neck and upper part of the chest. It is a triangular space with muscles on two sides and bone on the third side.

It is here that the rare thoracic outlet syndrome originates. Emphasis should be put on the word "rare." In this syndrome, the thoracic outlet is abnormally small and so compresses the nerves and the blood vessels in this area. This may cause pain and poor circulation in the arm.

Thoracic outlet syndrome is now another lesson for the medical and surgical community. Thousands of people had surgical procedures (to enlarge the outlet) with no benefit and some harm. In 1965, for example, W. W. Woods coined the term "cervicobrachial neurovascular compression syndrome." He felt that there was clear evidence that whiplash patients had compression of the nerves and blood vessels exiting the neck and passing into the arm. This entity became known as thoracic outlet syndrome.

What Woods could not realize at the time, however, was that the surgery he used to correct this problem has been shown, in proper follow-up studies, to be useless. Moreover, one often finds in normal subjects the physical examination sign he describes in patients. Many have denounced the entire concept proposed by Woods, including J. R. Youmans (1990).

The evolution of [thoracic outlet syndrome] is further clouded by concepts that at one time or another reached great popularity, only to fall into disfavor later. Examples include (1) the use of Adson's maneuver to confirm entrapment by the loss of the radial pulse with stretch of the scalenus anticus muscle, which is no longer considered a meaningful test (2) the popularity of the procedure of simple scalenus anticus muscle section, which later proved ineffective in most circumstances and (3) the more recent reliance on the concept that electrical slowing could be demonstrated across the thoracic outlet using standard nerve conduction velocity techniques, a concept that was recently disproved.

A careful review of neurologists' and neurosurgeons' expert opinions on this syndrome explains the reason one cannot easily accept this diagnosis in whiplash patients. L. P. Rowland (1989) notes:

How often [thoracic outlet syndrome] lesions are actually responsible for symptoms . . . [is] of intense debate. . . . When neurologists write about this neurologic disorder . . . the tone is always skeptical and the syndrome is described as exceedingly rare, with an annual incidence of about 1/1,000,000.

Among the more imaginative lesions are those ascribed to hypertrophy of the scalenus muscles. . . .

In the *true* syndrome there are definite clinical and electrical abnormalities.

Rowland (1989) also confirms that physical examination signs do not confirm the diagnosis on their own: "Attempts to reproduce the syndrome by abducting the arm (the Adson test) or other maneuvers have been cited repeatedly, but the same "abnormalities" can be demonstrated in normal people and have *no diagnostic value* [emphasis added]."

R. D. Adams and M. Victor (1989) concur: "One should be skeptical of the diagnosis unless rigid clinical and [electromyogram] criteria . . . have been met."

Finally, K. D. Sethi and T. R. Swift (1991) reaffirm the lack of diagnostic capability of physical examination maneuvers: "Various diagnostic maneuvers to demonstrate obliteration of the arterial pulse at the wrist with head turning, deep breathing and shoulder movement are of no value, being positive in up to 80% of normal subjects. Likewise, the scalenus anticus syndrome does not exist, and scalenotomy, formerly in fashion, is of no value in treatment."

A number of other authors (M. Cherington 1989, Cherington et al 1986, A. C. Cuetter and D. M. Bartoszek 1989, D. A. Nelson 1990, T. Smith and W. Trojaborg 1987, and A. J. Wilbourn 1990) have vehemently challenged this misdiagnosis and pointed out the many flaws made by those who believe they are diagnosing a legitimate form of tissue damage in these patients. Thus, one must always view skeptically the diagnosis of thoracic outlet syndrome in whiplash patients.

Instead, arm pain and a feeling of numbness in association with neck pain are referred symptoms. They are analogous to the arm pain or numbness experienced during a heart attack. Nerve injury is not required. The situation with back pain and leg numbness is also analogous, where it is often reported in the absence of any objective neurological findings to suggest a nerve injury (ie, loss or diminishment of deep tendon reflexes, objective muscle weakness, and sensory deficits in a specific dermatomal pattern).

In patients without objective neurological findings, there is no evidence that the acute whiplash injury also results in a neurological injury responsible for arm or leg numbness. Thoracic outlet syndrome is also not a viable alternative. The symptom merely reflects the common, benign, and as yet unexplained phenomenon of pain referral in those with neck or back pain (from a variety of causes).

SUMMARY

The use of neurologic tests over the past 40 years has not provided medical researchers with evidence for a site of chronic tissue damage that follows the acute injury. The same is true of the radiologic tests and the whiplash experiments. That the acute injury exists is accepted, but one must ask why researchers are having so much difficulty finding the site of chronic damage that continues to cause all of the symptoms to be reported, often for months or years. Our inability to find this source is one reason to look elsewhere for answers. The next chapters will address this topic in more detail.

The Psychology of Whiplash

O that you could turn your eyes toward the napes of your necks, and make but an interior survey of your good selves!

—William Shakespeare. *Coriolanus* Act II, Scene 1.

KEY POINTS

- There are two models that help explain why some whiplash patients report chronic pain and why some countries have whiplash cultures and others do not.
- In the first model, whiplash is a psychocultural illness. In the second model, whiplash involves adoption of the sick role. Together, the models can explain the behavior and symptoms of most whiplash patients.

This and subsequent chapters that address the "psychology of whiplash" will not argue that the chronic symptoms being reported by whiplash patients are "all in their head." Instead, understanding the psychology of whiplash means understanding why a whiplash patient in North America, for example, reports chronic symptoms after an acute injury whereas one in Lithuania does not. Understanding the psychology of whiplash cultures means understanding why volunteers in whiplash experiments act the same way as Lithuanian accident victims, each often reporting acute symptoms from an injury but not reporting chronic symptoms thereafter. This understanding allows one also to consider that not all (or even many) whiplash patients are malingering or interested merely in the monetary payoff at the end. There is no doubt that insurance fraud exists and that patients know full well that a monetary reward may wait at the end of the litigation. (See, for example, N. Baer 1997.) Just as there is still little evidence to support the notion that the acute whiplash injury leads to some form of chronic physical damage that causes chronic symptoms, there is equally little evidence that one can explain all whiplash patients with a model based on notions of malingering and greed. There is more to whiplash than accounted for by either of those models.

We have already considered that a biopsychosocial approach is necessary. Some biological factors include the acute neck or back sprain, development of poor posture (a source of pain in itself) following the acute injury, the adverse effects of medications, and as we shall further consider, a variety of physical sources of pain seen in the general population that are then being amplified and misattributed by the accident victim to the accident injury. These biological factors form the substrate upon which psychosocial factors act to create a whiplash patient with chronic pain. The biological factors indicate that there is a physical source to the pain but that the pain's severity has been increased by psychosocial factors.

The need for at least two models is apparent. The first model—whiplash as a psychocultural illness—accounts for the vast majority of whiplash patients. They tend to report chronic symptoms that diminish over time and will not report severe symptoms causing disability years after the accident. The second model—adoption of the sick role—accounts for a minority of whiplash patients. It is very important to consider this small minority, however. They often report disability even more than 2 years after the accident and seem unresponsive to therapy. They may even report chronic pain after litigation is complete. They consume great costs in therapy, disability pensions, and litigation.

These two models assign different degrees of relevance to pre- and postaccident psychosocial histories. This history is indeed relevant in both models (as it is in most illnesses). There is, however, a distinct preaccident history that is the quintessential contributor to the "adoption of the sick role" model and is the chief reason why the illness behavior has unique features. Table 8–1 lists the primary differences between the two models and (in its footnote) some important characteristics associated with nonorganic pain in patients.

If a patient exhibits 3 or more signs from each group listed in the footnote to Table 8–1, it is significant, worthy of further assessment. Alone, however, these lists do not identify the exact psychological factors involved. They do not separate psychocultural illness from what Waddell et al considered abnormal or inappropriate illness behavior (through adoption of the sick role, in this case), since some psychological factors are acting in each case. Moreover, one should not consider these to be signs of malingering. They were never studied or demonstrated to correlate with malingering.

Thus, health care providers should not immediately diagnose adoption of the sick role solely on the basis of the positive features or signs of nonorganic pain. Instead, they should identify a certain pattern and course of illness behavior as

Table 8–1 Comparison of Models 1 and 2 of Whiplash

Model	Psychocultural Illness (Model 1)	Adoption of the Sick Role (Model 2)
Incidence	Accounts for majority of whiplash patients when entire population considered	Accounts for majority of whiplash patients who claim disability 2 or more years after the accident
Preaccident personality and psychosocial history in relation to causation	Relevant, but not as abnormal as in second model	Essential
Would develop in an individual of "normal phlegmatic disposition"	Perhaps	No
Thin skull rule might be applicable	Yes	No
Symptom characteristics typical of nonorganic pain*	Few, decreasing with time	Many, often increasing with time
Signs of nonorganic pain*	Few, decreasing with time	Many, often increasing with time
Reported course of symptoms	Often improve steadily over weeks to months	Little improvement over time, often worsening with time, and usually labeled as totally disabled more than 2 years from time of accident
Reported response to therapy	Appear to have eventual steady improvement regardless of therapy chosen	Little or no response to therapy and may report worsening with some therapies
Reported working capacity	Often remain working or have more brief periods (weeks to months) of disability	Rarely continue working at preaccident level and often on total disability or other income support

- *According to G. Waddell et al (1989), features of the patient's pain (likely applicable to both neck and back pain) that suggest the patient's behavior is not likely explicable by physical pathology and is grossly infuenced by psychological factors include
  - constant pain
  - diffuse pain
  - whole limb pain or numbness
  - leg giving way
  - tailbone pain and back pain
  - intolerance to treatments
  - emergency hospital admissions for pain
  Signs on examination (Waddell's signs) that suggest the patient's behavior is not likely explicable by physical pathology and is grossly influenced by psychological factors include
  - pain behaviors (grimacing or extreme reactions with examination maneuvers of neck or back)
  - superficial tenderness (light touch or pinching of skin evokes significant pain response)
  - nondermatomal (not following specific nerve injury patterns) sensory changes
  - jerky, give-way muscle weakness
  - regional weakness (eg, whole leg or arm)
  - pain with simulation tests (eg, applied pressure down the spine from the top of the skull or hip rotation)
  - substantially improved straight leg raise with distraction (ie, compare straight leg raise in the lying and sitting position—the patient is not aware that straight leg raise is actually also being tested; in disease, the range of straight leg raising should be roughly equal in both cases)

well as specific preaccident profiles to make the diagnosis of adoption of the sick role, a matter discussed in Chapter 10.

But before we start, be sure your seat belts are still fastened and head restraints properly adjusted. It gets bumpy from here on.

Psychocultural Illness (Model 1)

KEY POINTS

- The psychocultural model accepts that it is possible for a variety of physical sources and processes to contribute to chronic pain. But, according to the model, psychosocial factors act to generate the clinical picture of chronic pain.
- Pre- and postaccident psychosocial profiles seem to contribute to perceptions and duration of chronic pain.
- Symptom expectation, amplification, and attribution may be important in the genesis and persistence of chronic symptom reporting in whiplash patients.
- Members of the therapeutic and legal communities as well as insurance companies contribute to this expectation, amplification, and attribution.

INTRODUCTION

As stated in Chapter 8, the psychocultural illness model applies to the vast majority of whiplash patients. It becomes somewhat less relevant for those patients claiming long-term disability. Then, the adoption of the sick role model seems more appropriate.

This first model does not consider the reporting of chronic symptoms to be strictly psychosomatic or psychogenic (as if physical disorders are not involved). It is tempting for many to leap to such conclusions when confronted with a patient whose pain seems inexplicable. Practitioners may state that the psychological factors actually produce pain. Yet resorting to labels such as psychosomatic or psychogenic has often been a poor choice in medicine.

That is not to say that such phenomena do not exist (indeed, somatization, as described in the second model, can be relevant in some contexts). But this first model considers such an approach unnecessary and hazardous. At one time, medical experts thought asthma, inflammatory bowel disease, diabetes, peptic ulcer disease, and other conditions were purely psychosomatic or psychogenic disorders (lacking the "bio" aspect of a biopsychosocial model). They were wrong. The physical disorders underlying these illnesses are now well known. But these practitioners were also somewhat right: How an individual perceives, registers, and responds to symptoms and the course of these "diseases" partly depends on some psychological and social (cultural) factors. These factors may make an illness more severe, more worrying, or more disabling. They may even alter the response to therapy. These factors alter the patient's behavior, symptom perception, and symptom reporting. They are important contributors to the final presentation of the illness.

Indeed, the psychocultural model of whiplash does not consider the cause of the symptoms being reported but the cause of the symptom reporting. They are not the same. Consider the possibility that the chronic pain of whiplash patients has a variety of physical causes with unknown origins (as is the case for most of the daily aches and pains we suffer). Consider that each source is being acted upon by psychological and cultural factors that alter the perception, registration, and reporting of these symptoms; how one behaves in response to them; what therapies one chooses; and how one responds to therapy.

It has been proposed that the culture influences how the individual with acute whiplash injury behaves. The culture affects, for example, whiplash victims' perception of the severity of the injury and prognosis, and their tendency to seek therapy or compensation. Cultural factors may encourage individuals to rest and recover, to seek intensive therapy, or to dismiss the injury as minor.

As stated above, to say that psychocultural events perpetuate symptom reporting does not mean that an initial physical injury did not occur or that there are no physical sources for the pain. It is not the acute injury that separates the Lithuanian whiplash victim from, say, a North American accident victim. It is how they and others respond to that injury that is different, and this is what the psychocultural model explores.

The psychological and cultural elements in this model include the following:

- Pre- and postaccident psychosocial profile. It may be that the accident victims' psychosocial profile increases their risk of being influenced by the factors cited below. Alone, these aspects would not likely account for the reporting of chronic symptoms.
- Symptom expectation. Cultural information suggests the possibility or even the strong expectation of chronic symptoms or disability.
- Symptom amplification. Patients become hypervigilant for symptoms, largely because of expected chronicity. Moreover, others repeatedly draw patients' attention to symptoms. The result is amplification of minor symptoms (they become more severe and more prolonged).

- Symptom attribution. Accident victims, because they expect chronicity and others reinforce that expectation, may attribute to the accident not just the initial symptoms. They also attribute symptoms arising from other factors like abnormal posture, occupations, the background frequency of musculoskeletal complaints in the general population, medication use, and so forth.
- The effects of the therapeutic community, the litigation process, and insurance companies.

One should not confuse this psychocultural illness with posttraumatic stress disorder. It is also not appropriate to call this psychocultural illness a psychological injury. It is chiefly the exposure of the individual to certain extraneous factors that have to do with the culture rather than the psychological "trauma" of the accident event itself that is important. An individual has a minor physical injury as a result of a minor accident, and one expects a minor, short-lived illness as a result. Psychological and cultural factors intervene to alter the behavior of some accident victims in their reporting of chronic symptoms. These factors are not a result of psychological trauma.

PRE- AND POSTACCIDENT PSYCHOSOCIAL PROFILE

The constitution of diseases is framed by the patterne of the constitution of living creatures.

—Florio J., trans. *The Essayes of Michael Lord of Montaigne.* Book III, chapter XIII. London: George Routledge & Sons; 1885:559.

Controversy

For some time many have debated whether the preaccident (and the postaccident) psychosocial profile is important in the reporting of chronic symptoms. Clearly, personality traits or other aspects of the psychosocial profile are insufficient factors alone to lead to symptom reporting. Lithuanians must share some of these personality traits with North Americans. It may be, however, that in certain cultures, personality traits and psychosocial factors interact to effect a certain illness behavior more readily: Cultures sanction certain illness behaviors. A more specific issue has been whether whiplash victims report chronic symptoms simply because they have neurotic and hypochondriacal tendencies.

A recent study by B. P. Radanov et al (reported 1994–1996) has suggested, at least in their study group, that chronic symptoms of whiplash can arise in individuals who are not necessarily hypochondriacal or neurotic. Their research thus presents an important finding. One must be cautious, however, and not extend this to mean that pre- or postaccident personality or psychosocial factors are not contributing to the behavior of reporting chronic symptoms following the accident. Neurotic or hypochondriacal personality traits may not be necessary for chronic symptoms to occur, but that does not eliminate other aspects of an individual's psychosocial profile from being relevant. From a legal viewpoint, some may argue that "one takes one's victim as one finds them" and that the psychological profile is irrelevant. To understand why some accident victims report chronic symptoms, however, both the medical and legal communities must consider these psychological profiles more closely. The issues have relevance in treatment, prevention, and statements of prognosis. (Until recently, most courts have been assuming that the basis for prognosis is the possibility of chronic physical damage from the accident.) Knowing more about what generates chronic symptoms may actually be quite relevant to the courts.

Reality

Some have quoted Radanov et al's work to indicate that the psychosocial profile is not at all important. On the contrary, the psychosocial circumstances surrounding the accident may indeed be relevant. Radanov et al's work, although seemingly impressive in its reported conclusions, does not eliminate this possibility. Whiplash as a psychocultural illness appears frequently to develop in what most would label "normal" individuals. The fact is that "normal individuals" have many stressors—a variety of dynamic relationships with family, friends, and employers as well as disappointments and struggles. Indeed, common sense tells us that our psychosocial profile is relevant in virtually every illness, whether it is a broken leg, a heart attack, the flu, or a neck injury.

There are many articles and studies dealing with psychology as the major factor in perpetuating or even generating patients' chronic pain. R. C. Grzesiak and D. S. Ciccone (1994) have written a text quoting much of this research. They consider the preinjury or preillness psychosocial history and other psychosocial factors after the acute onset of the illness or injury as not just important but fundamental to the development of chronic pain. They also indicate that these factors are relevant in a host of different chronic pain syndromes. There is a large body of literature dealing with these factors, for example, in patients reporting chronic, disabling low back pain after a work-related injury. Moreover, in chronic low back pain patients, the literature concludes that the psychological factors are not merely a result of the acute injury and its pain. They are instead what determines if the patient will report chronic pain thereafter. These factors are present before and after the injury.

The timing of an illness can affect recovery as much as the initial cause of the illness itself. Imagine getting the flu 3 days before you are leaving for a vacation you have long been planning. You are not going to let malaise and fatigue stop you. You force yourself out of bed. You use various remedies to try to cure yourself sooner, and you likely recover faster because you ignore symptoms that might otherwise inconvenience you. Imagine the same flu following your vacation, at a time when you were not looking forward to going back to your job. Do you force yourself (especially if you have the protection of your income) to recover as quickly? Do you seek out every possible remedy as eagerly? Do you simply ignore symptoms so you can get to your job sooner? It is likely that you do not, and yet you are not neurotic, not a hypochondriac, and not likely to rate abnormally on psychological tests. You are also not malingering. Rather, a relative lack of motivating factors to get well sooner is impairing recovery. Psychosocial factors have influenced the outcome.

For virtually any illness (injuries included), preoccupation with other matters, experiencing unhappiness, or enduring a greater-than-usual burden of responsibilities all affect the illness outcome. Who we are at the time of the accident is relevant.

There have been studies showing that how one recovers, to continue the example, from the "flu" (influenza or other viral infections) does not really depend very much on the infection itself. One might expect it to do so, but it does not. Rather, it depends on the individual's psychosocial profile before the infection. In 1961, J. B. Imboden et al elegantly demonstrated this. The aim of their prospective study was to determine what factors caused some individuals to recover from influenza within a few weeks and others to develop a chronic illness associated with fatigue. To answer this, they collected psychological profiles on 600 individuals in advance, knowing that an influenza epidemic was about to occur in 1957. Thus, they knew the psychosocial state of the individual *before* the infection, eliminating any biasing of this data by the illness that followed the infection. The researchers found that what best predicted whether the individuals would develop chronic fatigue was the psychosocial status before the infection. This meant that two individuals may have the same infection, be of the same age, and have the same symptoms, clinical findings, and laboratory findings from the initial infection, yet have different outcomes. (Since then, S. Wessely et al [1998] have reviewed a number of studies indicating that recovery from viral infections is often dependent on psychosocial factors.)

Problem of Study Design

Thus, while Radanov et al's study is important in indicating that not all whiplash patients have chronic symptoms because they were neurotic before the accident, to conclude that psychosocial factors are not a factor in symptom generation or do not alter outcome may yet be a premature statement. Indeed,

M. Karlsborg et al (1997) of Denmark found that the best predictor of reporting chronic symptoms was the occurrence of stressful life events that were unrelated to the accident. As stated by the authors, "The presence of stress unrelated to the accident did predict the number of complaints at the last . . . examination 6 months later."

Which study conclusion is correct? The mere fact that these researchers appear to arrive at opposite conclusions raises questions. Either psychosocial factors are very important in the reporting of chronic symptoms in whiplash patients, or studies that lack appropriate design cannot reliably explain the effects of psychosocial factors in whiplash patients.

It is worth considering in detail some of the potential sources of important bias and other deficiencies in studies that attempt to address this question. O. Kwan and J. Friel (1999) have indicated ways to reduce such flaws.*

- Patients should enter a study as they present consecutively in a defined time, to either an emergency department or a clinic that serves a given area. Researchers should not recruit them by advertising to the general population alone. Otherwise there is an immediate potential for a significant bias. What motivates a patient to respond to such an advertisement, and what motivates a patient not to respond?
- The number of patients entering the study after having presented consecutively should be a substantial proportion of the number available for study over the period of time the recruitment was conducted. Otherwise one wonders what the other sizable portion of the patients are like. What are their outcomes and characteristics? Why did they not enter the study? Although authors often state that they feel their study patients were "representative," it is one thing to hold that belief and another to demonstrate its validity. There must be an attempt to show that the method of recruiting patients did not lead to sampling bias. In cases, for example, where there is a national insurance scheme, the researchers have the opportunity of at least finding out more information (at least outcome) about patients who did not enter the study.
- If one does choose to use advertisement in the general population as a means of recruitment for an outcome study, it may be helpful to know how many different physicians cared for the patients. Were there few or many physicians suggesting that patients enter the study? This would again show whether there was a wide enough sampling distribution.
- There should be an attempt to control for different treatments. This is also true of information gained by different patients from the media, from rela-

---

Source: Adapted with permissiion from O. Kwan and J. Friel, A Comment on Radanov BP. Common Whiplash—Research Findings Revisited, *Journal of Rheumatology*, in press, © 1999.

tives or associates who may have had a similar injury in the past, or from therapists. While having thousands of patients may drive these confounding variables into randomness, it is unlikely that several dozen or even a hundred patients accomplishes the same.

- There should be a comparison between the study patients and the general population. Are they of the same psychosocial status as the general population? It may be that the patients in such studies present themselves psychologically as being more ideal than they really are. One way to detect this is to compare them to a demographically matched population of people who were not in accidents. One could then see if members of the study group are misrepresenting themselves, or are accurately representing themselves but are part of a highly selected group.

- There should be an attempt to ensure that (or examine whether) differences in outcomes are not due to things that may have nothing to do with the accident-related injuries. One should attempt to account for non–accident related factors, such as back or neck injury from work or recreational activities, that may alter outcome. Again, having thousands of patients may force this confounding variable into randomness, but a much smaller number may not. There should also be an attempt to determine if the symptoms are part of the base rate of symptoms in the general population. That is, neck and back pain occur in the general population, and some of the symptoms ascribed to the accident might have occurred in any case. It is useful to have a control population of non–accident victims like the Lithuanian studies did.

- In obtaining information about the patient's psychosocial history, there should be a collateral history with interviews of spouses or other family members to verify the accuracy of information. The study should not merely rely on self-reporting. It is understandable that individuals who are in a claim with an insurance company (and are concerned about being labeled as having an illegitimate basis for symptoms) might underreport certain aspects of their life.

How reliable is one's reporting of relationship difficulties, of childhood abuse, of performance problems in school? (Who wants to admit to these?)

Collateral information also helps to verify biases in self-reporting as family members may have noted little or no impairment, even though the patient feels symptoms severely hamper him or her.

Such assessments would require hours of interviewing. This renders the study a difficult task but one that befits the responsible researcher.

- Secondary gain should not be assumed to be only a matter of monetary compensation. One should also conduct a detailed analysis of the patient's family dynamics and other possible secondary gains: freedom from certain occupational and social obligations, sympathy for pain, and so forth. Grzesiak and Ciccone (1994, p 10) cite research that indicates that even the more subtle, insidious, and intermittent but unrelenting psychosocial stressors are important in the reporting of chronic pain. Clearly, a very exhaustive and detailed study is necessary to assess these stressors.

- There should be an accounting for job satisfaction as a factor deterring early return to work.
- If the original study group is relatively small, making further analyses and conclusions of subsets should be avoided, especially if "sweeping" conclusions are made.
- The study should be reproducible, preferably where similar insurance schemes exist. Is a study of a single group of patients in a single setting likely to resolve this very complex issue?
- There are rapid changes in the epidemiology of whiplash over even a few years (witness Australia and now Norway). Would the results found by a study in a country a few years ago be found in a study there today? If not, then cultural factors are indeed important.
- Before using the study results to explain the behavior of whiplash patients in other countries, one must examine if the outcome pattern is typical of other countries. Otherwise, before one generalizes about the results, an explanation is necessary. For example, one should offer an explanation of why chronic whiplash is so much more common in some countries and virtually nonexistent in others. If it is not a psychocultural illness, why do countries have such great differences in the prevalence of chronic whiplash?

Finally, P. F. Van Akkerveeken and A. A. Vendrig (1998) have added:

[Radanov et al's] main finding was that neither personality traits nor psychopathologic symptoms measured at baseline predicted patients' functioning in any respect . . . at follow-up. . . . Do these findings imply that psychological factors are not important for the development of chronic symptoms after whiplash trauma? The answer is no. . . . It is conceivable that other psychological factors or mechanisms, such as conditioning processes and the role of the patient's health beliefs, are significant.

Indeed, many factors may be significant, and Radanov et al addressed only very few in a potentially biased fashion. This is reiterated by M. Drottning et al (1995). Their study meets many of the aforementioned criteria for a high-quality study. They followed consecutive patients from hours after an accident to 4 weeks after an accident. The purpose was to examine the relationship between the acute emotional response to the accident and symptom reporting at 4 weeks. In a study of 107 patients, these researchers confirmed that the acute emotional response to the accident was the strongest predictor of ongoing symptom reporting 4 weeks later. As they note, "This seriously questions some authors' assumptions that psychosocial factors do not primarily influence the course of recovery from common whiplash."

Indeed, they go on to state that premorbid psychopathology and acute emotional response to the accident potentially explain Radanov et al's outcome results.

Nevertheless, Radanov et al do shed some light on a number of events that are operative in whiplash patients' behavior. They confirm that a multitude of external factors (eg, battling with one's insurance company, fear of disability) act at the time of the accident and thereafter to produce chronic symptoms. One does not necessarily have to be neurotic to have chronic symptoms. In 1996, B. J. Wallis et al reaffirmed that overt neurotic tendencies are not necessarily relevant in postaccident psychological distress. They examined psychological profiles by using the SCL-90-R tool on Australian whiplash patients.

This is not to say that neurotic or hypochondriacal tendencies have no effect on symptom reporting. Clearly they may.

Contribution of Personality Traits

Those with the psychocultural illness of whiplash may not carry the features of neurotics, hypochondriacs, or those with personality disorders, but they may still have psychosocial factors and personality traits that alter the illness course.

In 1993, for example, R. Mayou et al looked at the risk factors for developing psychiatric consequences after road accidents.

Almost a quarter of subjects described psychiatric complications at one year. It was particularly likely in those psychologically and socially vulnerable, but was also strongly associated with chronic medical impairment and social, financial, and work problems. . . .

18% of subjects . . . described an acute syndrome of emotional distress . . . associated with previous psychological vulnerability (neuroticism) and remaining conscious after the accident.

Their study results indicate that psychological factors acting at the time of and after the accident could generate considerable morbidity. The study included 74 whiplash patients and confirmed that these psychiatric consequences can occur in those with an essentially normal preaccident psychological profile. Those with a history of neuroticism, however, were at risk for more severe psychiatric consequences.

Physicians have long recognized that one cannot ignore what effect the preaccident psychological profile could have on symptom severity. As far back as 1930, for example, F. Kennedy (quoting Sir John Collie) stated that:

It is unfortunately the experience of most physicians that nervous people, who are given to self-examination, unconsciously foster subjective sensations which their stronger and better balanced neighbours would ignore. The idea of illness or a possible injury and its consequences obsess them. Their pains are real, but often psychic. Such people are victimized by their unstable nervous system. Too often they make no stand against morbid introspection. Frequent gossips with others who have found themselves in similar circumstances, continual rehearsals of the illness or the accident, and the oft-repeated recital of sensations, all act as cooperating factors in bringing about a condition of auto-suggestion.

In 1945, J. Ruesch and K. M. Bowman conducted a very detailed assessment of pretraumatic personality in patients with head injury, some of whom were in automobile accidents. By examining many aspects of the patients' pretraumatic life, the researchers realized that "the post-traumatic personality is more dependent on the pre-traumatic personality than on factors related to the injury."

Then M. M. Braaf and S. Rosner, in 1955, found most patients had social maladjustment and neurotic personalities before the head injury. They believed that this predicted the development of chronic symptoms after an accident. They did not have a control population (ie, people who had recovered completely after an accident), however, to see how many of them had abnormal pretraumatic personalities.

On the specific symptom of headache, A. P. Friedman and J. Ransohoff, in 1964, concluded that "present evidence indicates there is a high incidence of prolonged headaches among those patients who were considered to have been neurotic prior to a head injury."

Similarly, A. A. Farbman, in 1973, added:

A detailed study of many factors unrelated to the accident disclosed only four that were closely associated with an increased duration of symptoms: (1) strong emotional factors; (2) extensive medical history; (3) prolonged and frequent treatments, particularly with modalities such as neck collars, neck traction, manipulations, and adjustments; and (4) litigation. The most significant was the emotional factor.

Thus, while preaccident personality disorders may not be the actual cause of the symptoms, the duration and severity of symptoms may sometimes be related in part to the psychosocial profile near the time of the accident. An experiment volunteer and a Lithuanian accident victim are not going to be reporting chronic symptoms that they attribute to the accident. They are thus not going to have any chronic symptoms affected by their psychosocial status or personality. This, in turn, negates any possibility for propagation of their symptoms by these factors.

Yet because accident victims are not alone in their illness (many others become involved), one must also consider other factors that act on even relatively normal individuals to generate reporting of chronic symptoms. The discussion below deals with these factors.

SYMPTOM EXPECTATION, AMPLIFICATION, AND ATTRIBUTION

Symptom Expectation

How could the symptoms of whiplash patients continue to be somewhat similar from one individual to another and not be due to chronic damage? One step in the process is expectation. As explained previously, society has a certain amount of knowledge about the symptoms and course of certain illnesses, especially the common or well-publicized illnesses. There is a tendency for patients to expect certain symptoms or complications of any illness if they have sufficient knowledge of that illness. There are also fashions in medicine, and as will be explained later, the medical community can actually create a cohort with similar symptoms.

W. Mittenberg et al (1992) conducted a study to see if expectation could be an element acting in chronic symptom reporting. They asked subjects who had never experienced whiplash or concussion to select symptoms they expected from whiplash or concussion. They also requested a "checklist" of symptoms from patients who had a previous head injury. They revealed that expectation could produce a cluster of patients with the same symptoms, through "the anticipation, widely held by individuals who have had *no opportunity* to observe or experience postconcussion symptoms, that [postconcussion syndrome] will occur following mild head injury."

Their study revealed other important findings.

> Current results indicate common expectations of postconcussive headache, anxiety, depression, concentration difficulty, vertigo, diplopia, confusion, irritability, fatigue, and photophobia and memory difficulties. These symptoms are anticipated at relatively high levels of probability and form an internally consistent "syndrome".

> Moreover, the relative incidence of postconcussion symptoms reported by head trauma patients correlated substantially . . . with the relative frequency of postconcussion symptoms anticipated by uninjured controls. Patients with head injuries consistently underestimated the normal prevalence of these symptoms in their retrospective accounts compared with the base rate reported by normal controls. This result

suggests that patients may reattribute benign emotional, physiological, and memory symptoms to head injury.

That an imaginary concussion will reliably elicit expectations of a co-herent cluster of symptoms virtually identical to [postconcussive syndrome] implies that expectations share almost as much variance with the syndrome as head injury itself. A causative role is suggested.

The aetiological role of expectations may also explain why persistent [postconcussion syndrome] is uncommon following mild head injuries sustained by children and in athlete competition. Children are less able to appreciate the health risks of head trauma, and are therefore less likely to appraise any minor injury as a potential source of persistent symptoms. Children are also less likely to have developed specific expectations of postconcussion headache, anxiety, depression, memory, or concentration impairment. Participants in boxing, football, and other contact sports are repeatedly observed to sustain minor head trauma without obvious persistent ill effects. Being "knocked out" or "dazed" in the context of an athletic event is therefore less likely to elicit anticipations of persistent postconcussion syndrome than identical experiences that occur in the context of a motor vehicle accident.

Symptom expectations, selective attention, and anxiety can, under certain circumstances, interact to produce syndromes that mimic essentially any pathological process.

A similar study by J. B. Aubrey et al (1989) showed that physical symptoms, more than any other, were an expected result (80% of the time). This indicates that the general public is quite aware of whiplash symptoms. Certainly, as stated by L. Keiser (1968), "Some patients . . . have pain because they know they have had an accident and feel that pain must be associated with it."

Or less formally:

There was a faith-healer of Deal
Who said, 'Although pain isn't real,
If I sit on a pin
And it punctures my skin,
I dislike what I fancy I feel.'

—Anonymous. Mind over matter. In: Meynell F, ed. *The Week-End Book.*
London: The Nonesuch Press; 1955:217.

Shorter (1992) explains that the development of a similar illness among whiplash patients does not require a conscious effort.

In psychosomatic illness the body's response to stress or unhappiness is orchestrated by the unconscious. The unconscious mind, just like the conscious, is influenced by the surrounding culture, which has models of what it considers to be legitimate and illegitimate symptoms. Legitimate symptoms are ascribed to an underlying organic disease for which the patient could not possibly be blamed. Illegitimate ones, by contrast, may be thought due to [malingering]. By defining certain symptoms as illegitimate, a culture strongly encourages patients not to develop them or to risk being thought "undeserving" individuals with no real medical problems. Accordingly there is great pressure on the unconscious mind to produce only legitimate symptoms.

Symptom Amplification

Beyond symptom expectation and fashions, it is also probable that symptom amplification plays a role in whiplash patients.

Amplification of symptoms may explain the severity of neck pain, for example, after an accident even though the mechanics of the event do not suggest the symptoms should be so severe. Recall that M. E. Allen et al (1994) showed that accelerations involved in everyday events such as sneezing or "plopping" into a chair may be similar to those experienced by whiplash patients in low-velocity collisions. It may be that some people do have episodes of neck pain after "violent sneezing," but there does not seem to be an epidemic of them in physicians' offices. It may be that the circumstances (benign) in sneezing are different from the circumstances (serious or dangerous) in an accident and that the individual's recognition (even preconscious) of this may influence symptom severity.

As further indicated by A. J. Barsky (1992), "Symptoms are intensified when they are attributed to a serious disease than to more benign causes such as . . . lack of sleep, lack of exercise, or overwork."

The very nature of an accident may thus potentiate symptom amplification. How severe the impact seems to the occupant is not entirely reliable as a measure of its actual severity in engineering terms. The occupant's clues come largely from the unexpectedness (which amplifies the perception) and the sound. In a study by G. P. Nielsen et al (1997), one of the authors (a physician) participated in the experimental collisions. As noted in Chapter 5, this physician was struck by how loud and emotionally jarring a relatively minor accident was. He concluded that some individuals could have symptoms because of this fright alone.

A further example of how the circumstances in which one develops pain affect the outcome is that of "head banger's whiplash," discussed by M. R. Kassirer and N. Manon (1993). "Head banging" refers to a dance activity in which the head and neck move violently and repeatedly in flexion and extension. They found that this group of individuals had neck pain lasting for 1 to 3 days whereas the same age group, when in a motor vehicle accident, could have pain for weeks or months. The circumstances in which the pain occurs may explain why the "head bangers" had less neck pain even though they may have undergone more trauma. As explained by Kassirer and Manon, there is no associated negative emotional reaction to the event that precipitated the whiplash syndrome, as there may be in even mild injuries from rear-end collisions.

Beyond this effect of the circumstances on acute symptoms, there are chronic effects of symptom amplification. That is, another aspect of the aforementioned symptom expectation is that the overwhelming information in certain cultures regarding the potential for chronic pain outcomes leads the individual to expect disability and become hypervigilant for symptoms. They register normal bodily sensations as abnormal and react to bodily sensations with affect and cognitions that intensify them, making them more alarming, ominous, and disturbing (Barsky et al 1988).

Amplification of symptoms further occurs when the accident victim must repeatedly draw attention to the symptoms. This occurs every time the patient sees a therapist, or if the patient keeps a detailed diary of symptoms, prepares for legal discovery, and so forth. Barsky (1992) notes that "attention to a symptom amplifies it, whereas distractions diminish it. Thus the more frequently . . . patients are asked to rate their pain, the more intense they rate it."

Indeed, A. Arntz and P. De Jong (1993) conducted studies and reviewed others that show that even if one controls for anxiety levels, simply having attention focused on pain amplifies the pain or lowers the threshold for perception of pain. Thus, minor symptoms appear more severe and of greater duration. Neck and back pain are easily "aggravated" because of a lower pain threshold in the setting of an individual who has his or her attention focused on pain. Many factors draw attention to the pain.

It is perfectly understandable that individuals who are establishing a claim would want to have all of their perceived injuries and suffering documented. Others ask them to maintain such a focus on symptoms. Yet this very activity may amplify the symptoms. Most individuals in the general population cannot recite the details of any symptoms they may have experienced over the past, say, 3 years, but accident victims often can—others compel them to do so. A pattern thus ensues. Benign sensations are regarded as more serious than they would be in another setting. This further promotes emotional distress, which causes further amplification of bodily sensations. With increased attention to those sensations, there is then a series of maladaptive coping methods (reduction in activity, development of poor posture, etc). Then the response of others to the symptoms generates even more attention to bodily sensations. Thus, there are many factors that amplify the symptoms of an accident victim, both acutely and chronically.

Symptom Attribution

We do not know the exact cause of most neck and back pain associated with occupational activities, recreational activities, and daily life. A variety of tissues (eg, annulus of the disc, facet joints, muscles and ligaments, skin) in the neck and back have pain receptors. In most cases of neck or back pain in the general population, however, one cannot identify what particular structure initiates the sensation of pain. Pain is a perception, and reporting of pain is clearly dependent on more than the activity of sensory receptors. Yet we accept that these episodes are genuine in most people and that they are a relatively common aspect of human existence. For the most part, most people do not remember how many times they had neck pain in the past 3 months, how many days it lasted, and so on. Accident victims *do* appear to remember a great deal of their pain history since the accident.

We know from numerous epidemiological studies that all of the symptoms of whiplash are common in the general population on a chronic and intermittent basis. In many cases, spontaneous neck or back pain may develop after an accident but be completely unrelated to the accident, because there is a certain incidence of these spontaneous symptoms in the general population. D. Obelieniene et al (1999) studied Lithuanian accident victims prospectively. They found that neck pain and headaches, besides being very frequent in the general population, occur spontaneously and fluctuate over short periods of time at the same rate and pattern of the Lithuanian accident victims. In other words, some neck pain would have occurred in any case had the individual remained a part of the nonaccident general population.

Presumably, the accident victim may have been and will continue experiencing this background incidence of neck, back, and other symptoms. Yet there is a tendency to ignore this possibility in many whiplash patients. In 1995, P. D. Marshall et al confirmed that minor neck symptoms are common in individuals who do not report a history of neck injury. Patients who attribute their current neck pain to an accident or injury tend to forget their preaccident history of neck pain. This could partly be due to patients' concern that such information may negate their claim. Another possibility is that accident victims become more aware and register minor symptoms (symptom amplification) that they would not report to a physician or others before the accident. They had no amplification or other reason to do so before the accident.

There is also a large body of literature that more specifically addresses the recognition of a high incidence of symptoms such as neck and back pain in association with many occupations (see, for example, reviews by M. Hagberg 1996, C. Hartigan et al 1996, M. I. Jayson 1996, T. J. Stobbe 1996, S. R. Stock et al 1996, and S. Yamamoto 1997). Presumably, some portion of whiplash patients belong to these occupations. They are at risk for developing symptoms from their occupations in the future, yet again there may be a tendency instead to assume such symptoms arise from the accident. When asked, some accident victims state that they do not recall having neck or back pain from their work activities before the accident. They find it difficult to conceive that their work is responsible for symptoms after the accident. That they do not recall a history of work-related symptoms before the accident may not necessarily (as some would assume) mean the patients are denying these symptoms for fear of influencing compensation outcomes. The patients may simply be more aware of symptoms after the accident than they were before, even though in each case the symptoms arise from work-related activities.

In the setting of expectation of chronic pain, patients may assume that all symptoms of pain following an accident arise from the accident. Preaccident sources of pain thus become more noticeable in this setting of hypervigilance, and symptoms that patients previously viewed as benign and largely ignored are now registered. The accident victim may thus misattribute symptoms to the accident.

Accident victims also behave as if they expected to remain perfectly asymptomatic throughout their lives. In actuality, it is probable that even if the accident had not happened, they would eventually experience at least some component of their symptoms from other sources. Had they not been in a state of symptom amplification, the individuals would do as most do and ignore them. After an accident, however, all new symptoms register and remain registered, especially for one involved in a claim.

This phenomenon of misattributing symptoms to the accident can occur even in the experimental setting. J. R. Brault et al ("Clinical response of human subjects to rear-end automobile collisions," 1998) subjected 42 volunteers to low-velocity rear-end collision. About 30% of the subjects reported minor symptoms, even with a change in velocity (ΔV) of as little as 4 km/h (2.4 mph). This is contrary to all prior experiments. Should minor symptoms being reported after collisions that produce no greater head accelerations than sneezing does be blamed on the collision? The symptoms reported by Brault et al's subjects may not have come from the collision. It may be that these individuals were hypervigilant about symptoms, experienced minor aches as part of daily life, and attributed these minor aches to the collision. (See Chapter 21.)

Summary

Thus, symptom expectation (resulting in part from medical fashions and cultural information), symptom amplification, and symptom attribution may be important in the genesis and maintenance of chronic symptom reporting in whiplash patients. To understand why whiplash patients report chronic symptoms, one has to consider that in some cases the symptoms and their duration are being mistakenly attributed to the accident. It is a natural mistake for the patient to make.

Take Lithuanian accident victims, for example. They have not heard that a whiplash injury often causes chronic pain, and so they do not expect disability. This influences their behavior. They feel they have had a minor injury. They will have no symptom amplification because they view the injury as benign. They will not have their attention excessively drawn to their pain, and they will carry on with their usual activities, which will distract them from any residual pain. They will have no tendency to be vigilant of symptoms in the future and will not attribute future neck pain to that original injury; they have no reason to make such a link.

THERAPEUTIC COMMUNITY

It is clear that other individuals contribute to the process of symptom expectation, amplification, and attribution. Physicians and other therapists can have a significant impact on patients' view of their health and the outcome of their illness. As has already been shown, there is no evidence that most whiplash patients have anything more than a muscular or ligamentous sprain. There is no evidence that one may develop "degenerative disc disease" or arthritis after such a sprain. Excluding the exceedingly rare fracture, radiological findings on neck X-ray are of no significance in the patient's outcome or prognosis (see "Radiology of Whiplash" in Chapter 5). Yet physicians and other therapists may lead patients to believe many myths regarding these issues. A lack of education, or worse, inappropriate advice can create significant anxiety and worry about chronic pain (symptom expectation and amplification). To tell people they are at risk for arthritis is tantamount to telling them they have a crippling disease. Equally, to tell them that the accident "moved their vertebrae out of alignment" or "tore ligaments that take a very, very long time to heal" may further promote illness or disability worry. Appearing unsympathetic or dismissing patients' complaints instead of letting them know that one understands that their pain is real and why they want help may be just as harmful. Many recognize that the therapeutic community can induce pain as well as relieve it.

In 1959, for example, K. H. Abbott explained the effect the physician may have on the patient's symptoms.

> Often the problem begins when the patient consults the doctor after injury and is told that nothing is wrong with him; however, he may actually have a neck sprain and be extremely fearful of severe damage to his neck that could threaten paralysis. When the patient knows he has pain in his neck and he is not given appropriate attention, he becomes

extremely apprehensive, tense, and anxious; thus he develops a pattern of neurotic reaction to his injury. On the other hand, an overzealous doctor may make statements that will frighten the patient and thus further condition the person who is susceptible to suggestion.

In 1977, N. Parker alluded to similar iatrogenic factors.

Doctors feel the need to do something tangible, and this is reinforced by the patient's expectations. It is extremely difficult to leave the healing process to nature—a tablet, an injection, a bandage, an appliance, a test, something has to be given and this can be the first step on the road to psychiatric invalidism. The more treatments and investigations are undertaken, the more impressed is the patient that something is seriously wrong, particularly if we are dealing with a migrant who is not told, or misinterprets what is happening. Many of these patients have been turned into psychiatric casualties when confident reassurance at the outset would have been all that was necessary. However, it is easy to be wise in retrospect and the doctor of first contact is not to know that x-ray films will show negative results or that treatment may lead to iatrogenic illness. Some unnecessary orthopaedic procedures, however, could be avoided by earlier referral for psychiatric assessment. The litigation process itself may aggravate symptoms—the repetition of the history as the patient goes from one specialist to another for reports, the critical, even hostile atmosphere in which some of these examinations are undertaken, and the long delay in settlement all add their contribution to the final picture.

F. J. Wilfling and P. C. Wing (1984) commented as well on how physicians can, quite unintentionally, produce a patient with chronic pain: "Specific professional mismanagement following trauma may have a profound effect on even the client with well above average personal and environmental adjustment, resources, and reserves. If such an individual following injury . . . is subjected to lengthy investigation, over-medication, and perhaps even exploratory surgery, he too may succumb."

Therapeutic failures are equally distressing to patients, may increase anxiety about future health, and may affirm a possibility of future disability. Because physicians often treat the chronic symptoms reported by whiplash patients as being due to some form of chronic damage from the accident injury, the treatment they recommend will fail. Thus, therapists use medications, collars, various passive therapies such as ultrasound, heat, electromagnetic therapy, massage, and physical manipulation. This all happens with the misguided notion that these are appropriate because the therapist assumes the symptom reporting is from some physical damage that is "healed" by these means. When a form of treatment fails, however, this may have an important adverse psychological effect on the patient. Patients do not usually consider that the therapy failed because it was inappropriate for the mechanism of their pain. They instead assume that if therapy fails it can only be due to a resistant or more severe physical injury than the physician must have realized. This can only raise their fear about their future health. Every therapy for physical injury that one exhausts and that fails will only drive patients further toward the conviction, along with frustration, that they are incurable.

Therapists may also increase patients' anxiety about long-term outcome, affecting their illness course by failing to provide accurate and reassuring information to the patient. As Mayou (1993) has stated, "The patients' illness behaviour must be seen alongside medical behaviour. Many patients find it difficult to tolerate uncertainty and ambiguity. They readily misinterpret medical information, drawing erroneous conclusions from past experience, the media, and the reaction of friends and relatives." Thus, physicians and therapists may, despite good intentions, be responsible for some of the psychological factors that generate chronic pain reporting.

Consider the examples of experiment volunteers and Lithuanian accident victims. A physician on the research team will probably examine an experiment volunteer and immediately reassure that volunteer that he or she is fine and requires no further attention. The volunteer then carries on with his or her usual activities. And in virtually all cases, the Lithuanian accident victim does not seek contact with the therapeutic community, so the therapeutic community has no opportunity to influence the outcome.

LITIGATION, COMPENSATION, AND INSURANCE COMPANIES

What if the very doubt and inquisition woundeth our imagination and changeth us?

—Florio J., trans. *The Essayes of Michael Lord of Montaigne*. Book III, chapter XIII. London: George Routledge & Sons; 1885:557.

Introduction

In concert with the iatrogenic factors are the adverse psychological effects of being involved with insurance companies and the litigation process. As part of this process, others subject the patient to numerous examinations that merely draw more attention to symptoms (symptom amplification). The litigation process and insurance companies may affect illness development in both models of whiplash. Even patients not involved in litigation, when they merely have to deal with an insurance company, may find this process frustrating. It can generate considerable anger and anxiety.

Studies of the psychological effects of engaging in litigation are few in whiplash. A recent study by L. C. Swartzman et al (1996) did find that being involved in litigation influenced the reporting of pain (pain was reported as more severe) in current litigants. This was not because of a more severe injury or other physical factors that could influence pain severity. Beyond this, the authors admit to the limited attempt to assess the psychological status of the study group. It is not surprising that litigants may "under report psychological difficulty for fear that their pain would be viewed as a psychological as opposed to a physical problem." It is surprising that the litigants should not have more distress if they truly have more pain (and they said they did). Underreporting of distress may indeed be a factor in that study.

Certainly, a measure of how stressful the process can be is the finding by P. R. Lees-Haley and R. S. Brown (1993). They note that litigants with no history of illness or trauma suffer from similar physical, emotional, and cognitive problems as do whiplash patients.

Lawyers

In 1990, H. N. Weissman reviewed the effects of protracted litigation, looking well beyond issues of monetary compensation. He indicated that the litigation process causes intensified symptom expression (symptom amplification) and inaccurate attribution and false imputation of symptoms. It also leads to anger and resentment from the process others force upon the accident victim. This may lead to depression or other psychological distress that is not due to the accident but to the choice to enter this process.

The statement that "you had better wait a few years before settling your claim because you never know what might become of you" may perhaps be a necessary one for the plaintiff's lawyer to make. Yet, it can hardly instill an expectation of a good recovery in the patient. B. P. Radanov et al (1995) indicate that when patients fear the possibility of long-lasting symptoms or disability early in their course, they have symptoms for longer than if their attitude is one of less worry about these possibilities. The group of patients (21) with ongoing symptoms at 2 years had "initially showed significantly more concern with respect to the possibility of long-lasting symptoms or disability (for example, illness or disability worry), and reported a greater variety of subjective complaints at the initial examination.

Finally, being told by a lawyer to keep a diary of all symptoms and to bring any such symptoms to the attention of therapists can only amplify patients' symptoms. To be questioned repeatedly by physicians and lawyers about symptoms, their severity, and their significance also amplifies them. Others compel the patient to focus on their symptoms, not on their recovery.

Those who are quick to blame personal injury lawyers for the behavior of whiplash patients, however, should also note that lawyers acting for the insurance companies have an adverse effect on patients as well. When one feels injured, it is not a pleasant experience when others imply malingering, and when one must undergo repeated examinations to prove one is telling the truth. Recall that when patients become hypervigilant for symptoms, amplify symptoms, and misattribute symptoms from preaccident sources, occupational sources, and so forth to their accident, they may honestly believe their symptoms come from the accident. When they amplify symptoms from poor posture, they again may believe that they are telling the truth about the origin of their symptoms. Yet they feel others are accusing them of malingering. They may decide that ensuring that they receive compensation by a court of law ruling is the only way ultimately to prove to everyone that their symptoms are indeed real. In doing so, they focus even more on their "injury" and their symptoms. Again, while the defense lawyer may have a duty to be on guard for malingering, there is little doubt that in some cases, this process promotes chronic symptom reporting.

Insurance Companies

Although most aim concerns about the effects of litigation at the legal process, insurance companies may also have a very negative effect on the patient's outcome. Insurance companies are of course concerned with costs of therapy and with paying disability benefits to injured parties while they are recovering. Patients may worry about chronic pain and want therapy. They also want reassurance of income maintenance while they are recovering for injuries that are, after all, not their fault. Yet patients find themselves in a battle to recover expenses for therapy and disability income while in therapy. The insurance companies appear, to the patient, to have more concern about how much the therapy is going to cost and if the patient's symptoms are "real" or not. Whenever a patient is not working, the insurance company is repeatedly pressuring the patient and often his or her physicians to state the date when the patient will be able to return to work. Insurance companies will go as far as to obtain details from the employer to find out the work requirements. Then they demand that the patient undergo an independent medical examination (a physician hired by the insurance company to provide an objective assessment). This is to determine the optimal therapy and if there is true disability.

Injured parties develop frustration and resentment. After all, why do they have to prove their injuries and justify therapy? Meanwhile the liable party is often uninjured, does not have to go for therapy, does not have to battle with insurance companies, and does not undergo multiple examinations. In some insurance schemes, the patient's insurance company is responsible for initial therapy and disability income, while the patient seeks compensation from the liable party's insurance company. Ironically, patients find they are also being poorly treated by the company to which they have been paying insurance premiums for years! The patient encounters resistance, not assistance. This can only reinforce the feeling of victimization.

As such, one needs to consider the broader aspects of the litigation and compensation process, and the battles with insurance companies. The issue of monetary gain is just one of these considerations.

All these examples show the effect the process can have, regardless of the goals. Clearly, too many have been focusing the debate on the issue of monetary gain as the key psychological element.

Symptoms and Settlement

In 1956, N. Gotten reviewed 100 cases of whiplash after settlement of litigation.

> We were forced by the survey to draw certain definite conclusions in regard to psychosomatic symptoms that had developed in a considerable number of these patients . . . the possibility that the illness had been used as a means of implementing psychological or other adjustments that had previously been postponed or that, because of financial difficulties, the patient had not been able to fulfill. Our survey indicated that some patients who complained seemed to have developed through the injury an outlet or excuse for avoiding unpleasant tasks and a means of securing recognition from other members of the family and attention from neighbours, friends, and children. This was not thought by the examiner to be entirely on a conscious level. The apprehension, nervous tension, and anxiety that these patients developed subsequent to the injury, as a result of fear for future health and as a result of the litigation, tended to accentuate the formation of a profound post-traumatic neurosis.

Commenting further on Gotten's study, Abbott (1956) noted that:

> Many patients have a fear of legal matters, particularly of "going to court." Of course, this is the fear of the unknown or unfamiliar. But this is just as real as the fear he also holds (1) that no punishment will be meted out to the driver of the other car (and these people do exhibit extreme hostility toward the driver of the other car) and (2) that no compensation will be received for the pain, anxiety, and loss of time that they have experienced.

Mayou (1995) confirmed that accident victims do indeed have such concerns and anger. He noted that studies of many types of road accident victims show that:

Those who saw themselves as innocent victims were often angry that those responsible had not been charged and that even if convicted the sentences had seemed to them to be inadequate and the offenders had shown little sign of regret. Several described being present at court hearings in a state of physical discomfort and disability and being outraged to see those who had been convicted as having caused the accident leaving the court looking pleased with the minor penalty and showing no sign of remorse.

And Abbott, in his panel discussion with R. T. McIntire et al (1957), reminds us of an issue in legal circles for decades, even before whiplash: "All emotional or neurotic reactions should be carefully examined and their proper place in the syndrome brought out in the physician's testimony. It is then the judge's or the jury's prerogative to decide whether or not such a reaction to an injury (or incident in life) is compensable."

Then came a controversial article in 1961 by H. Miller. He made the simple observation that *some* patients with whiplash had a tendency to improve significantly after settlement of their litigation. He looked at 50 patients whom he identified as being neurotic. There were undoubtedly a number of patients in the 4,000 cases of litigants he reviewed who did not improve after settlement of litigation, but Miller did not make this point clear. Others misinterpreted his work to mean that all patients had "litigation neurosis," whereas clearly this is not the case, and most would agree that litigation is but one factor affecting a patient's outcome.

Later, other authors would criticize this article because they could show that resolution of litigation did not always relieve a patient's symptoms. It is certainly incorrect to apply Miller's conclusions to all whiplash patients because desire for compensation is only one psychological factor. It would be equally incorrect to assume that desire for compensation played no role. In any case, the process of litigation would continue in debates.

In 1973, I. MacNab tried to assess the effects of litigation settlement on outcome. This was one of the early studies arguing against desire for compensation being the cause of whiplash symptoms. MacNab did reveal that about half of such patients remain symptomatic after settlement. Beyond that revelation, R. D. Goldney (1989) noted that little else could be confirmed: "The study of MacNab (1973) is difficult to evaluate as no clinical information is given other than the fact that 121 of 266 subjects still had symptoms two years following settlement of litigation. No data is given to indicate the work status of those subjects, and comparison in terms of employability is therefore impossible."

Then, in 1981, R. Kelly and B. N. Smith noted that clearly not all patients with whiplash improve after litigation settlement. This demonstrates that other factors, such as illness behavior, use of the illness as a psychological escape, and so on were more important in some patients. He was critical of the article by H. Miller in 1961, which selected 50 patients to show that the majority resumed work after litigation. G. Mendelson (1982) explains the reasons for this discrepancy: "A possible reason for this discrepancy may lie in the fact that Miller saw a group of litigants preselected for referral by the insurers and their legal advisors, and that for his follow-up he selected 50 patients showing 'gross neurotic symptoms.'"

It was clear that a number of factors decide what symptoms a patient with whiplash would have and for how long those symptoms would be present. In some individuals, one factor predominated. Sometimes it was the desire for compensation, and clearly in many cases it was not.

SUMMARY

One can understand why a Lithuanian accident victim or an experiment volunteer would have the same behavior after the acute injury. There are clearly profound effects of symptom expectation, symptom amplification, exposure to the therapeutic community, and engaging in the litigation and compensation process. If these influences were not present, the illness after a minor accident would be what one expects of a minor injury. Instead, these psychological and cultural factors may alter the natural history of the acute minor injury. Note that this model does not attempt to pinpoint the cause of every episode of neck or back pain. (Medical science has yet to provide a clear explanation of what exactly causes many of the daily aches and pains we experience.) Instead, this model attempts to explain why some individuals will suffer an acute injury and then report chronic symptoms (whatever the cause), attributing these to the accident.

The pain of whiplash patients likely has a variety of physical sources, but the pain severity, its attribution, and the patient's behavior depend on psychosocial factors.

This biopsychosocial model of psychocultural illness after an accident presents a unifying explanation for many patients reporting chronic whiplash symptoms. Figure 9–1 illustrates the complex interplay of factors that contribute to reporting of chronic symptoms, according to the psychocultural illness model.

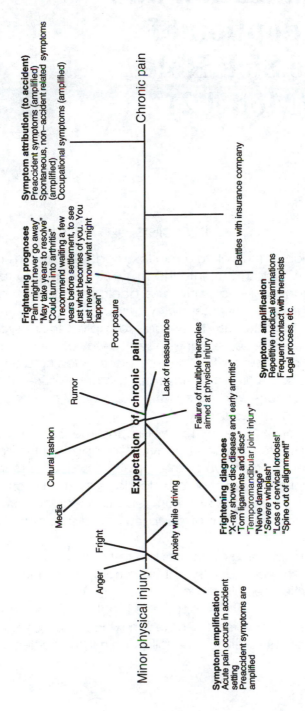

Figure 9–1 The Pathway to Chronic Pain

Somatization and Adoption of the Sick Role (Model 2)

CHAPTER 10

KEY POINTS

- The adoption of the sick role model (model 2) explains chronic pain in the whiplash patient who has been unable to return to work for months or years after the accident and has failed to make any great improvement with therapy.
- Certain risk factors cause individuals to express their psychological distress from life as pain and to seek a way out. A person seeking the sick role must present in a manner suggesting a no-fault illness. At the same time, the sick role can only work—producing secondary gains—when the patient is clearly pursuing all avenues back to full health.
- Labels matter. One needs to explain the mechanism of illness when using the terms "illness behavior," "adoption of the sick role," "chronic benign pain syndrome," "pain disorder," or "somatization." The central implication of each label is that psychological mechanisms can lead to symptom reporting that then provides a socially acceptable form of disability and grants entry into the sick role.
- Fibromyalgia following accidents is a result of psychological and cultural mechanisms, and symptom amplification and adoption of the sick role affect fibromyalgia.
- Though experts sometimes apply the labels "posttraumatic stress disorder" and "conversion disorder" in whiplash cases, these two conditions are not likely to arise following minor accidents.

INTRODUCTION

This second model—somatization and adoption of the sick role—deals with symptom reporting in whiplash patients who not only report symptoms for long periods but report total disability more than 2 years after the accident. The model applies to a small percentage of whiplash patients overall but probably to the vast majority claiming chronic disability. One reason for the lack of detailed study of this phenomenon in whiplash patients is simply that these patients are relatively rare. One would have to study thousands of whiplash patients to identify this subset for further study. Alternatively, one would have to study patients still disabled after 2 years and compare them with the nondisabled, being sure to have a large enough population for study (ie, at least 100 patients). Nevertheless, researchers have developed concepts of illness behavior and adoption of the sick role. With these concepts, and studies of illness behavior in back pain patients by G. Waddell et al in the 1970s and 1980s, there is sufficient reason to consider this second model.

The symptom reporting in these patients arises in part from the same factors cited in the psychocultural illness model, but these play a small role compared to the factors that lead these patients to somatize (express psychological distress or disorder as bodily symptoms) and then behave in response to their symptoms by adopting the sick role.

There have been many diagnostic (but general) labels for the behavior of such individuals, including abnormal illness behavior, inappropriate or maladaptive illness behavior, somatoform disorder (called simply pain disorder), fibromyalgia, and chronic benign pain syndrome. Somatization is the mechanism by which the illness behavior manifests, and adoption of the sick role is the goal.

These various terms all include the recognition that the patient is displaying features of pain that are beyond explanation by physical disorder. What is also common to each label is a recognition that there is a certain pattern of illness behavior and course that is distinctive in these patients. These patients show little or no improvement even after months and indeed may worsen with time. They continue to report total disability even years after the accident, and they inevitably have a very significant preaccident history that motivates them to adopt and maintain the sick role. To understand this illness behavior, one must consider a few definitions.

ILLNESS AND DISEASE

What is an illness? The simplest answer would be a condition with which an individual feels "ill." This definition is perhaps too broad, in that few people feel well all the time, and yet they do not consider themselves to have an illness. The definition implies that illness has very much to do with the individual's perception of health and nonhealth and that this perception varies widely among the population.

> If the man thinks about his physical or moral state, he nearly always discovers that he is ill.
>
> —Goethe J. W. *Sprüche in Prosa* (Aphorisms in Prose). Fricke H, ed. Frankfurt, Germany: Deutscher Klassiker Verlag; 1993.

According to C. V. Ford (1983), disease is "the objective anatomic deformations and pathophysiologic conditions. These changes can be objectively demonstrated or inferred (although sophisticated diagnostic equipment may be required) and may be caused by such varied etiologic factors as degenerative processes, trauma, toxins, and infectious agents."

Illness is the experience of perceiving a symptom (or symptoms) and then attributing that symptom to a disease or some "disorder." Illness is thus dependent on what the individual perceives and how he or she responds to that perception.

One can, of course, have a disease without an illness (ie, feel well even though the disease is present). An example of disease without illness is hypertension, otherwise known as high blood pressure. This condition, if untreated, even when the patient feels well, will eventually cause heart disease, narrowing of major arteries, and possibly eye and kidney disease. The patient is likely to experience symptoms eventually. Physicians often have to explain to patients that although they do not perceive symptoms at the moment, they must take medication to control their high blood pressure, or someday they will feel ill. Most people with high blood pressure have had it for weeks, months, or even years without having an illness. They are asymptomatic (no symptoms). When told they have high blood pressure, a few develop headaches that they attribute to the high blood pressure, even though they never had headaches before. They now have an illness. They have perceived a symptom and have attributed that symptom to the high blood pressure (the disease). Illness is therefore an experience, modified only in part by the underlying disease process. The individual's interpretation of the significance of those perceived symptoms also alters the illness experience. Clearly, many factors (biological, emotional, intellectual, psychological, and cultural) affect what type of illness will develop in an individual. It is likely that the illness experience can exist even without disease.

Members of the medical community use "illness" to cover both physical and psychological disorders. They have artificially divided illnesses into organic and nonorganic. That is, when there appears to be primarily a physical (biological) cause for the patient's behavior (eg, a bacterium, a laceration, or damage to a joint), an organic illness (disease) is said to be present. When it appears that the cause of the patient's ill feeling is mostly psychological, then a nonorganic illness is said to be present. In reality, all illnesses have biological and psychological aspects that determine the behavior of the patient. If biological aspects are considered dominant, an illness is called organic. If psychological aspects seem dominant, the illness is called nonorganic.

SICK ROLE AND ILLNESS BEHAVIOR

There is a close relationship between illness behavior and the meaning of the sick role to some whiplash patients.

In I. Pilowsky (1969), T. Parsons is credited with developing the concept that illness can be a socially constructed idea. Pilowsky quotes Parsons, who said that the sick role is "a 'partially and conditionally legitimated state' which an individual may be granted, provided that he . . . recognizes his obligation to cooperate with others for the purpose of 'getting well' as soon as possible. Furthermore, he is expected to make use of the services of those whom society regards as competent to diagnose and treat illness."

Although the sick role infers illness, an undesirable experience, being granted the sick role means being granted certain gains that may have many benefits for the individual.

> How sickness enlarges the dimensions of a man's self to himself!
> —The convalescent. In: Lamb C., ed. *Essays of Elia*. London:
> Grant Richards Publishing; 1901:250.

The sick role does, for example, absolve individuals from fault for their failure to meet social and work obligations (Pilowsky 1969).

Under certain circumstances, as Ford (1983) explains, the sick role offers a psychologically attractive option: "The sick role is more attractive when (1) it is more culturally acceptable; (2) the social support system is perceived to be inadequate; (3) the individual feels under psychological stress; (4) the sick role resolves personal and social problems; (5) the individual is less self-reliant; and (6) coping skills are decreased."

It is suggested that the sick role can be used to solve certain problems in living but that society does not accept emotional disorders or difficulties in coping with life problems to be an acceptable entry into the sick role.

Some patients may hope the sick role will solve all their problems.

> Oh yet we trust that somehow good
>
> Will be the final goal of ill.
> —Tennyson A. In memoriam A. H. H. In: *The Works of Alfred Tennyson*.
> Canto LIV. London: C. Kegan Paul & Co; 1881:301.

Yet how does one attain the sick role? It is granted by others on certain conditions. Pilowsky (1978) indicates that the sick person's incapacity is not regarded as something for which that person can be held responsible. It is therefore not considered his or her fault, which is critical to being granted the sick role by others. In most societies, illnesses with biological (physical) factors held as the significant mechanisms (ie, organic illnesses) are considered "no-fault" illnesses. The sick role may be granted under such circumstances. Implicit in this is the belief that a person cannot fully control how a disease influences his or her behavior. If one has knee inflammation, one has knee pain. The pain is not under one's control and not one's fault. In contrast, many people in general, health care gatekeepers, and patients view psychological illness or disability as partially the patient's fault: his or her moral fortitude is often called into question.

The practical effect of this stigmatization has been readily demonstrated by Aaron et al (1997). They compared two patient groups given exactly the same diagnosis (fibromyalgia), having the same symptoms, and having the same physical examination findings. One group claimed that their fibromyalgia began after physical trauma. The other group claimed that their fibromyalgia began after emotional trauma. Members of the groups were not treated the same way. The group claiming onset of fibromyalgia after emotional trauma had a very difficult time having their disability recognized and were routinely turned down for disability applications. The members of the group claiming onset after physical trauma had a much easier time. It appears that a person seeking the sick role (and hoping to be successful) must therefore present in a manner suggesting a no-fault illness.

The definition of illness can be linked to the sick role (Pilowsky 1978): "An illness is a state of the organism which fulfills the requirements of an appropriate reference group, for admission to the sick role." This fulfillment of the role requires certain behavior. As defined by D. Mechanic and E. H. Volkart (1961), illness behavior is "the way in which symptoms are perceived, evaluated, and acted upon by a person who recognizes some pain, discomfort, or other signs of . . . malfunction."

The sick role is thus a phenomenon during which one is granted secondary gain. Without the secondary gain, the sick role would have no value. The sick role is also a social contract, for there is the proviso that the sick role is granted so long as one recognizes the obligation to cooperate with others for the purpose of "getting well" as soon as possible. Thus, the individual must be fully motivated to become well. Once the individual shows a lack of motivation to get well, then the contract is broken. In its most extreme form, the lack of motivation to get well (or motivation to remain ill) is considered malingering. In malingering, one consciously plots to maintain the sick role. Is there another way to carry out one's desire to maintain the sick role? To answer this question, it is worth examining more closely the concept of secondary gain in the sick role.

SECONDARY GAIN

Today, "secondary gain" is largely a legal concept. It can be understood as arising out of a social construct—the sick role. Special rights and privileges are granted to individuals who become ill. They may be relieved from work and social obligations and other civic duties. When it benefits an individual, being relieved of duties is a secondary gain. It should be noted that these "advantages" always exist in one's environment and are awarded as part of the social contract.

Hence, secondary gain is readily available to the individual fulfilling the criteria for the sick role. The secondary gains are not merely financial. This is one reason why patients do not improve despite receiving disability pensions providing lower incomes than they may have had previously: there are many other secondary gains driving the illness behavior. A. J. Barsky and G. L. Klerman (1983) consider secondary gain as

> the acceptable and "legitimate" interpersonal advantages that result when one has the symptoms of a physical disease. The somatically distressed individual is excused from certain responsibilities and obligations and can avoid challenges and duties. The physically symptomatic person also garners sympathy, attention, support, and many types of concrete assistance. . . . All of this occurs without a loss of pride or self-esteem and without a sense of failure, fault, or defeat. This is because the patient cannot be blamed for his or her inability and is not held responsible or culpable.

From D. A. Fishbain (1994), one can list common examples of secondary gain.

- gratifying preexisting unresolved dependent strivings
- gratifying preexisting unresolved vengeful strivings (the employee felt unappreciated or was engaged in a risky job but is now being paid for not working, or revenge against insurance companies or adjusters who gave the patient a hard time)
- obtaining one's entitlement for years of struggling and dutiful attention to responsibilities
- converting a socially unacceptable disability (psychological disorder) to a socially acceptable disability (injury or disease beyond one's control)
- displacing the blame for one's failures from oneself to an apparently disabling illness beyond one's control
- eliciting caregiving, sympathy, and concern from family and friends
- avoiding work or obtaining preferential work
- withdrawing from an unpleasant or unsatisfactory life role or activity
- maintaining status in the family or domination of family
- avoiding sex

- communicating with and relating to others in a new, socially sanctioned manner
- obtaining drugs
- gaining financial awards associated with disability

ECONOMY OF SECONDARY GAIN

Most people believe that being ill is not desirable; although there are gains to being ill (in this instance, secondary gains), there clearly are losses. But why would anyone pursue secondary gain if illness also brings losses? What is the net gain if illness brings losses?

Illness brings the greatest losses to individuals not otherwise distressed or already suffering in other ways. What if individuals are distressed, overburdened, and suffering in a way that gives them no option for a socially acceptable reprieve—without losing honor, without abandoning their work ethic, and without being blamed if they fail? What if the losses that most people experience (such as loss of income, loss of enjoyment of family life, loss of opportunity and hope of achieving one's goals) are already present or relatively unimportant before the illness? What if one's circumstances become so intolerable that abandoning them all might be a viable alternative for psychological survival? Does the illness really bring so much loss that it is inconceivable to adopt the sick role? Perhaps not. Besides, there are the secondary gains. Perhaps it is this balancing that determines whether individuals adopt the sick role. Most people find that illness carries too many losses, but some might see illness as a net gain.

Some individuals who are suffering psychologically may hide their symptoms, perhaps even from themselves. They may have suffered many stressors, miseries, and disappointments yet have to cope with these losses and burdens because society will not grant them any freedom to do otherwise (only the sick role grants this freedom from burdens). They are forced to continue in their miserable lives. Why not suffer with all those difficulties and receive the benefits of the sick role?

There are ways other than frank malingering for this transition to the sick role to occur. Fundamental to this process is somatization.

SOMATIZATION

Somatization is the means by which the patient maintains the symptoms of chronic pain and the illness behavior. Z. J. Lipowski (1988) defines somatization as "a tendency to experience and communicate somatic distress in response to psychosocial stress."

That is the simplest definition, in which somatization is a process, but there are many contexts in which somatization may operate. To understand the significance of somatization in a given individual, one must consider the context in which it occurs. As adapted from Pilowsky (1997), contexts in which somatization may occur include the following:

- Somatization as the bodily aspect of emotion. Here the term refers to the bodily changes that are part of emotion (ie, anxiety and sweating, breathlessness, palpitations, tremor, etc).
- Somatization as communication. Complaining of bodily symptoms can be a way of letting others know that one feels abandoned, rejected, or in need of attention. Bodily symptoms, for example, are more likely to receive such attention.
- Somatization as an idiom of distress. Some sociocultural differences between patient and physician, for example, may make it difficult for a patient to express distress. Bodily symptoms communicate this distress more readily than verbalization would.
- Somatization as a means of expression in those with an inability to express emotion or for whom emotional expression is undesirable.
- Somatization as attention and attribution. Somatization may be a state in which excessive attention is paid to bodily sensations that most people would not notice. A term often used is "somatosensory amplification."
- Somatization as a response to health care systems. Many health care systems, by their nature, influence the sort of symptoms that people consider a legitimate use of the resources. Such systems do not as readily treat psychological symptoms.
- Somatization as entry into the sick role, as discussed above. Bodily symptoms are a more socially acceptable reason for entry into the sick role. Thus, there is a preconscious and conscious motivation to report and emphasize bodily symptoms rather than psychological ones.

Somatization (in a certain context) can be considered the process by which inappropriate illness behavior occurs. It is thus important to explicitly define the role of somatization in each case. As long as the context of somatization is explicitly stated, there should be little confusion.

The pattern of this behavior has been described by Lipowski (1988).

> Somatizing patients . . . complain of physical symptoms that either lack demonstrable organic bases or are judged to be grossly in excess of what one would expect on grounds of objective medical findings. . . .

> Individuals so predisposed tend to adopt somatization as a mode of coping with life's vicissitudes, psychological needs and conflicts, feelings of guilt and anger, and low self-esteem. By adopting the sick role they seek to gain attention and support and to avoid social and family

obligations and demands. The responses of family members and doctors may reinforce this somatizing tendency and help to maintain it indefinitely.

As explained by Ford (1983), discussing an accident victim:

> The sick role may be used by the person to rationalise personal failures or inadequacies, particularly of a characterologic nature, or the need to accept welfare by using the explanation that one cannot be blamed for illness nor expected to perform at the same level as a healthy person.

> An accident serves to transform psychological disability into a [physical] disability and therefore an unacceptable disability into an acceptable disability.

As more diagramatically explained by A. H. Hirschfeld and R. C. Behan (1966):

> Personality difficulties + Troubled life situation = Unacceptable disability

but then,

> Unacceptable disability + Accident = Acceptable disability

They explain that an individual experiencing general dissatisfaction with life may eventually develop disabling emotional responses.

> People are often highly motivated by what they feel others think of them. But still more vital is the fact that these opinions are reflected in the person himself and he finds that certain disabilities must be totally rejected by his own conscience, or sense of pride.

> The person who has the unacceptable disability finds himself hiding it. He does not wish to share it even with the physician. He does not want to stop work because of it, not only because he will be unpaid, but more significantly because he will think so poorly of himself. The resolution of this problem must therefore await the appearance of an excuse which will make it face-saving to the patient.

An accident provides a solution to this dilemma—a socially acceptable form of disability adopted by the patient. This is accomplished through somatization.

Lipowski also emphasizes, as does Pilowsky, that somatization is not strictly the result of conscious thought processing. It is the further processing of one's symptoms (their meaning) by goal-oriented thought processing that generates the behavior accompanying somatization (see also Chapter 23).

MECHANISM OF ADOPTION OF THE SICK ROLE

There are four essential conditions needed for adoption of the sick role.

1. Individuals must have experienced events that create psychological distress, disorder, or simply failure to cope with their life miseries and disappointments. These individuals have a struggle, but they need a socially acceptable way out.
2. A socially acceptable opportunity that is not the individuals' fault, in this context an accident, must arise. As noted above, society will grant the sick role when individuals are unable to control the "disease," but when individuals present with psychological disorders, in most cases, they are held partially at fault. Illnesses presenting as chronic pain, for example, may resemble disease and thereby are given no-fault labels such as late whiplash syndrome, fibromyalgia, and so forth.
3. The individual must present with the chief symptoms being pain, fatigue, numbness, and so forth—all symptoms that emphasize a disease process and minimize psychological symptoms. Somatization, as discussed below, is one fashion in which this may be accomplished.
4. The individual must find an enabling no-fault gatekeeper, someone who will minimize the role of psychological factors as well and label the patient with a syndrome that appears to have an organic basis. This is one of the reasons some patients must seek out a number of physicians until they find one who will finally let them through the gate. As described earlier, these enabling no-fault gatekeepers (usually physicians) act as they do for a variety of reasons. They may simply want to avoid the response they will get from the patient if they explore psychological factors. Besides this, there is tertiary gain. Tertiary gain is the personal advantage others gain from an individual's illness. This gain can be simply monetary (ie, "You have a serious injury, and you will have to come see me for therapy every week for a year"), but it can present in other ways. Physicians who explore psychological factors with a patient are sometimes called "stupid and crazy." On the other hand, gatekeepers who give patients the label they need for a no-fault entry are "wise," "sympathetic," "finally the one who knows what my pain is due to." They are given the role of advocate. It is a very rewarding role to play, even without the monetary aspect. Indeed, such gatekeepers can become "international experts," touring the world speaking to patient support groups and glorified for their wisdom

and compassion. Some of these professionals actually have the same malady, so they receive the tertiary gain of lending legitimacy to their own "disease" by supporting others who have the same. Tertiary gain may thus be a very powerful force. By whatever mechanism tertiary gain proceeds, the enabling gatekeeper is an important element in adoption of the sick role.

Somatization is the chief mechanism by which the individual appears to present with the necessary no-fault entry into the sick role.

And so we have, in brief, the following conclusions about the sick role:

- The sick role has criteria. Those criteria are well known and presumably overlearned.
- Secondary gains are available to those with the sick role. These gains are also presumably overlearned.
- The sick role is available to those with no-fault entry (a no-fault illness).
- The no-fault entry is thus available to those presenting with specified types of symptoms and syndromes.
- One presents with those symptoms that may lead to a no-fault diagnosis (and minimizes any symptom that might lead to an at-fault diagnosis).
- Behavior that perpetuates the sick role is maintained through somatization.

DIAGNOSIS OF SOMATIZATION AND ADOPTION OF THE SICK ROLE

In 1969, Pilowsky defined abnormal (or inappropriate) illness behavior. This behavior is expected to be encountered in the patient adopting the sick role. Pilowsky developed this concept to delineate the relationships among the sick role, illness, behavior, and disease. Originally, the intent was to help understand the patient who reports physical symptoms for which no adequate organic origin is apparent. In 1978, he expanded this concept. He included essentially any circumstance wherein the patient reports certain symptoms and perceives those symptoms in a fashion that the physician considers inappropriate.

In 1978, Pilowsky defined abnormal illness behavior as "the persistence of an inappropriate or maladaptive mode of perceiving, evaluating and acting in relation to one's own state of health, despite the fact that a doctor (or other appropriate social agent) . . . has offered a reasonably lucid explanation of the nature of the illness and the appropriate course of management to be followed."

Pilowsky has stated that this definition assumes that the physician is in an ideal circumstance in which to recognize and then report to the patient this explanation for his or her illness. In many practice settings, and certainly in the medicolegal setting, however, physicians are seldom able or willing to offer an explanation to the patient. They may be loath to do so for a number of reasons. First, there is tremendous controversy over the cause of chronic symptom reporting in whiplash victims. It can be very difficult for the physician to be confident about the cause of the symptoms and reassure the patient, for example, that there is no serious physical disorder. Whatever view a physician has, a patient can go to another physician and receive an opposite view. Second, a physician may attempt to explain that there is nothing *physically* wrong with the patient or that the symptoms relate to "stress." In response, the patient may become angry or violent, feel accused of being "crazy," consider the physician ignorant, or report the physician to a governing body, all of which discourage the physician from attempting to make a diagnosis of abnormal illness behavior again. In the setting of a personal injury claim, the patient may be upset that this diagnosis will affect the way others (particularly the courts) view the symptoms and compensation.

Physicians tend to be cautious even of what they write in the patient's file because patients, lawyers, and others will see that file, and the physician may again face an unkind response. There may even be physicians who never want to be seen as anything but a patient advocate. They will tell the patient what the patient wants to hear. They may indeed enable adoption of the sick role. It is thus not surprising that physicians or therapists seldom render a diagnosis of abnormal illness behavior, especially in the medicolegal setting.

To diagnose inappropriate illness behavior, physicians may not specifically have to see that the patient has been given a sufficient explanation of a condition, yet to recognize that a patient perceives, evaluates, and acts in an inappropriate or maladaptive mode. Preaccident risk factors that predispose one to adopt the sick role, symptoms and signs of nonorganic features, and a view of the illness course and patient's behavior may be sufficient to make this diagnosis. One may be able to recognize that the illness behavior is inappropriate for the degree of injury.

This diagnosis should be made on the basis of a number of fundamental positive findings. One certainly suspects adoption of the sick role in those reporting total disability long after the accident, especially when there is no ongoing damage from the acute injury to explain chronic pain reporting in the first place, but this is not enough to establish a diagnosis. Psychological disorder or mechanisms of illness should be diagnosed on the basis of positive findings.

History

As the risk factors for adoption of the sick role are in part the risk factors for somatization, one begins with identifying in the history the risk factors for somatization (R. Ferrari, O. Kwan et al 1999). One looks for the risk factors shown in Exhibit 10–1.

Ferrari, Kwan et al (1999) offer a more detailed discussion of how one checks for each of the risk factors listed in Exhibit 10–1 and understands their relevance in the patient's illness behavior.

Exhibit 10–1 Risk Factors for Somatization

1. **Genetic factors and early childhood experience**
   - Family history of depression, alcohol abuse, or dependence or antisocial personality disorder
   - Role model in family of chronic illness
   - Experience of abuse, parental abandonment, serious physical illness, or other traumatic experience
2. **Personality traits or idiosyncrasies and personality disorders**
   - Excessive preoccupation with maintenance of health
   - Distortion of minor symptoms
   - Frequent medical consultations and allied professions
   - Rigidity of being (or in adjustment)
   - Chronic giving-in and giving-up attitudinal state
   - Habitual pessimistic explanation style
   - Alexithymia
   - Histrionic, antisocial, and borderline personality disorders
3. **Scapegoating motive and convenient focus**
   - History of dissatisfying life or repeated miseries
4. **Object loss and pathological grieving—look for**
   - The inability to speak of the deceased without intense and fresh grief
   - The triggering of intense grief reaction by minor events
   - A prevailing theme of loss in the individual's verbalization
   - The inability to move or dispose of the possessions of the deceased
   - The subjective experiencing of the physical symptoms of the deceased, particularly around the anniversary of the death
   - Radical life changes or avoidance of friends, family, or former activities
   - A prior history of subclinical depression with guilt, low self-esteem, or false euphoria
   - The imitation of the mannerisms or personality of the deceased
   - Self-destruct impulses
   - Unaccountable sadness at certain times of the year
   - Phobias regarding illness or death
   - The avoidance of death-related rituals
   - Associations marked by themes of loss
5. **Negative affectivity**
   - History of anxiety disorder or depression
   - History of divorce or features of inhibited anger
6. **Prior episodes of somatization behavior**
   - Previous work-related injury claims
   - Previous personal injury claims

continues

Exhibit 10–1 continued

> • History of irritable bowel syndrome, fibromyalgia, chronic fatigue syndrome, chronic pelvic or chronic benign chest pain, "allergic to everything" or "multiple chemical sensitivities," or similar somatoform disorders
>
> *Source:* Adapted with permission from Ferrari R, Kwan O, Friel J. Illness Behavior and Adoption of the Sick Role in Whiplash Claimants. Forensics: *The Online Journal of the American College of Forensic Examiners*, *www.acfe.com.* © 1999 American College of Forensic Examiners.

It is important to note, however, that adoption of the sick role does not apply exclusively to individuals with what may be generally perceived to be unsatisfying social or occupational lives. Adoption of the sick role is recognized even in individuals who appear to be leading rewarding lives.

The observations of D. S. Ciccone and R. C. Grzesiak (1992) indicate that:

> Many patients who go on to develop chronic pain following an acute injury or illness report a premorbid pattern of excessive self-sacrifice, hyperactivity, or overachievement. They often have a history of going to work at an early age, putting in frequent overtime hours, and holding more than one job at a time. They may have permitted or encouraged others to rely upon them excessively and, as a result, were routinely called upon and expected to perform special tasks or favors. These tasks were often burdensome in nature or at least not intrinsically rewarding for the patient. Following the onset of pain, this pattern of unrelenting self-sacrifice and overachievement typically comes to an abrupt halt with the patient becoming the recipient of special care instead of the provider. . . . The onset of physical injury or illness apparently offers these patients an opportunity to relieve themselves of their occupational and social obligations without any need for self-reproach and without any loss of social approval.

The demands they were expected to meet "only apply so long as the patient is physically fit." Similar observations are made by D. Blumer and M. Heilbronn (1982).

The individual who adopts the sick role following an accident thus has a preaccident history with the motivation to adopt the sick role in a socially acceptable fashion, so as to legitimately be granted the secondary gains of the sick role. Chronic pain is a socially acceptable basis of disability. Somatization can be considered to be the mechanism of inappropriate illness behavior and adoption of the sick role, wherein the patient's psychological disorder or distress is manifested via somatization as pain.

Having identified the preaccident motivations for adoption of the socially acceptable reason for disability and the risk factors for somatization, one must then identify that the illness course is one of little or no improvement, or even decline. That is, even though individuals may have reasons to adopt the sick role, this does not mean that they will. Even with the model of psychocultural illness, most accident victims report that symptoms steadily improve over several weeks or months, with often a relatively early return to work. When a patient shows little improvement over this period or worsens and reports disability more than a year after the accident, one can suspect, if the preaccident history is appropriately identified, that inappropriate illness behavior and adoption of the sick role are occurring.

Nonorganic Signs

With the history noted, one should identify in the examination the symptoms and signs of abnormal illness behavior. These are noted by, for example, the signs of nonorganic pain indicated by G. Waddell et al (1989). They offer a definition of this illness behavior as "maladaptive overt illness related behaviour which is out of proportion to the underlying physical disease and more readily attributable to associated cognitive and affective disturbances (which are morbid in degree) than to the objective physical disease."

The comments from an examining physician may include such observations as:

- The patient's symptoms are bizarre, and his behavior is out of keeping with the nature of his injuries.
- The patient shrieked when light pressure was applied to her back or even the slightest movement of the spine made.
- The patient is preoccupied with his symptoms and the notion that he has been utterly disabled by the accident.
- There were numerous inconsistencies during the examination, with the patient demonstrating exaggerated responses to examination.

The patient may also use histrionic or melodramatic terminology (eg, the pain is described in terms of "red hot pokers" or "hot needles driven through the body"). Experience is not the basis for these descriptions, and these descriptions are absent in routine painful disorders like arthritis.

Besides the general observations of the patient's behavior, it is sometimes possible to cite more specific examples of the patient's abnormal illness behavior. These are unexpected in organic illness. According to G. Waddell et al (1989) and as noted in Table 8–1, features of the patient's pain (likely applicable to both neck and back pain) may include

- constant pain
- diffuse pain

- whole limb pain or numbness
- leg giving way
- tailbone pain and back pain
- intolerance to treatments
- emergency hospital admissions for pain

Signs on examination (Waddell's signs) include

- pain behaviors (grimacing or extreme reactions with examination maneuvers of neck or back)
- superficial tenderness (light touch or pinching of skin evokes significant pain response)
- nondermatomal (not following specific nerve injury patterns) sensory changes
- jerky, give-way muscle weakness
- regional weakness (eg, whole leg or arm)
- pain with simulation tests (eg, applied pressure down the spine from the top of the skull or hip rotation)
- improved straight leg raise with distraction (ie, compare straight leg raise in the lying and sitting position—the patient is not aware that straight leg raise is actually also being tested; in organic disease, the range of straight leg raising should be equal in both cases)

If a patient has 3 or more of the signs listed in each group, it is considered significant and worthy of further investigation. Alone, however, this does not identify the exact psychological factors involved. Certainly, Waddell's signs should not be considered simply signs of malingering, as that has never been validated. Instead, Waddell's signs indicate the presence of psychosocial barriers to recovery (see Ferrari 1999).

The recognition of this illness behavior and the reasons the patient is motivated toward this behavior is important not only in providing therapy but in determining (for legal purposes) whether the symptoms are related to the accident. As will be considered later, accidents play different roles in individuals presenting with chronic pain. Since each diagnostic term should imply a mechanism, and since the courts consider mechanisms when considering causation, one must be careful how one uses diagnostic terms. Because these terms are sometimes used loosely by nonpsychiatrists, it is important that one explicitly state the mechanism being implied when using terms such as "abnormal illness behavior," "adoption of the sick role," "conversion disorder," or "pain disorder." The legal implications are obvious.

Specific terms, particularly if their mechanisms can be specifically defined, are more useful than general terms. Although, for example, the phrase "chronic pain syndrome" is sometimes used to describe the "end product" in certain illness behaviors, it is less useful in a legal sense because medical experts (and legal experts) use the term differently. Some intend it to mean an illness that is maintained through psychological mechanisms, whereas others use it to refer to some as-yet-unexplained form of disease that can, for example, be linked causally to a physical injury. Vague terms such as this should be used only when the underlying mechanism can be described, so that confusion does not arise. (See also "Chronic Benign Pain Syndrome" below.) Indeed, definitions are critical to usage of such diagnostic terms in considering whiplash patients.

ILLNESS BEHAVIOR AS A CHOICE

This illness behavior, where the end goal is adoption of the sick role, may appear to be almost automatic for some of these patients. The question is, Can they control their behavior? This question has important therapeutic and legal implications. These considerations and what is meant by "preconscious," "conscious," "unconscious," and other terms in the context of illness behavior are discussed in detail in Chapter 23.

Pilowsky has suggested that both unconscious and conscious motivations and thought processes contribute to adoption of the sick role. Strictly speaking, one should consider the motivations here as enacted preconscious and conscious thought processes. (This is described in detail in Chapter 20.) Motivation is a form of readiness. Motivation thus implies that the individual is prepared for an action and is waiting for the opportunity to take the action. Motivations reach into the individual's environment. Unconscious thoughts come to consciousness, in the strictly Freudian sense, only through psychoanalytic processes such as dream analysis, hypnosis, and so on. For motivations to be present and then acted upon, they must lie within the realm of the preconscious and conscious. The preconscious is different from the unconscious; the preconscious deals with mental events, processes, and content that are capable of being brought into conscious awareness.

Preconscious information processing has an "automatic" nature to it, but for complex behavior the maintenance of goal-oriented information processing still requires intent and conscious input to remain effective and use this more automatic thought processing. Clearly, there is a spectrum of information processing (from preconscious motivations to conscious ones) in these patients. Whether motivations are preconscious or conscious, one can choose whether to act on them.

How motivation drives our behavior is evident in everyday life. Most people, for example, have learned that placing their hand in a fire hurts. They avoid getting too close to a fire, not because they consciously think about the possibility of getting burned. Instead, the thought process is now preconscious. Yet a person could alter this behavior if there were reason to do so (eg, someone reached into a fire to rescue a friend who had fallen into it). One can ignore or undo learned behavior. One makes a choice. The recognition of this ability is the basis for behavioral psychotherapy. As explained by S. C. Wooley et al (1978), "adoption of the [sick] role . . . is shaped by three sets of influences: vicarious learning through models, especially in childhood; (2) direct social reinforcement of illness behavior by family, friends, and physicians; and (3) avoidance learning."

These researchers argue (and there are studies that support their argument) that:

> Illness behaviour, like any other learned behavior, should be responsive to environmental stimuli. Patients should be able to distinguish when pain or illness behavior will be rewarded—viz., in the presence of a potential care-taker—and when it will not. . . . It is likely that not only the expression of pain and social elicitation of care-taking, but attention to painful stimuli, and by extension the experience of pain itself, is subject to stimulus control.

Their studies demonstrated that individuals can change their illness behavior if they choose to relinquish or to remove themselves from stimuli that encourage secondary gains. Thus, in adoption of the sick role in this setting, the individual is capable of stopping that behavior. There is a choice not to do so.

OTHER LABELS FOR ADOPTION OF THE SICK ROLE

Some other labels used for adoption of the sick role include pain disorder and chronic benign pain syndrome. These are each discussed briefly below. Note that while the label is different in each case, it still refers to a pattern of a similar, recognizable illness behavior.

Pain Disorder

Pain disorder is a specific subtype of somatoform disorder.[1,2] By definition, "psychological factors are judged to have the major role in the onset, severity, exacerbation, or maintenance of the pain."[2(p458)] Pain disorder is a recognized psychological disorder in which:

> The predominant disturbance . . . is severe and prolonged pain for which there is no adequate medical explanation.[1(p1021)]

> The predominant feature . . . is a preoccupation with severe and continuous pain . . . that has no adequate medical explanation.[1(p1023)]

Inappropriate illness behavior is a fundamental feature of pain disorder. Thus, despite the absence of organic disease, "patients . . . are often severely disabled, living the life of an invalid . . . [with] long histories of medical and surgical care, visiting many doctors."[1(p1023)]

The illness behavior includes:

> an implicit appeal to the physician to take responsibility for a cure, be-
> haviours that sustain the sick role, environmental rewards that maintain
> the sick role, and avoidance of healthy roles.[3(p176)]

> [Somatoform patients] are completely preoccupied with their pain, cit-
> ing it as the source of all their misery . . . and devoutly maintaining that
> the rest of their lives is blissful. Somatoform pain patients . . . are intent
> on having their physicians accept their pain as completely organic in
> origin.[1(p1023)]

Nevertheless, it should be noted that to say patients have pain disorder is not to
say they did not have an acute injury. It is recognized that pain disorder may
occur in the setting of "medical disease." In the whiplash patient, the acute injury
resolves, but the reporting of chronic, severe pain does not.

Chronic Benign Pain Syndrome

Others use the term "chronic benign pain syndrome" to describe this illness
behavior in whiplash patients. It is synonymous with "somatoform pain disorder."
As described by G. F. Gregory and D. J. Crockett (1988):

> Chronic benign pain syndrome . . . is associated with various com-
> plaints of poor sleep habits, sexual dysfunctions, gastro-intestinal
> upset, and visual difficulties such as blurring of vision. . . . Frequently,
> the patient focuses on pain complaint to such an extent that the patient
> may seem to be unaware of, or indifferent to, other possible sources of
> [psychological] distress. . . . Evidence of exaggeration of symptoms is
> often observed.

They comment on the behavior that allows this diagnosis to be made.

> The pain patient may exhibit a great deal of emotional behaviour when
> describing his problems including crying out when the painful area is
> stimulated, demonstrating noticeable grimaces when asked to engage in
> diagnostic maneuvers.

> Chronic benign pain syndrome may be an unconscious process.

Others who have discussed this syndrome after accidents include F. J. Wilfling
and P. C. Wing (1984). They describe how chronic benign pain syndrome may
allow entry into the sick role and "being 'sick' . . . may sanction failure in work,

school or relationships, and enable the individual to receive otherwise unavailable care and nurture."

They emphasize, as well, that the symptoms may be genuine: "It is extremely important to point out that the continuation or elaboration of pain disability behaviours is not evidence of malingering or conscious manipulation. . . . It can be argued that these behaviour changes will take place unconsciously."

An important adjunct to the use of the chronic pain syndrome diagnosis is the description of the mechanism of this pain. The view that the chronic pain syndrome arises by the mechanism of physical damage is, of course, not scientifically sound. There is no physical damage from the acute injury that continues to lead to symptom reporting. If one uses chronic pain syndrome to indicate psychological disorder, then "chronic benign pain syndrome" is the more appropriate term. Otherwise, confusion will arise in the courts regarding mechanism and the issue of a causal link to the accident. The term "chronic pain syndrome" also applies to patients with terminal cancer, for example, untreatable osteomyelitis, structural brain disorders, and so forth. The term is not useful unless one defines the mechanism. Gregory and Crockett (1988) explain the confusion that has already arisen in the courts with the use of "chronic pain syndrome" without defining the illness mechanism explicitly.

> What is not clear is whether the Judges in the decisions which hold that "chronic pain syndrome" is fully compensable use the term in the same way as [those who consider it noncompensable]. If they are referring to different conditions, then the fact that the results are different is not surprising. If they are referring to people suffering from the same type of problems, then the difference in the result is more disturbing.

It is thus more important to define illness mechanisms than merely to apply illness labels.

SUMMARY

There is a small subset of whiplash patients whose behavior is very different from that of most whiplash patients. We can understand their illness by understanding the sick role, the secondary gains of the sick role, and the preaccident history that places them at risk to use an accident as a socially acceptable basis for achieving the secondary gains of the sick role, which they then adopt.

It really does not matter what labels one chooses. One needs to explain the mechanism when using the terms "illness behavior," "adoption of the sick role," "chronic benign pain syndrome," "pain disorder," or "somatization." The central implication of each label is that psychological mechanisms can lead to symptom reporting that then provides a socially acceptable form of disability and grants entry into the sick role.

This model also helps to explain why some patients continue to report disability even after settlement of their litigation.

- The psychological disorder arose because of many factors besides a desire for monetary compensation. As long as the psychological disorder remains untreated, the settlement will not resolve the patient's symptoms.
- Patients have developed a pain identity. That is, they have been in this mode of pain behavior for a long time. Their entire social structure has adjusted to accommodate them as an ill individual, and now they cannot relinquish a role that is part of their identity.
- There are other secondary gains that encourage maintenance of patients' symptoms.
- New causes are creating symptoms, but because these new causes have not yet been identified, the original disorder appears still to be causing symptoms.
- Individuals have been out of the work force for so long that returning is difficult. They might have to retrain, might have to struggle to find a job after being rejected several times, and so forth. Rather than deal with feelings of inadequacy and failure or struggle to enter the work force again, individuals may remain ill, and that is socially acceptable. The individuals will not lose honor or be blamed by others (or themselves) for their failing, because it is the injury that disables them.
- One might not want to return to the preaccident work. Living off the settlement, even if it yields a lower income overall, may be more desirable than returning to an undesirable job.
- In some cases, there may be resentment about having received too little compensation, and this may promote somatization. The individuals have been expressing psychologically based symptoms as pain. They are likely to follow this learned behavior when psychologically distressed in the future. It is more acceptable because one has an "injury" as a cause of disability, not simply depression and resentment.
- In some cases, individuals actually had a conscious interest in financial gain and do not want to improve suddenly after the settlement, as they do not want to reveal their true motivation. They may choose to improve slowly over a longer period that appears more "natural."

ADOPTION OF THE SICK ROLE—HISTORIC OBSERVATIONS

As early as 1930, F. Kennedy noted that patients sometimes used a traumatic event to, preconsciously or consciously, cope with preaccident difficulties. Physicians noted then that patients held the strictest belief about being physically damaged, seldom attributing their symptoms to psychological factors. If patients did admit to psychological disorder, they insisted that it was only secondary to the experience of chronic pain.

Kennedy recognized that many individuals were adopting the sick role. Kennedy described this as "assumption of the disease picture." The accident was not responsible for the patient's illness behavior; rather, it offered individuals an opportunity to obtain the rewards of the sick role through more acceptable means. Kennedy specified that the psychologically challenging nature of the event was irrelevant. The capacity of the accident to cause serious injury or death was immaterial to the patient (unlike in posttraumatic stress disorder). Indeed, individuals exhibited this form of behavior even after minor accidents.

Others have long recognized that there was a psychological basis for symptom reporting in these cases. In 1927, F. Buzzard noted the general characteristics of this illness behavior.

> It rarely develops when a really serious physical disability, such as a broken limb, has been sustained. [It] does not develop after hunting accidents for which only the rider or his horse is responsible. When [it] follows an accident, the site of injury is immaterial. It is common after blows on the head or spine because injuries to these parts are in the lay mind associated with the idea of particularly terrible forms of disablement. It is met with after injuries to any part of the body.

J. F. Rosenbaum (1982) added further observations on the relationship between chronic pain reporting from an apparent injury and the psychological state of the individual.

> The event which begins the cycle of pain and sanctuary in the sick role may be a specific traumatic injury, yet may well be trivial, but for an overdetermined, multiplicity of reasons, the moment is seized. A variety of factors appear to enhance the unconscious quest to maintain the experience of pain and its access to the sick role: nurturance or gratification by family for sick role or pain behaviour, financial compensation or relief, resolution of unconscious conflicts about aggression or success, other family dynamics, and depression. One problem in having only pain, as opposed to, for example, arthritis and pain, as the access to sick role benefits is that there are no visible signs and no definitive diagnoses to validate the claim of illness. Hence, suffering and distress are the only markers of illness, a circumstance serving to exaggerate the degree of disability. The evaluating psychiatrist, therefore, must review early history and current living situation to identify factors rendering the patient vulnerable to and reinforcing the sick role.

P. G. Denker (1939) also recognized the predisposition that may lead patients to adopt the sick role (quoting C. H. Huddleston).

Whatever his personal and family histories have been, any individual may find himself in a situation that tends to become progressively more unbearable and so predisposes to psychoneurotic conduct. A man working at tasks beyond his intellectual or physical capacity, or his emotional endurance, and harassed by obligations to carry on exhausting work without being able, from whatever ultimate maladjustments, to derive satisfaction from his work, this man is becoming predisposed toward a neurosis. Bare failure is intolerable; but failure camouflaged and compensated for by an illness that brings attention, sympathy, rest, and often an indemnity or wages without work is far from intolerable.

Further explaining this, J. Ramsay (1939) wrote:

In such cases the soil is ready for the seed; in other words, that some mental conflict or maladjustment to life was already present and that the injury acted as an exciting cause of the psychoneurotic symptoms. . . . Such a man will say, and will believe the statement to be perfectly true: "I was all right until the accident, and look at me now." As a matter of fact he was, from a psychological standpoint, far from all right before his injury; the latter has merely brought to light his preexisting intrapsychic difficulties.

Finally, in 1964, J. R. Hodge (quoting A. H. Hirschfeld and R. C. Behan) stated that:

Symptoms do not develop fortuitously. . . . The accident is therefore only a single event in a continuing dynamic process. Before the injury several events occur. . . . The process is started and carries on to increased anxiety, tension, and often guilt. It explodes in catastrophe and then continues, capturing the pain and incapacity resulting from the accident for its own purpose.

The development of the accident itself, and of the subsequent symptoms as well, represent a solution to the life problems of these patients. Without this solution, financial and psychological bankruptcy faces them and the accident paradoxically represents both an emotional boon and a self-destructive psychological process. Such patients, therefore, come to physicians because of their acute pain, but not for the purpose of being cured. In these instances total relief of symptoms represents a loss of the economic and psychological solutions to their life problems.

"Whiplash injury" is in style and begins with an actual physical disability. The patient does not produce the initial symptoms by psychological means, but instead captures the physical symptoms for psychological purposes. Today the patient does not simulate an illness; he has an illness, and he may hold on to this illness for secondary gains even after psychotherapy has helped with the presenting emotional symptoms.

This model of adoption of the sick role is thus not new. Only the label has changed. One of the recent labels, fibromyalgia, has entered the legal arena of accident victims and is thus worth discussing further.

FIBROMYALGIA AND MOTOR VEHICLE ACCIDENTS*

Some consider fibromyalgia an illness behavior with somatization, with both preconscious and conscious motivations to adopt the sick role being operative. If one views "fibromyalgia" as another term for "adoption of the sick role," then clearly the accident is not the cause of fibromyalgia. Rather the accident is an *opportunity* to adopt the sick role through the label of fibromyalgia.

In 1996, a consensus report on fibromyalgia (see F. Wolfe) concluded that "overall, then, data from the literature are insufficient to indicate whether causal relationships exist between trauma and [fibromyalgia]."

The consensus was that there is a need for further study. In 1997, D. Buskila et al compared the incidence of fibromyalgia after whiplash injury with the incidence of fibromyalgia following leg fractures. They found that fibromyalgia was 13 times more frequent following neck injury than it was following lower extremity injury, even though the groups studied were equally likely to have insurance claims pending. The authors cautioned, however, that "the present data in the literature are insufficient to indicate whether causal relationships exist between trauma and [fibromyalgia]."

This is an important consideration. First, demonstrating an association is not equivalent to demonstrating a causal relationship. To do this is often a difficult task. One can reasonably accept that trauma caused a fracture because the two events are in close temporal relation. On the other hand, as the diagnosis of fibromyalgia is usually several months or years following the trauma, the temporal relationships are not close. There is thus the possibility that other factors have intervened, leading to the diagnosis of fibromyalgia.

Source: Adapted with permission from R. Ferrari and A. S. Russell, Neck Injury and Chronic Pain Syndromes: Comment on Article by Buskila et al., *Arthritis and Rheumatism,* Vol. 41, No. 4, pp. 758–759. © 1998, Lippincott Williams & Wilkins and R. Ferrari and O. Kwan, Perceived Physical and Emotional Trauma as Precipitating Events in Fibromyalgia: Comment on Article by Aaron et al., *Arthritis and Rheumatism,* © 1998, Lippincott Williams & Wilkins.

Another means by which to demonstrate a causal association, in a scientific sense, would be to reproduce the exposure experimentally. There has never been anyone who developed a chronic pain syndrome despite 4 decades of simulated "whiplash" collisions with volunteers, even though the collisions render acute symptoms.

There is no physical basis for diffuse, chronic pain in whiplash patients (as the medical literature attests), so describing the physical chain of events is difficult. The other possibility is that psychological factors are responsible for the symptoms and findings of fibromyalgia.

First Consideration

Ferrari and A. S. Russell ("Neck injury and chronic pain syndromes: comment on article by Buskila et al," 1998) have offered an explanation for the findings of Buskila et al. The reporting of pain upon pressure at specific points (as compared with the reporting of pain with pressure at control points) is fundamental in the American College of Rheumatology diagnostic criteria. One could reword the findings dealt with in the study by Buskila et al as a question: "Why do tender points appear to be more painful in neck injury patients than they are in leg fracture patients?" Tender points appear to reflect a lowered pain threshold. Barsky (1992) has suggested that this could be mediated by psychological factors. Such factors include the setting in which the symptoms develop, the amount of attention to (or distraction from) the symptoms, levels of anxiety, and so on. Tender points are found even in individuals without complaints of regional or diffuse pain but with measures of psychological distress. In these individuals, fatigue, poor sleep, and depression correlate with the presence of tender points irrespective of the absence or presence of regional or diffuse pain (P. Croft et al 1994). Thus, the "tender points" of fibromyalgia are merely an amplified pain response in areas where all of us feel some mild discomfort if tested (see also M. L. Cohen and J. L. Quintner 1993).

If amplification is a result or sign of psychological distress, then why would people with leg fractures develop this finding less often than people with neck injuries? Both suffer the initial distress from fright at the time of the accident, as well as anger at the other driver, inconvenience, and the initial pain from the injury. Beyond this initial period, however, the psychological distress may actually be greater for the whiplash (neck injury) patient. Buskila et al showed that neck injury patients had more anxiety, fatigue, sleep disturbance, and depression, all of which produce tender points, independent of pain complaints.

In most cases, for example, leg fracture victims have injuries that are known to have a good outcome. There is very little media attention about a need for prolonged casting and surgery. These patients see a physician who shows them the fracture objectively on X-ray and reassures them that they will do well. The patients are even more reassured weeks later when they can be shown the objective sign of fracture healing on another X-ray. They will not be sent to a multitude of therapists, all using approaches that are bound to fail, and they will not battle with an insurance company (a patient with a fracture, unlike a whiplash patient, is unlikely to be considered a malingerer). When their cast comes off, they will be told that the period of casting caused muscle stiffness and weaknesses. Normal bone healing requires that they begin walking even if it initially causes pain. (That is, they are told that the initial pain they feel is normal, not harmful, and that it would be more harmful to stop using the leg than to use it.)

Compare this to whiplash patients. They are part of a culture that circulates information about whiplash injury leading to chronic pain and disability. These patients may be told by their physician that the injury could take a long time to "heal," be sent to many different therapists, suffer repeated therapeutic failures, develop the impression that to be active with pain may cause more harm, and battle with an insurance company whose representatives doubt the legitimacy of the symptoms. In most cases, one would expect the whiplash patient to become more distressed with time than does the leg fracture patient. Their outcomes are different because of what they know or expect about their injury and how they are treated thereafter. If tender points are more often identified in the more distressed individual, and if this is the key to the diagnosis of fibromyalgia, then it is not surprising that such a diagnosis is more often made in the whiplash patient than in the leg fracture patient.

Second Consideration

Ferrari and O. Kwan (1999) have explored in part the alternative mechanisms by which a diagnosis of fibromyalgia arises following an accident. Although they agree that the factors involved in the model above apply as well, they also consider that fibromyalgia symptoms represent a result of somatization as the mechanism of adoption of the sick role. Yet one should ask why, if one believes that fibromyalgia is simply adoption of the sick role following the accident, the accident being an opportunity for secondary gains, this does not occur just as frequently with leg fractures. The reason is simple: when adoption of the sick role occurs, the preconscious and conscious motivations must lead to symptoms that mimic organic illness. Organic illnesses are more often considered a socially acceptable reason to enter the sick role. How psychological distress is expressed to others is culturally determined. As psychological disorder is considered an unacceptable form of disability, the preconscious mind produces bodily symptoms from that distress, and the conscious mind will focus on those symptoms, reducing attention to any psychological symptoms. To carry out this task, the preconscious and conscious mind require information, at some point, as to what is acceptable as a symptom of organic disease.

As E. Shorter (1992) has explained, the symptoms of fibromyalgia are what they are because in the twentieth century, the symptoms of pain, fatigue, numbness, and so on can yet mimic organic illness. Consider a questionnaire asking people which symptoms can be considered physical in origin and which can be considered psychogenic. Many would be able to separate these. They would accept, for example, headache, fatigue, pain, numbness, swelling, sore throat, feeling of fever, and so forth as possibly being from physical disorders. People would not accept a feeling that the skin is leaking black fluid, that one's foot is unattached to one's body, or that one has a large facial cancerous growth (that no one else can see) as physical disorders.

Even if individuals with leg fractures had preconscious and conscious motivations to adopt the sick role, they have little knowledge that whole body pain is the expected outcome of leg fracture. The preconscious mind is unlikely to produce such symptoms.

On the other hand, the information that diffuse whole body pain and a multitude of other chronic symptoms can and do follow an accident has long been available. The observation that this form of illness behavior should follow accidents even predates the automobile. In the nineteenth century, people worried about railway spine (see Chapter 2).

An accident victim with a leg fracture or other objective injury with a well-defined course does not know that the injury can lead to whole body pain. That is another reason why a diagnosis of fibromyalgia more often follows minor collisions with neck pain and not leg fractures.

By either consideration, clearly a diagnosis of fibromyalgia may follow an injury of certain types because of the factors that render tender points, or that render a socially acceptable reason for disability in an individual motivated to adopt the sick role.

DIFFERENTIAL DIAGNOSIS

One must be careful not to confuse the two models of whiplash with some other labels used for accident victims. As stated before, however one chooses to label whiplash patients, it is imperative that one specify the mechanism being implied by the label. This has a critical impact on therapy considerations and legal issues. Two other examples of psychological disorder labels that physicians and others tend to use with whiplash patients are posttraumatic stress disorder and conversion disorder (hysteria). If one understands these diagnoses to be a form of psychological disorder resulting from exposure to extreme "mental trauma," these two diagnoses are rarely applicable to whiplash patients. It is worthwhile to consider the mechanism of posttraumatic stress disorder and conversion disorder as a result of an accident. One can then see why they rarely occur in whiplash patients.

Posttraumatic Stress Disorder

According to the *Diagnostic and Statistical Manual of Mental Disorders (DSM)*:[2(p427)]

> The essential feature [of posttraumatic stress disorder] is the development of characteristic symptoms following a psychologically traumatic event that is generally outside the range of usual human experience. The characteristic symptoms involve reexperiencing the traumatic event: numbing of responsiveness to, or reduced involvement with, the external world and a variety of autonomic, dysphoric or cognitive symptoms.

As a personal injury, posttraumatic stress disorder may be a compensable injury. One may demonstrate that the psychological disorder followed an accident that exposed the individual to severe mental trauma. The first clear link between psychological disorder and accidents came with railway spine. Traumatic neurosis was the diagnosis used then. Unfortunately, many have used traumatic neurosis in other ways since. Again, one must always ask what mechanism of illness is implied by those using traumatic neurosis as a diagnosis. Otherwise, most avoid this diagnostic term altogether in favor of more standardized and well-defined diagnoses such as posttraumatic stress disorder.

Physicians introduced the concept of traumatic neurosis in the latter part of the nineteenth century. Adolf Strümpell defined traumatic neurosis as a set of symptoms characterized by "purely psychical origin" as a result of accidents producing "violent mental emotion."[4(p.313)] While fear is a normal response to any accident, certain accidents were more likely to produce a greater fear response and could produce a psychological disorder even after others reassured the individuals of their safety. Even if there is no physical injury but a clear recognition that potentially severe or life-threatening injury could have happened, a profound change in the individual's psychological behavior may develop. This leads to neurosis or psychosis.

In the early literature on traumatic neurosis, physicians considered certain accidents that may generate this illness. These included falls from heights (recognized by most individuals to be capable of serious injury or death) and severe head blows.[4] Others included being thrown from a carriage,[4] railway accidents of a grave nature, often including dead bodies and flames,[5,6] severe electrical shock,[5] and exposure to battle (shell shock).[7] Patients with traumatic neurosis, like patients with posttraumatic stress disorder, recognized their psychological disorder.

They complained of fear about ever entering an automobile or train again and recurrent nightmares. Thus, traumatic neurosis did in some cases represent what is now called post-traumatic stress disorder and was thought to be a result of the accident.

Since its identification in the 1950s, posttraumatic stress disorder has long been a foreseeable result of certain accidents.[1,8–10] According to the medical literature, "minor motor vehicle accidents" do not often cause this disorder, but "severe automobile accidents" may.[10] It is very apparent that otherwise normal individuals seldom develop such chronic symptoms after the typical accidents producing whiplash patients. Posttraumatic stress disorder tends to occur only when the individual has perceived a definite risk to his or her life. This is not the description most patients will give of their accident that produced whiplash. Most do not have recurring nightmares about the accident or complain of the same psychological disturbances as did railway spine patients. Railway accidents were severe and common. It was not uncommon for a train to be traveling at 30 miles an hour and suddenly hit a parked locomotive in the London fog. Numerous deaths, flames, and screams were the consequence of such accidents. Even in a physically uninjured individual, the mental trauma could produce a profound psychological disorder, one that included physical symptoms.

Thus, it is easy to distinguish posttraumatic stress disorder from either of the two whiplash models described earlier. As described by Gregory and Crockett (1988):

> In post traumatic stress disorders, the patient must present with signs of: subjective depression; sleep disturbed by nightmares involving repetitions of the traumatic event; avoidance of activities associated with the original trauma; and emotional withdrawal. Although the trauma does not necessarily imply physical harm, a post traumatic stress disorder must be in response to a traumatic event which by its very magnitude would cause disturbance in the majority of people exposed to it. By definition, post traumatic stress disorder will arise only in accidents involving extreme threat to the well-being of the victim. It will not occur in the majority of traffic accidents.

Note that there is a specific mechanism of illness involved in a diagnosis of posttraumatic stress disorder. It is clear that the accident is an essential cause of the disorder. Without a severe accident, the illness could not develop. One must of course determine that the continuation of the disorder is not motivated by other factors (eg, malingering of posttraumatic stress disorder, adopting the sick role via claimed posttraumatic stress disorder after a relatively minor accident if there is an enabling gatekeeper to allow this, or stress from unrelated life events being attributed to the accident-related disorder).

Conversion Disorder

"Conversion" is an often misused, abused, and poorly understood word in many psychological reports. Used as part of the vernacular, it would be (and was years ago) acceptable to say that somatization is the "conversion" of psychological distress into bodily symptoms. But this is not commonly used now because somatization and conversion disorder are thought to arise in very different contexts. It is thus confusing and incorrect now to use these terms together. Some attempt to use the word "conversion" or "conversion reaction" to state that the accident caused a great deal of distress and the pain is thus a "conversion reaction"—implying that it is part of the compensable injury. One should question anyone using the term in this way. Conversion symptoms and conversion disorder do not, by the *DSM IV* definition, include pain as the major or significant feature.[1(p1013)] They are primarily sensory and motor disturbances such as blindness, loss of sensation in part of the body (for no physical reason), and paralysis of a limb (for no physical reason). A further feature of a conversion symptom is that it often bears some symbolic relationship to the emotional conflict that causes it (eg, an individual watches people being consumed in a burning building, cannot save them, and wakes up the next morning with blindness).

One should avoid the use of "hysteria" because its meaning has been so much distorted over time. Hysteria would now be listed in *DSM IV* as conversion disorder.

The basis for conversion disorder (and hysteria) is primary gain, and this is seldom expected to be the case in most accident victims, especially not with chronic pain. Primary gain involves the unconscious mind and is achieved when a bodily symptom relieves the anxiety or inner conflict of the unconscious mind. Once the symptom appears, individuals are at greater peace with themselves and the world, even though they have an obvious loss or disturbance of function from this symptom. Consider a man who strikes his wife and nearly causes her serious head injury. He now feels tremendous guilt for what he has done to his wife, anger at having lost his temper, anxiety about what he may become, and so forth. He is in great turmoil, perturbed by shame and guilt. The next morning he wakes up with his right arm (the arm he hit his wife with) paralyzed. He is being punished, and his guilt is relieved. The symptom has just gained him a sense of peace and atonement. This is the primary gain. Unlike most of us who would run shrieking to the nearest hospital, these patients are surprisingly not very disturbed at having a paralyzed arm. They show "la belle indifference."

One should always question a diagnosis concluding that a patient's chronic pain is due to primary gain. It is sometimes unfortunate that some expert witnesses may attempt to label the patient as having conversion disorder or the like, simply because they know that most agree primary gain has to do with the unconscious mind. If it is unconscious, it is not under the claimant's control. If the claimant cannot control it, it might be compensable.

This contention is of course readily refuted. For primary gain to be achieved, relief of distress and anxiety must occur. The symptom must put the individual at peace with him- or herself and the world, at least to some extent. That is the gain. Clearly, chronic pain patients are very distressed and anxious and are not at peace with anyone (except their lawyer). If chronic pain is a symptom of primary gain, patients should no longer have great distress. They should not be bothered by a life of pain, just like the man who hit his wife is surprisingly not too bothered by his paralysis. Since the chronic pain causes more distress than it resolves, it cannot achieve the primary gain of creating inner peace. In fact, the patient with primary gain with conversion disorder does not actively seek out secondary gains.

One expects conversion disorder to arise only after exposure to an accident that is sufficiently challenging to the individual's psyche. An individual who witnesses the death of others in a horrifying accident may develop blindness as a response.

REFERENCES

1. Barsky AJ. Somatoform disorders. In: Kaplan HR, Sadock BJ, eds. *Comprehensive Textbook of Psychiatry*. 5th ed. Baltimore: Williams & Wilkins; 1989:1021–1023.

2. American Psychiatric Association. *Diagnostic and Statistical Manual of Mental Disorders*. 4th ed. Washington, DC: 1994:458.

3. Kellner R. *Psychosomatic Syndromes and Somatic Symptoms*. Washington, DC: American Psychiatric Press; 1991:176.

4. Strümpell A. Traumatic neuroses. In: Stalker AM, trans. *Clinical Lectures on Medicine and Surgery*. Third series. 1894:303–325.

5. Knapp PC. Traumatic neurasthenia and hysteria. *Brain*. 1897;20:385–406.

6. Lind JE. Traumatic neurasthenia, especially "railway spine." *Medical Record*. 1937;146:65–71.

7. Sharpe S. Discussion on traumatic neurasthenia and the litigation neurosis. *Proceedings of the Royal Society of Medicine*. 1927;21:353–364.

8. Napier M, Wheat K. *Recovering Damages for Psychiatric Injury*. London: Blackstone Press Ltd.; 1995.

9. Davidson JRT. Posttraumatic stress disorder and acute stress disorder. In: Kaplan HR, Sadock BJ, eds. *Comprehensive Text of Psychiatry*. 6th ed. Baltimore: Williams & Wilkins; 1995:1227.

10. Davidson JRT, Foa EB, eds. *Posttraumatic Stress Disorder*. Washington, DC: American Psychiatric Press; 1993.

Causation by Way of the Accident

KEY POINTS

- Understanding causation by way of the accident means understanding why patients are behaving the way they are. Given the lessons of the psychocultural illness and adoption of the sick role models, it is important to consider what role the accident (the defendant's actions) plays in the chronic pain being reported.
- The thin skull rule (as well as some relevant exceptions to the rule) guides some whiplash cases.

INTRODUCTION

Medicolegal matters demand an interaction between members of the health profession and members of the legal profession. Whiplash cases are often complex, and although there exist well-defined rules and concepts of law regarding proximate cause, the thin skull rule, and so on, the courts are often limited by the lack of more explicit opinions regarding the mechanism of the claimed injury. The forensic examiner or expert must not merely provide diagnostic labels but ask and explain why the claimant is behaving in a certain way. A statement of the probable mechanism of illness would make it easier for the courts to apply their rules and concepts. Perhaps judgments that arise from similarly presenting cases would become more consistent.

Clearly, the first step is understanding the mechanism of the patient's symptom reporting. Through this approach, one can ask what role the accident plays in the mechanism and thus determine causation by way of the accident. As stated previously in this text, a temporal relationship between the reporting of the patient's symptoms and the accident does not prove that the accident caused those reported symptoms. Causation generally requires some conception of the mechanism by which the illness was a result of the accident. To determine causation, therefore, one must determine what mechanism is operative and what role the accident plays in that mechanism. One could begin the determination of causation by first identifying a diagnosis that also reflects the mechanism of the reporting of symptoms. Thus, once one has made the determination of either psychocultural illness or adoption of the sick role, the task of determining causation is underway.

MATTER OF CAUSATION

One must appreciate that cause in fact and proximate cause are not necessarily the same. Cause in fact is simply the probable cause that can be arrived at by identification and assimilation of the chain of events following the negligent action. Proximate cause is the event that is said to represent the limit of the liability for the damages alleged to arise from the negligent event. Proximate cause is thus an issue of remoteness from the negligent action. The cause in fact considers only that the negligent action is the factual basis for the assertion of liability, but proximate cause determines the extent of liability for that action.

Cause in fact is determined by the presentation of evidence that, in personal injury cases, is usually brought forward by expert testimony. When an accident occurs as a result of negligence, for example, the sequence of events following the accident is detailed, and claimed symptoms are then attributed to a specific disorder. The cause-in-fact link between the injury disorder and the accident is then presented by expert witnesses. In such considerations, other causes (both pre- or postaccident) are, to various extents, also dealt with by the expert witnesses and through other miscellaneous sources of such facts. On the balance of evidence (51% or more probability), the admitted negligent event may be considered to have played a role in that cause in fact. It is in assessing the accident as a proximate cause, dealing with remoteness, and dealing with the thin skull after the admitted negligent event, however, that the complexities arise.

Establishing proximate cause is an arduous task when the disorder being claimed is of a chronic nature, often years after the negligent action occurred. An accident may have, for example, caused an initial injury such as a neck sprain or an acute anxiety disorder. It is more difficult, however, when chronic pain is presented and one must determine if the negligent action remains the proximate cause. Added to this, the chronicity or severity of the disorder may be claimed to have stemmed from preexisting vulnerabilities (ie, the thin skull rule—see below) that predispose the person to a more prolonged disorder. In many cases, in fact, issues of proximate cause and application of the thin skull rule must be simultaneously addressed. These two issues require in advance a consideration of illness mechanism before they can be adequately addressed.

THIN SKULL (OR EGGSHELL SKULL) RULE

Individuals with neurotic or hypochondriacal tendencies may develop more severe symptoms than individuals without these tendencies. Yet even without these tendencies, these neurotic or hypochondriacal individuals might have developed symptoms following an accident. Symptoms develop in most whiplash patients, the majority of whom one would not label as hypochondriacs or neurotics.

Preaccident hypochondriacal or neurotic tendencies may make symptoms more severe or prolonged, even though the tendencies are not the actual initiating *cause* of the symptoms. In such cases, one must consider the "thin skull rule," also called the "eggshell skull rule." The courts apply this rule to protect victims who happened to have some preexisting weakness that would predispose them to a more severe injury.

As explained by M. Napier and K. Wheat (1995, quoting a case), "One takes one's victim as one finds him: 'If a man is negligently . . . injured in his body, it is no answer to the sufferer's claim for damages that he would have suffered less injury, or no injury at all, if he had not an unusually thin skull or an unusually weak heart.'"

It is thus not the foreseeability of the *severity* of injury that is necessary, but rather if the *type* of injury is foreseeable. If some type of physical injury is foreseeable in a normal individual, then some type of physical injury is foreseeable in the thin-skulled individual, even if the severity is not.

The thin psyche rule would parallel this notion in stating that if some type of psychological injury (be it anxiety or depression) is foreseeable in a normal individual, then some type of psychological injury or reaction is foreseeable in the thin psyche individual. It is not necessary that the severity of the psychological injury be foreseeable.

Before one applies the thin skull rule, however, there is still the issue of the illness mechanism. Whatever mechanism is deemed the probable mechanism for the chronic disorder is then the mechanism upon which these rules will be applied. Without an illness mechanism, these rules cannot be properly applied.

PSYCHOCULTURAL ILLNESS

If one accepts the psychocultural illness model, then the courts have a tremendous challenge in awarding compensation. Until now, the courts have often been proceeding on the assumption that the reporting of chronic pain, for example, is due to some persistent chronic damage that came from the acute injury. They have also been assuming that this damage is permanent or slow to resolve. This model of psychocultural illness challenges that entire conception. The psychological factors involved are producing the reporting of chronic symptoms that are not related to any ongoing physical damage from the accident. One must then ask if the chronic symptom reporting is compensable.

If patients are reporting symptoms that are being misattributed to the accident injury, is that behavior compensable? If they are amplifying preaccident symptoms, or the minor aches and pains in the general population are being amplified, is this part of the compensable injury? What factors that cause symptom amplification should one link to the accident? Can the psychologically adverse effects of the litigation process or battling with one's insurance company be part of the compensable injury? One could merely conclude that the individual, being a part of a certain culture, may have behaviors that stem from that culture. Since the liable parties take their victims as they find them, are the parties liable for the victims' behavior? Is the defendant liable for the behavioral effects insurance companies, lawyers, and therapists have on the plaintiff? Here proximate cause becomes an issue: how remotely will events be considered caused by the defendant's actions? It is the proximate cause that deals with all these distant events and actions. (See also F. J. Wilfling and P. C. Wing 1984.)

These are all difficult questions and issues. This model does at least lead to the realization that the physical injury itself has a good outcome—like that of whiplash patients in Germany, Greece, or Lithuania. The compensation for the physical injury alone should be small since the individual has had a minor injury from a minor accident. There remains the more difficult issue of how to compensate for the rest of the symptom reporting.

ADOPTION OF THE SICK ROLE

Recall that an understanding of the mechanism of illness behavior is paramount to understanding causation by way of the accident. Here the key factor is the individuals' preconscious and conscious motivations to adopt the sick role (and their recognition of the opportunity to do so). Again, these individuals may have indeed experienced an initial physical injury, fright, and inconvenience from the accident event. Yet what happens afterward is not due to the accident, even though the symptoms appear to follow the accident. By understanding the mechanism of the illness behavior, it will be easier to determine what role, if any, the accident has in that mechanism.

Thin Skull Rule

As R. Ferrari, O. Kwan et al (1999) explain, the thin skull rule and the "but for the accident" argument are not applicable under certain circumstances. The general principles are as follows:

- In cases where the court is satisfied the *continuation* of pain from the accident is attributable to preexisting or other psychological factors not attributable to the defendant's actions, it is not sufficient that the defendant's actions caused the *onset* of pain.
- The defendant's actions cannot be held as the cause of the psychological factors or disorders if they arise from a desire for secondary gains (including care, sympathy, and other secondary gains cited below).
- The defendant's actions cannot be held as the cause of the plaintiff's symptoms if the plaintiff could be expected to overcome them by his or her own inherent or internal resources (ie, "willpower").
- If the operative psychological factors exist or are maintained because the plaintiff is motivated to maintain them or wishes that they not end, the cause of such factors is said to be subjective or internal.
- It is not sufficient to ask whether the pain syndrome is compensable. It may or may not be. The determination is dependent on having an understanding of the mechanism of the pain.

Clearly, with adoption of the sick role, the accident does not cause the behavior but merely presents the opportunity for the patient to select a more attractive solution. If one attempts to link the accident event and the patient's symptoms, one recognizes that the essential ingredient is that the individual be motivated to adopt the sick role. Without this, the patient will not be preconsciously or consciously motivated to report symptoms that appear to be part of an organic disability. Whether the patient adopts the sick role following an accident depends not on the psychological or physical trauma of the accident event itself. Instead, it depends on whether the individual considers such an event to be a socially acceptable reason for chronic disability.

Recall the model described by R. C. Behan and A. H. Hirschfeld (1966):

Personality difficulties + Troubled life situation = Unacceptable disability

but then,

Unacceptable disability + Accident = Acceptable disability

Thus, the argument that "were it not for the accident, the patient could not have developed this illness behavior" does not confirm a mechanism of causation by way of the accident. Even if one accepts that the accident was responsible for the onset of symptoms (physical injury and psychological effects), the fact that the illness mechanism is a continuation via adoption of the sick role satisfies one of the exceptions to the thin skull rule above. Some use the Latin rubric *novus actus interviens* to indicate this phenomenon, the individual not recovering any further because of the intervention of these motivations (see also G. F. Gregory and D. J. Crockett 1988).

The reason the patient developed this illness behavior after the accident is not that the accident was a *cause* but rather that it was an *opportunity*. If the individual belonged to a culture in which whiplash was not recognized as an acceptable form of chronic disability (eg, were the individual a Lithuanian), this opportunity would not be available even though the accident happened.

Put another way, one could consider why adoption of the sick role after an accident exists in relatively great frequency in North America but not Lithuania. Consider two individuals, one from North America and one from Lithuania, each with a history of psychological distress, adverse life events, failure to cope with psychological stressors, great disappointments, and so forth. One would expect that such individuals exist in both Lithuania and North America. Both individuals could be motivated (even preconsciously) to adopt the sick role and to seek a socially acceptable reason to enter the sick role.

Imagine they have similar accidents. Current experience and evidence indicate that the North American may report chronic disability and the Lithuanian will not. Why the difference in outcome? They both have similar risk factors. Both are involved in similar accidents. Both could have had a physical injury. Both could be preconsciously or consciously motivated to adopt a socially acceptable form of disability. If the accident is the cause of the illness behavior, then it should be just as likely to lead to this behavior in the Lithuanian as it is in the North American.

But the Lithuanian does not live in a society where neck pain after a car accident is considered a socially acceptable reason for chronic disability. The medical community does not tell Lithuanians that chronic pain is an expected outcome of such accidents. Thereby, as previously discussed in Chapter 10, the enabling gatekeeper is not available. The Lithuanian cannot consciously or even preconsciously recognize the accident as a socially acceptable reason for disability. The North American (or individuals of other whiplash cultures) can.

It is thus not important what exactly the event is, be it accident, infection, or other agent. As long as the individual recognizes event X as an event associated with a socially acceptable reason for disability, then it will appear to be an opportunity. The event is not the cause; it is the opportunity. The choice to seize the opportunity is one the patient makes, and the behavior that follows is one that the individual could stop, but he or she has reasons (preconscious and consciously enacted motivations) to continue. See Chapter 23.

Convenient Focus

Tied in with the thin skull rule is convenient focus. This is a legal concept, but it is equivalent to psychologists' concept of scapegoating. It means that an individual seizes an event as the source of all his or her miseries; the individual claims that life before the event was not necessarily perfect but was "coped with well."

It is likely that many of these patients have psychological distress or disorder in much of their lives, but clearly they do not always have a disability syndrome while suffering in such states. They will not express openly their misery, as this is socially unacceptable. They may remain in this state for some time, however, because they are waiting for a socially acceptable reprieve. More than this, however, many of these individuals appear to be "coping well" with their lives, for a simple reason: they have no choice. They carry an "at-fault" illness until an opportunity arrives for transforming it into a no-fault illness. Such opportunities (eg, motor vehicle accidents) usually arrive by chance. The patients can then seize that event in their state of misery and somatize to transform their distress into the no-fault symptom picture of chronic pain. Then they have to seek out the no-fault gate-keeper who will give them entry and allow adoption of the sick role.

There are many reasons for the timing of adoption of the sick role, including difficulty in finding a willing gatekeeper (which may delay use of an opportunity). Illness is associated with secondary losses as well as gains. Depending on the appeal of the secondary gains (how desperately one needs a reprieve from work and social opportunities, for example), the secondary losses may be affordable. When an individual's existence is most miserable, adoption of the sick role is most likely to occur.

Thus, an accident may come at the right time, when an individual is most distressed and most needs a way out. How is it that these individuals suffer a series of emotionally traumatic events in their life without apparent disability, but then a minor accident disables them? The quantum of damage in the minor accident is small; the quantum of opportunity is great.

Notwithstanding these considerations, before the courts resolve the issues of causation in these illnesses, it is certainly essential that reporting of chronic symptoms be recognized as not being a result of ongoing physical damage from the original acute injury.

Assessment, Treatment, and Prognosis

KEY POINTS

- There are some specific issues that come up with assessing whiplash patients, particularly those in a claim. The first is "Did an injury likely occur?" The second consideration is "How long after the accident can the symptoms (whether headache, neck stiffness, or neck pain) first appear?" "Can people who claim the symptoms started 3 days after the accident claim they had a whiplash injury?" Data from the engineering studies and studies of Lithuanian accident victims help to answer these questions.
- The examining physician or therapist should obtain certain important information about the patient's history and look for certain useful signs when considering what is causing the patient's pain. Specific pain descriptions by the patient may lead a practitioner or therapist to suspect the patient is motivated to adopt the sick role.
- Sometimes, a forensic examiner in psychology or psychiatry should be involved in the assessment. Radiologic assessment also has value in some instances.
- Effective treatment or prevention requires a drastic change in practitioners' understanding of why whiplash patients report chronic symptoms. Practitioners need to move away from the "healing an injury" approach. Without such a change, patients reporting chronic symptoms have little hope.

INTRODUCTION

This discussion will not give a detailed checklist of things to ask on history or look for in physical examination. This very much depends on, for example, what one believes whiplash is and what one plans to do with that information. There are plenty of review articles and texts for such broader purposes. Instead, this discussion will focus on specific issues arising in the assessment and treatment of the whiplash patient.

Further, this discussion deals with Grade 1 and Grade 2 whiplash-associated disorders. That is, the Quebec Task Force (QTF) classification cites Grades 1 to 4. Grade 1 is a complaint of neck stiffness only, with no abnormalities reported on examination. Grade 2 is reporting of neck pain and sites of tenderness, and a reduced range of spine motion. Within this grade, patients may be reporting other symptoms, including back pain, jaw pain, dizziness, and so forth. Grades 3 and 4 are distinguishable by the requirement of clearly objective findings. Examples include loss or diminishment of deep tendon reflexes, objective muscle weakness, and sensory deficits in a specific dermatomal pattern reflecting nerve injury (Grade 3) or X-ray findings of fracture or vertebral dislocation (Grade 4). These latter two grades apply to a small minority of whiplash injury claims. In contrast, Grades 1 and 2, which account for most claims of whiplash injury, are diagnosed purely on the basis of symptom reporting. There are no truly objective findings (ie, findings that are independent of the patient's input).

Considering results of experimental collisions as well as data from Germany, Greece, and Lithuania on the natural history of the acute injury, one would arbitrarily define chronic symptom reporting as that persisting over 3 to 6 weeks. These data show us that the acute injury may produce symptoms of neck pain, headache, and possibly back pain. Other acute symptoms include those generally relating to an accident, including the initial fright and momentary "dazing" or minor disorientation. There is strictly no relationship between these other symptoms and acute neck or back injury. There is no further discussion of these here. The discussion here does not deal with temporomandibular joint examination, given the discussions that have previously occurred in this text (see Chapter 6, for example).

If one accepts the two biopsychosocial models of whiplash, then one focuses the history and physical examination on identifying what factors (biological/physical and psychosocial) are responsible for symptom reporting.

HISTORY

Did a Physical Injury Occur?

It is worth noting the characteristics of the accident, which the patient may be able to report—or information will be available through engineering analysis. A rear-end collision is highly unlikely to have caused an acute physical injury in certain cases. An acute physical injury is unlikely with less than $500 damage to the struck vehicle (a crude measure), a striking vehicle (of equal mass) velocity less than 12 km/h (7.2 mph), or a change in velocity (ΔV) of the struck vehicle less than 8 km/h (5 mph). If any are the case, then one considers other mechanisms of symptom reporting. In such cases, no matter what symptoms the patient is reporting or for how long the patient reports them, a link to a *physical* injury from the accident is highly questionable. Fright might be a factor, as G. P. Nielsen et al (1997) noted (see "Whiplash Experiments" in Chapter 5).

If one *does* accept that a physical injury occurred, one must carefully consider which symptoms are due to the accident, especially when the patient is being assessed weeks or months after the accident. Recall that there is a tendency for the accident victim to assume or report that all the symptoms are due to the accident, no matter when they begin.

Timing of Symptoms

First, one must consider how much time can elapse from the accident to the accident victims' first report that they experienced neck or back pain. Obviously, some have tried the circular (and very unscientific) approach to answering this question by asking a group of whiplash patients when they first noted pain. Researchers then report the results in a "study" and state, for example, "15% of whiplash victims do not develop their first symptom from the accident injury until 48 hours after the accident." Of course, the real question remains unanswered. All one demonstrates is that some whiplash claimants report symptoms in a delayed pattern, not that an acute injury should lead to this pattern of symptom reporting. It would be more scientific to ask a whiplash victim from a volunteer experiment or a Lithuanian accident victim. They are least likely to have ulterior motives or other confounding variables involved. According to that data, some symptom of headache, neck or back stiffness, or pain always occurs within 12 hours. One caution is that patients may report headache in the first 12 hours and the next day refer to it as neck pain (ie, they are simply labeling it differently). In such cases, one can accept that the neck pain did occur within the first 12 hours but was simply perceived as headache by the patients. At least they report a pain symptom (whatever the label) within the first 12 hours.

To argue that the delay can be longer than this is to argue that there is an unusual type of injury in, say, a North American accident victim. One is arguing that this injury never occurs in the volunteer experiments and does not appear to occur in Lithuanian accident victims. In a minority of cases, feeling very anxious and "dazed" for the first several hours may be a factor in delayed symptom perception. Such a phenomenon of delayed symptom reporting, however, should not be a cause of symptoms first being perceived more than 12 hours from the accident event.

Second, if one attempts to link symptoms occurring weeks later to the accident, one should define a mechanism; otherwise one suffers from the same malady of symptom attribution as the patient! Back pain that starts 6 months after the accident, for example, is not likely attributable to the accident, unless one can identify a very specific mechanism that is sufficiently plausible. The scientific literature does not appear to demonstrate any such mechanism.

If one can indicate the mechanism for a delay in such symptoms (there may be some) and demonstrate what evidence there is in the literature, it may be reasonable to argue that such delays are acceptable. Otherwise, these other symptoms are probably being misattributed to the accident. They may have existed before the accident and are now being amplified and registered, or they may develop after the accident for unrelated reasons. These symptoms do exist in the general population. Rather than just assuming that whatever symptoms the patient presents with are due to the accident, practitioners should take a more scientific approach. This is especially true because of the great potential for misattribution (often innocent) and for insurance fraud (not innocent).

Psychosocial Aspects

M. Karlsborg et al (1997) showed that one could predict chronic symptom reporting at 6 months and correlate this with new life events. They recommend a detailed psychosocial assessment in the individual still reporting symptoms after 6 weeks. Of course, many physicians, for a variety of reasons, are reluctant even to broach psychosocial issues with the patient, and some simply are not very adept at such an approach. That is likely why insurance companies often have the patient assessed by someone with experience at detailed psychological assessments. This is of particular importance in individuals at risk for adopting the sick role. In such cases, they may very well leave the room when the physician or therapist asks questions in an attempt to understand their preaccident history.

A history of the patient's psychosocial circumstances, past and present, is vital (see Chapters 9 and 10). More specific questions about the nature of the pain may be revealing, as discussed below.

Nonorganic Features

When chronic pain is being reported, one can obtain a measure of the likelihood of nonorganic factors either being responsible for the pain reporting or greatly modifying pain reporting (see Chapter 10). One asks about features such as constant pain (especially severe), diffuse pain, whole limb numbness or pain, tailbone pain, leg giving way, intolerance to treatments, and emergency admission to the hospital for pain management. G. Waddell et al (1989) suggest that the finding of at least 3 of these features makes it probable that psychological factors are significantly altering pain reporting. Obviously, the more of these features the patient has, the more important psychological factors probably are. (See Ferrari 1999 for a more detailed discussion of the clinical applications of Waddell's signs.)

PHYSICAL EXAMINATION

Regardless of whether one defines whiplash as a mechanism of injury, an injury, or a clinical syndrome, it is generally impossible objectively to prove or disprove an underlying pathological basis of the injury.

Lack of Objectivity in Most Cases

Indeed, while it may seem surprising, the precise anatomical cause of spontaneous episodes of acute neck or back pain in the general population remains unclear in most cases. In Grade 1 or 2 whiplash-associated disorders, there are no tests that readily or reliably determine if pain reporting stems from lesions of facet joints, discs, muscles, ligaments, or all or none of the above. Equally, there is no evidence to support the idea that attempts to make such a distinction have any therapeutic relevance.

As such, there is tremendous potential for these two grades to be influenced by noninjury events, and they are most susceptible to simulation. H. A. Smythe et al (1997) demonstrated, for example, that normal individuals can be trained to represent patients with chronic pain syndromes such as fibromyalgia (for teaching and other exercises) so well that experts will not be able to distinguish them from real patients. (Claimants can therefore probably train themselves too and belittle our attempts to "objectively prove" an injury does or does not exist.)

Looking for Specific Signs

One may be able to note a head-forward posture and a flexed posture of the spine as a whole. This may be important in prescribing specific measures for posture correction (see "Treatment" below). It is possible to have acute injuries to other body parts along with a whiplash injury. One should therefore examine all the sites where the patient reports pain; these sites may show objective signs of physical disorders.

It is also prudent to look for neurological abnormalities, as might be seen in Grade 3 or 4 whiplash injury. Of course, neurological abnormalities can be objective and subjective. Asking patients if they have less sensation in some parts of their fingers than they do in others is not very objective. Demonstrating loss of reflexes and what an experienced examiner will recognize as true muscle weakness, however, is very objective.

Some therapists believe in pressing on specific tender spots so that they can make a diagnosis of a "specific" disorder, whereas others feel this is a meaningless maneuver.

Again, the purpose of the examination as discussed here is to understand the mechanism of the patient's symptom reporting, not to search for chronic neck damage that is not there.

Nonorganic Findings

Here again, nonorganic findings do not necessarily mean the patient is malingering. In many cases, nonorganic findings represent part of the pain behavior of an individual in whom psychological factors are largely responsible for symptom reporting. There are many descriptions and labels for these signs. One is looking, for example, for pain behavior (the patient is grimacing or leaping when touched, cannot sit through the interview, etc) and the other signs listed by Waddell et al (1989). These include marked superficial tenderness, back pain reporting with axial skull loading, back pain with mild hip rotation, significant differences in straight leg raise when distracted, nondermatomal sensory loss, and jerky, give-way weakness.

RADIOLOGICAL ASSESSMENT

Radiological studies (including magnetic resonance imaging [MRI] scans) are of no value in the acute or chronic setting, other than in excluding a fracture or dislocation or for confirming nerve root compression in Grade 3 or Grade 4 whiplash-associated disorder.

Straightening of the cervical lordosis, for example, has for decades been claimed to be a sign of whiplash injury. H. E. Crowe (1958), who coined the term "whiplash," was among the first to dispute the significance of this finding. Indeed, studies indicate that this finding is frequent in the healthy population. When comparing whiplash patients to asymptomatic controls, there is no greater frequency of this finding in those claiming acute whiplash injury (A. G. B. Borden et al 1960, D. R. Gore et al 1986, P. S. Helliwell et al 1994, and H. R. Zatzkin and F. W. Kveton 1960). Straightening of the cervical lordosis is not likely even to be attributable to muscle spasm (Helliwell et al 1994).

Further, studies have shown that abnormalities on X-ray such as minor degrees of forward angulation of the cervical spine or kyphosis are not found any more frequently in those claiming acute whiplash injury than they are in asymptomatic controls (Borden et al 1960, Gore et al 1986, J. H. Juhl et al 1962). Even a few millimeters of subluxation (gliding of one vertebra relative to those above and below) is common in otherwise healthy individuals (J. O. Lottes et al 1959). That is not to say that an acute injury does not occur, merely that these specific radiological abnormalities are not a reliable sign of such an injury.

In addition, there is little evidence that having an abnormal X-ray at the time of the acute injury affects outcome of symptom reporting. The few studies quoted to suggest that there is such a correlation between the X-ray and outcome have many potential flaws. These include low rates of follow-up (M. Hohl 1974), inclusion of patients with fractures (S. H. Norris and I. Watt 1983), and small patient numbers (B. P. Radanov et al 1995). A study lacking these flaws and biases reveals that having signs of disc degeneration, angulation, and kyphosis on X-ray at the time of the X-ray findings does not predict a worse outcome (C. Hildingsson and G. Toolanen 1990). This is not surprising. In 1988, J. I. Balla and R. Iansek, with a review of 5,000 cases, found a very poor correlation between neck X-ray findings and the symptoms of headache, neck pain, neck stiffness, and arm pain. That is, the presence of these symptoms in whiplash patients did not predict the finding of an abnormal X-ray. Equally, an abnormal X-ray did not predict reporting of these symptoms.

Finally, there is a relatively low incidence of whiplash claimants from older age groups, while the aforementioned X-ray abnormalities are increasingly prevalent with increasing age. This is in keeping with the view that X-ray signs of disc degeneration at the time of the accident are not a significant risk factor for acute injury.

Thus, radiological findings are not useful in the assessment of the vast majority of whiplash patients.

ANY OTHER INVESTIGATIONS?

In patients reporting dizziness, vertigo, hearing disturbances, or visual disturbances, it is highly improbable that there is any evidence of neurological injury to be found. As such, no specific investigations are required in those without head injury and loss of consciousness, or who do not present with any objective neurological findings. One thus tests reflexes and strength in the limbs as well as the cranial nerves. Objective evidence of abnormalities here is a reason to refer to a neurologist or consider other investigations including MRI of the spine and computed tomography or MRI of the head. Yet, again, with Grade 1 or 2 whiplash-associated disorder, one does not expect any of these symptoms to be related to any nervous system injury.

Some practitioners wish to reassure patients, so they order hearing tests and a more detailed ophthalmologic assessment, depending on the patients' symptoms. One has to be prepared, however, for normal results in virtually all cases, or for abnormalities that have nothing to do with the accident injury. Patients will still expect an explanation for their symptoms. One must then look at medications, anxiety, the effects of neck pain on balance control and visual function, and simply the existence of these symptoms in daily life. Patients may find it hard to believe that their change in hearing, for example, might be coincidental if they noticed it only since the accident. But then, that is what "coincidental" means.

Table 12–1 lists the possible sources of various symptoms. In whiplash cases, practitioners can use this list to cite for patients and others the most probable causes of symptoms.

MALINGERING

> When ye git 'urt, say it's yer back; the doctors can't never get 'round yer back.
>
> —Collie J. *Malingering and Feigned Sickness*. 2nd ed. London: Edward Arnold; 1917:258.

I have already stated that I believe most whiplash claimants' symptoms to be genuine. Many may argue about the etiology of these chronic symptoms, but many can at least agree that most claimants have some genuine form of suffering.

Yet it is as true today as it was for Sir John Collie at the turn of the century (see quotation above): malingering does occur in injury claims. Through much of this book, the assumption has been made that the symptoms are genuine. Even those who disagree with each other on the mechanism of chronic symptoms consider most claimants to be genuine. But malingering does exist (N. Baer 1997). Malingerers take advantage of controversy about illnesses.

Indeed, for perhaps a few centuries, claimants have had to add little sophistication to the claims they make, for the very reason Sir John Collie states: Doctors are notoriously poor at detecting malingering, or at least find themselves in circumstances that make such diagnoses less appealing, for the same reason as abnormal illness behavior is seldom diagnosed. While Sir John Collie regularly used electricity to test the veracity of some malingerers who claimed they had lost all sensation in their limbs, this is currently not an acceptable practice. Hence, examiners in forensic psychology are often asked to conduct "malingering detection."

Malingering is defined in the *Diagnostic and Statistical Manual of Mental Disorders*, 4th edition (*DSM IV*), as the intentional production of symptoms of a physical or mental disorder motivated by external incentives such as avoiding military duty, avoiding work, obtaining financial compensation, evading criminal prosecution, or obtaining drugs. There are other behaviors that may also be considered malingering, each entailing actions that are intended to help achieve a consciously desired goal.

- having genuine symptoms but claiming that they arose from a motor vehicle accident even though the symptoms were there before the accident (also known as transference; F. D. Lipman 1962)
- having genuine symptoms that arise from another source in the time period after the injury from the accident, yet claiming they are a continuation of the accident injury (also known as false imputation; P. J. Resnick 1984)

Table 12–1 Sources of Symptoms over Time

Symptom	Timing	Probable Sources (Malingering Considered in Each Case)
Neck or back pain (collision probably above injury threshold)	Few hours to few weeks Thereafter	Acute whiplash injury Postural abnormalities, misattribution of amplified symptoms from sources such as pattern of preaccident symptoms, spontaneous and occupational sources in general population, anxiety
Neck or back pain (collision probably below injury threshold)	Within hours of the accident All times postaccident	Anxiety, fright, and anger acutely Misattribution of amplified symptoms from sources such as pattern of preaccident symptoms, spontaneous and occupational sources in general population, anxiety. Postural abnormalities may develop if the individual responds to these nonaccident sources as if they represent injury. Patients then slouch to reduce symptoms and may become inactive.
Dizziness, vertigo, and other sensations of balance difficulties	Within hours of the accident Thereafter	Initial disorientation effects of head acceleration and fright Medication use, effects of neck pain on posture control, anxiety, misattribution of amplified symptoms from sources such as pattern of preaccident symptoms, spontaneous and other sources in general population Medication use, anxiety, misattribution of amplified symptoms from sources such as pattern of preaccident symptoms, spontaneous and other sources in general population

Hearing disturbances, tinnitus	All times postaccident	Medication use, effects of neck pain on posture control, anxiety, misattribution of amplified symptoms from sources such as pattern of preaccident symptoms, spontaneous and other sources in general population
Visual disturbances with no objective neurological abnormality	All times postaccident	Medications, anxiety, depression, pain, spontaneous and other sources in general population
Cognitive symptoms	Usually weeks to months after accident	Seat belt injury via confusion
Limb paresthesiae without objective neurological abnormalities	All times postaccident	Myotomal pattern of referred symptoms from neck or back pain, anxiety, spontaneous and other sources in general population
Chest pain without fracture or other intrathoracic lesion	Hours to weeks Thereafter	Postural abnormalities, anxiety, medications causing chest discomfort via indigestion, gastritis, esophageal spasm, etc

- having genuine, minor symptoms and knowingly exaggerating them (Lipman 1962)
- agreeing to receive treatment for symptoms not for the purpose of getting better or because the symptoms are really that bothersome but to help legitimize one's claim of injury
- having genuine symptoms but intentionally avoiding therapy in the hope of making the outcome worse, for the purpose of securing gains

Malingering is all about secondary and tertiary gains, which have been defined previously (see Chapter 10). While secondary gains are important in adoption of the sick role, they are also consciously sought by the malingerer. The tertiary gains are the personal advantages that others receive from the claimant, whether the claimant is genuine or not. The tertiary gain is also consciously pursued, albeit by others, sometimes with the claimant's knowledge, sometimes not. To avoid overlooking malingering, one must realize that it does not always stem from a desire for money.

Others malinger to achieve many other forms of secondary gains. Secondary gain may be pursued consciously (frank malingering) or preconsciously (individuals do so through learned behavior and are not always consciously planning out their pursuit of these gains). See Chapter 23 for more information about the thought processing.

Detection of Malingering

Forensic distortion analysis refers to the process of analyzing claimants and their circumstances not only to detect "classic" frank malingering (they have no symptom but report that they do) but also to see if the claimants are distorting their symptoms (they are exaggerating their symptoms). Malingering, therefore, encompasses a spectrum of distortion from having no symptoms to having a distortion of symptoms—hence forensic distortion analysis. In looser terms, detecting malingering means looking for inconsistencies or discrepancies between what is claimed and what is then found to be true.

According to R. J. Sbordone and C. J. Long (1995), a fundamental principle underlying examination of an injury claimant is ecological validity. "Ecological validity" is really a new term for an old concept in assessment of claimants. This concept simply means that one must consider whether the information gathered from assessment can provide a valid prediction of the individuals' behavior elsewhere in their life. One might test patients in some fashion in a "testing environment" and find they perform well, but this may not mean that they will perform just as well in their usual work environment. The reverse is also considered. Patients may fail a test in front of an examiner but do very well outside the testing environment—a possibility when malingering is being considered. Ecology is the relationship among various systems in an organism or between various organisms. If a deficit is claimed in one system, it is bound to show up in a related system within that ecology. That would be ecologically valid. Consider that the human being is like a pond. If there is a disturbance in one part of the pond, one can readily predict that a disturbance should appear elsewhere—the ecology demands that. Thus, if one claims to have disturbed the pond, and I find other disturbances I predict from that claim, then the claim is ecologically valid. If one claims to have disturbed the pond, but I do not find what is expected, the claim is ecologically invalid.

Sir John Collie used the concept of ecological validity. If an accident claimant reported, for example, no sensation in his legs, then Collie predicted (in keeping with known physiology of the time) that the patient would not feel electricity. If he applied electricity to the patient's feet and the patient screamed, inconsistent with the prediction of what should happen if the claimant were telling the truth, the claim was ecologically invalid.

Similarly, when surveillance is used, ecological validity is also employed. If a claimant reports an inability to lift 5 kg because of back pain, one would predict this would affect all aspects of his or her life. If the surveillance shows the patient lifting a sledgehammer, this discrepancy from the prediction indicates the claim is ecologically invalid.

One must appreciate, however, that the forensic examiner is merely providing evidence, not making the ultimate judgment about whether the patient is malingering. Unless one has a signed confession, one cannot prove malingering. G. Mendelson (1987) suggested that although the expert witness may draw attention to certain inconsistencies, lack of motivation, and poor treatment compliance, the ultimate question of veracity is a legal one. He considered that these principles in criminal proceedings could also be applicable in civil proceedings, citing a judgment:

> We do not consider that . . . in all cases psychologists and psychiatrists can be called to prove the probability of the accused's veracity. If any such rule was applied in our courts, trial by psychiatrists would be likely to take the place of trial by jury and magistrates. We do not find that prospect attractive and the law does not at present provide for it. . . . This is recognised in DSM-III, which specifically states that malingering is not a disorder but an act, and thus not a matter for diagnoses, but for a judicial finding on the facts of the case.

Illustrated below are three brief examples of how one uses this principle of ecological validity in accident claimants.

Malingering of Pain

Pain is subjective (ie, it is a symptom reported by the claimant). However, one can malinger when reporting the severity of pain via exaggeration, transference, or false imputation, to name just a few.

Ecological invalidity is most easily detected when patients claim to have so much pain that they cannot lift this or do that and surveillance shows otherwise. The competent forensic examiner can detect ecological invalidity even when the pain complaints are not as extreme. The details of these procedures are beyond the scope of this book, but what one should understand is that the forensic examiner spends a great deal of time asking patients what they cannot do, how limiting their pain is, and so forth. With that established, examiners can decide where to look for ecological validity. The dilemma for the malingerer is that to appear ecologically valid, the pain complaint would have to be very mild. Yet the point of malingering is to obtain a secondary gain. If one claims very minor symptoms and impairment, the gain is not likely to be achieved. Malingerers must therefore make more extreme claims, and this is what the forensic examiner feeds on.

Malingering Cognitive Dysfunction

Cognitive dysfunction is often reported after trauma. The primary symptoms reported include deficits in concentration, attention, and memory. Although specific neuropsychological tests may be useful, performance while taking them can be faked.

Discrepancies are sought here by simply comparing the patients' claims to their daily functioning. There may be evidence in the history (eg, if a working company manager states that she has severe memory problems, how is she capable of managing her job?). For the most part, however, ecological validity is sought through formal testing.

Forensic examiners use a variety of written and verbal tests. They are all based on the concept that the general public does not really know how memory and concentration functions work and that cognitive tasks require the coordination of a variety of separate processes. Malingerers may have no idea how a person with poor memory really acts.

Some believe, for example, that someone with brain injury would get most of the answers on a written test wrong. They might try to feign a brain injury by randomly entering their answers. Tests are designed to detect that very act, to show that a certain pattern of answers can only result if the answers are deliberately chosen at random. Some try to get every third or fourth question wrong. They do not realize that the test is designed intentionally to ask the same question in a slightly different way in several different places. When there are 500 or more questions, malingerers will lose track of how they answered similar questions. They will thus be likely to answer two similar questions in different ways.

Finally, other tests end up being a measure of intellectual functioning. Malingerers believe that if they simply say "I do not know" to most questions, this will show they have a brain injury. Actually, it will show they are so severely mentally impaired that they should not be able to dress themselves. Or it may show that the malingerers—despite having been in an accident where they bumped their head, had no loss of consciousness, and did not require hospitalization—are showing the same level of function as someone who had a head injury and remained in a coma for a month in the intensive care unit, requiring surgery to treat the intracranial hemorrhage.

Malingering Psychological (Mental) Disorder

Posttraumatic stress disorder is one of the few "no-fault" disorders in *DSM IV*, and the individual who has it is an instant victim. The problem is that the diagnostic criteria are so well publicized and subjective that they are often faked. In addition, the diagnostic criteria are quite loose and include individuals who merely "heard about the trauma." Even psychometric tests for posttraumatic stress disorder can be faked (L. A. Neal 1994).

Pursuing ecological validity, however, the competent forensic examiner in psychology can be useful. Posttraumatic stress disorder is the most severe form of anxiety disorder. As such, it creates havoc in the patient's life. To maintain the diagnosis of posttraumatic stress disorder, the malingerer must claim to have a severe disorder. Surveillance and a competent history allow the examiner to note how many examples there are of this individual actually leading a fairly normal life despite having the world's most severe anxiety disorder: ecological invalidity.

Moreover, it is known that nontraumatic anxiety disorders and substance abuse disorders can present with the appearance of posttraumatic stress disorder. The forensic examiner in psychology thus looks for these disorders as well.

Summary

In the end, suspecting malingering is much easier than detecting it. Detecting malingering is often arduous and expensive, but the cost of insurance fraud is even greater, with the capacity of physicians to "get 'round" such problems being limited. The role of the forensic examiner in psychology is thus of increasing importance.

But assuming patients are telling the truth, and I believe most of them are, one can turn to treatment issues.

TREATMENT

Lack of Proof of Effectiveness

The QTF on Whiplash-Associated Disorders (1995) pointed out how few studies there are to support most therapies used with whiplash patients. Nevertheless, many prescribe these expensive therapies without adequate data to support their use. For example, there are no studies to support the use of soft collars, muscle relaxants, narcotic analgesics, surgery, rest, cervical pillows, transcutaneous nerve stimulation, ultrasound, short wave diathermy, heat, ice, or massage. From the few studies available, there is no evidence of benefit to the use of traction, manipulation (chiropractic), acupuncture, electromagnetic therapy, steroid injections, and sterile water injections in whiplash. There is weak evidence that specific manual mobilization techniques (a therapist moves the patient's head through a range of motion) may be helpful (see A. Bonk et al 1999, H. Brodin 1985, K. Mealy et al 1986). These studies, however, compare outcomes to those of patients given passive therapies, collars, and so forth, so it is not clear what was the beneficial modality. The use of nonnarcotic analgesics and antiinflammatories is not of any proven benefit after 3 days. The lack of data to support the use of these therapies in the face of their ever-increasing usage seems bizarre. Indeed, there are few areas in medicine with so many different, costly therapies unsupported by reasonable efficacy studies.

Controlled Studies of Active Therapy

There are a few studies that examine the effects of exercises, stretches, posture advice, and psychological support. The studies that exist combine many of these therapies, so it is difficult to know which is the most effective. Bonk et al (1999), L. A. McKinney et al (1989), and Mealy et al (1986) showed that combining therapies that encourage early mobilization and posture advice with specific exercises or stretches is more effective than rest or passive therapies. In 1996, L. Provinciali et al also demonstrated that posture advice, exercises, and psychological support were more effective in reducing disability than modalities such as ultrasound, electrical stimulation, and electromagnetic therapy. In 1998, G. E. Borchgrevink et al examined the specific effects of prescribing a collar and rest. They compared the outcomes of a group treated with advice to "act as usual" with no collar and no sick leave to outcomes of a group given 14 days' sick leave and a collar. At 6 months, the act-as-usual group had a better outcome in many respects.

Rational Prescription to Therapy

What is the optimal therapeutic approach? One should be striving to reproduce the behaviors of those who suffer an acute whiplash injury in Lithuania. One is attempting to kindle a view of the injury as relatively benign. In this way whiplash victims would not expect chronic disability and would not let the initial symptoms alter their activity. They can then realize the natural history of this minor injury. This is what happens in Lithuania. A change of approach must take place in the culture, and this can occur only through an understanding of what causes chronic symptom reporting in whiplash cultures.

As in many illnesses, education is the first goal of therapy. Patients have heard or will hear many things about whiplash. It seems unreasonable simply to tell the patient "this is a minor injury, and do not worry about it." This is contrary to so much of what the patient has heard or will hear elsewhere. Instead, it seems more reasonable to explain to the patient that "while it is true that many people do go on to report chronic pain after an acute whiplash injury, the damage from the acute injury does not cause the chronic pain. Other things do, and you can prevent them from acting to cause chronic pain for you."

The patient may then perceive the injury as more benign and recognize that there are opportunities to prevent chronic pain. Reducing the expectation of chronic pain may reduce symptom amplification. It is also reasonable to let the patient know that following acute injury, especially if that injury seems severe, one becomes much more aware of one's body than ever before. This may actually be a protective mechanism, but whatever the cause, it means that one is going to notice every little ache and pain and experience it as more severe. It is not a crime to let the patient know this. Patients may then view future pain episodes as not necessarily signifying "damage."

Not surprisingly, patients are heavily influenced by how physicians and therapists discuss conditions. Telling patients to rest, to withdraw from activities, or to change their lifestyle is telling them they are sick. Telling them to keep the same activities as part of their therapy, to not withdraw from work or activities, and to "push through the pain" is telling them they are still healthy. Many patients are afraid to be more active because they associate pain with disease or damage. They may not realize that the longer one spends away from normal activities, the more likely one will have pain when attempting to resume those activities.

It may thus be that "successful" therapy for whiplash does more to change a patient's behavior than to "heal" an injury (Borchgrevink et al 1998, McKinney 1989). One repeatedly encourages the patient to behave as one would for any other minor injury, by not changing one's activity level after the first day or two of rest. (In fact, the QTF does not recommend prescribing rest beyond 4 days.) This will alter accident victims' behavior so that they behave as one who has a benign injury, who can partake in normal activities, and who need not rest to heal the injury. One should avoid the treatments such as medications, collars, and passive therapy, as they give the patient the opposite impression and encourage "injury" behaviors. Simply discussing the natural anxieties and potential misconceptions patients may hold may be helpful (Provinciali et al 1996).

Many recommend using exercises such as posterior neck muscle stretches and encouraging good posture, both of which have some benefit (G. D. Giebel et al 1997, McKinney 1989, Mealy et al 1986, Provinciali et al 1996). This is perhaps again because these therapies impress upon the patient that rest and "caution" are not necessary for what is after all a minor injury. It is likely that a patient's experience of persistent symptoms (even though they may not later be due to the acute injury) lead the individual to develop poor posture or "slouch" as a way of reducing symptoms (A. Cesarini et al 1996, R. A. McKenzie 1990). These posture correction measures may be helpful for this reason: poor posture itself may cause symptoms (K. Harms-Ringdahl and J. Ekholm 1986, T. P. Hedman and G. R. Fernie 1997, S. Middaugh et al 1994, D. H. Watson and P. H. Trott 1993, M. M. Williams et al 1991). This merely adds another factor that leads to chronic symptom reporting long after the injury has healed.

By prescribing active therapy and avoidance of rest, one is just suggesting that patients behave like Lithuanian whiplash victims.

Thus, with a great deal of reassurance and education, the prescription for the whiplash patient could be the following:

- Educate patients as noted above, emphasizing that patients can decide whether they go on to have chronic pain.
- Advise patients that it is not harmful to be active when symptoms are present and that staying at work is an important part of their active treatment.
- Advise patients to maintain (or correct to normal) their seated posture—to sit with a cushion along the upper part of their low back to prevent slouching in response to the pain. One should encourage this habit while therapy proceeds for the next few days or weeks, but it is likely less essential in individuals who do not substantially reduce their activities.
- Prescribe neck retraction exercises (10 per hour) and back extension exercises (40 to 60 a day). One way to do a neck retraction is by sitting in a chair with a cushion or lumbar roll along the upper part of one's lower back. In this seated posture, one retracts the chin back horizontally, without dropping the chin to the chest or raising it up away from the chest. This retraction may actually reproduce some discomfort. One holds that position for 3 seconds, relaxes, and repeats the exercise 10 times every hour (generally when at home because it looks like an odd activity). One can do a back extension in a number of ways. One way is to lie face down, with the arms resting at the sides, and use the upper and lower back muscles (neck relaxed) to arch the back, lifting the chest and face from the floor. The patient holds this for 3 seconds, and then repeats it 10 to 20 times, 3 or 4 times a day. See McKinney (1989) and McKenzie (1990) for more details.

One matter the QTF did not extensively address is the patient who has had passive therapy for a year, say, and has had a marked reduction in activity. If this patient's symptoms are relatively mild, and if his or her job is not very demanding physically, one could simply have the patient return to work with specific posture correction methods and ergonomic advice. In other cases, however, and particularly when the individual believes that pain with activity is harmful or that his or her work is physically demanding, this may be more difficult. Individuals with prolonged inactivity and passive therapies often have poor flexibility and weakness of the trunk muscles. They have now developed a new problem. They are not physically as fit as they were for their preaccident physical demands. Such individuals now need a more comprehensive set of exercises to mobilize and strengthen. They also need a reeducation to change how they view their activity level in response to pain. Such programs usually take from 4 to 6 weeks, mostly supervised. Following such a program, even if the patient still has symptoms, the approach is to return to normal activities, including full work activities. This is the last part of the therapy. It is an approach recommended by such experts as Hall, Nachemson, Waddell, and others. In fact, there is no evidence of harm to the back in returning to such activities with pain alone, once appropriate therapy has been received. Those who return without any restrictions placed on the type of duties do better than those who are given restrictions. The same can be said of patients with neck pain.

Finally, identifying that individual who is exhibiting or at risk for adoption of the sick role may be helpful. If the patient has not already developed this illness behavior but has a psychological history that may put him or her at risk for adoption of the sick role, now would be the time to determine how that individual is coping with his or her psychological stressors and station in life. This could be an opportunity for counseling and avoiding the road to disability. Otherwise, the treatment of someone who is adopting the sick role is difficult. This is not surprising, as the patient is trying to achieve the sick role. A few patients may respond to education and have sufficient insight into their psychological difficulties that they might accept psychotherapy, but these are few indeed. Patients are certainly capable of changing their behavior, but the economy of secondary gain behavior often weighs down any motivations to change behavior.

Summary

Effective treatment or prevention requires a drastic change in our understanding of why whiplash patients report chronic symptoms. We need a complete shift in our approach away from "healing of an injury." Without such a change, patients reporting chronic symptoms have little hope.

> Diseases desperate grown, by desperate appliance are relieved, or not at all.
> —Shakespeare W. *Hamlet. Prince of Denmark.* Act IV, Scene III.

PROGNOSIS

The prognosis in whiplash patients depends on the mechanism of their symptom reporting. If their symptom reporting is due to adoption of the sick role, then the prognosis is poor. This is understandable since it would be pointless for them to develop an illness with a good prognosis, as they would then lose the sick role.

The prognosis in individuals with psychocultural illness depends on their exposure to a number of factors that generate their illness and on the individuals themselves as well as the psychosocial circumstances. Obviously individuals with a tendency toward anxiety and hypochondriasis who have symptom expectation and contact with the therapeutic community, insurance companies, and litigators will have the worst prognosis. As one removes each factor, the prognosis improves. For example, removing litigation (see Radanov et al) in Switzerland improved patients' prognosis, even though other factors may not have changed.

If one removes most or all the factors responsible for the psychocultural illness, the prognosis is even better. In Lithuania, accident victims often do not even attend therapy, and their symptoms resolve.

The prognosis from the physical injury is thus excellent in cases of muscle or ligament sprain (Grade 1 or 2 whiplash injury). Both the whiplash experiments and the Lithuanian experience indicate that the symptoms from the physical injury alone would subside within days or weeks.

There is otherwise little point in discussing the prognosis of symptom reporting, because the prognosis is then not dependent on the initial injury, but rather on all the other factors that promote chronic symptom reporting. It is worth repeating that radiological abnormalities are not relevant to prognosis. Radiological abnormalities, however, may lead patients to believe that they now have or will have permanent damage. Without proper education, this anxiety may indeed appear to be altering the prognosis of chronic symptom reporting.

SUMMARY

Assessment, treatment, and prognosis depend on one's understanding of why some whiplash victims report chronic symptoms and others do not.

Literature Review

Annotated Bibliography— Alphabetically by First Author

This bibliography cites the vast majority of the English language medical literature available on whiplash and the relevant literature about related topics. I have collected and read all the literature cited.

One has to appreciate that the interpretation of a study changes with time. Critical response to a 1961 article probably will be different in 1962 and in 1998. Too often, experts do not reevaluate an older article considering more recently acquired knowledge and experience about an illness. Instead, experts simply quote that older article, as if its conclusions are as valid today as they were in 1961, for example. Too often, authors do not themselves repeat the critical review process every time they cite an article.

Readers should never assume that authors have critically reviewed or even read the articles they quote. Instead, they should review those articles for themselves.

I have added a brief note below some of the bibliographic entries to elaborate on specific points not dealt with elsewhere in this book or to provide more information about the entries. The comments within this bibliography are not intended as criticisms of particular researchers. These comments merely remind readers to be aware of certain important issues when considering the conclusions of published scientific literature.

We have all our faults. . . . Thou censurest me, so have I done others, and may do thee. . . . Go now, censure, criticise, scoff, and rail.
—Burton R. [Democritus Junior]. *The Anatomy of Melancholy.*
Chatto & Windus: London; 1898:8.

Where I have added no comment to the bibliographic entry, the reference does not appear to add much information that is not already addressed in the text or other citations.

Finally, Chapter 14 groups various articles from this section for ready referral when readers need articles on particular subjects.

Aaron LA, Bradley LA, Alarcon GS, et al. Perceived physical and emotional trauma as precipitating events in fibromyalgia. *Arthritis and Rheumatism.* 1997;40:453–460.

Aaron LA, Bradley LA, Alarcon GS, et al. Authors' reply. *Arthritis and Rheumatism.* 1998;41:379–380.

Abbott KH. Whiplash injuries [letter]. *Journal of the American Medical Association.* 1956;162:917.

This author writes in support of N. Gotten's study conclusions.

Abbott KH. Neck sprain syndrome. *Medical Arts and Sciences.* 1959;13: 139–153.

The author reviews the psychological aspects of whiplash in the early days.

Abel MS, Wagner RF. Moderately severe whiplash injuries of the cervical verte-brae and their radiologic diagnosis. *American Medical Association Scientific Exhibits.* 1957:287–295.

These researchers show that if one exerted tremendous forces on cadaveric cer-vical spines, fractures could result.

Acres SE. Whiplash injury and traffic accidents. *Medical Services Journal of Canada.* 1966;22:813–814.

Adams MA. Biomechanics of the cervical spine. In: Gunzburg R, Szpalski M, eds. *Whiplash Injuries. Current Concepts in Prevention, Diagnosis, and Treat-ment of the Cervical Whiplash Syndrome.* Philadelphia: Lippincott-Raven; 1998:13–20.

This author gives a theoretical explanation of what might happen to a whiplash victim, including phrases like "very high forces." The injuries he refers to, how-ever, are seldom seen in whiplash claimants (they occur in only Grade 3 or 4 whiplash-associated disorders). Indeed, some whiplash claimants in low-velocity injuries have experienced a magnitude of force comparable to sneezing (see M. E. Allen et al and Chapter 5, "Whiplash Experiments"). As such, the discus-sion in this chapter is not applicable to most whiplash claimants.

In considering biomechanics, the author has not discussed any of the human volunteer experiments but focuses on less relevant and less appropriate cadaver experiments.

Adams RD, Victor M. *Principles of Neurology.* 4th ed. New York: McGraw-Hill; 1989:174.

Alexander E Jr, Davis CH Jr, Field CH. Hyperextension injuries of the cervical spine. *Archives of Neurology and Psychiatry.* 1958;79:146–150.

Alexander MP. In the pursuit of proof of brain damage after whiplash injury. *Neurology.* 1998;51:336–340.

A useful review of the issue of brain injury in whiplash patients. See also A. Otte et al.

Algers G, Pettersson K, Hildingsson C, Toolanen G. Surgery for chronic symptoms after whiplash injury. *Acta Orthopaedica Scandinavica.* 1993;64: 654–656.

Allen ME, Weir-Jones I, Motiuk DR, et al. Acceleration perturbations of daily living. A comparison to 'whiplash.' *Spine.* 1994;19(11):1285–1290.

These researchers demonstrate that forces or accelerations on the head and neck generated in everyday life are of the same magnitude as some low-velocity rear-end collisions. Yet these events in daily life do not cause symptoms.

Alund M, Ledin T, Ödkvist L, Larson SE. Dynamic posturography among patients with common neck disorders. *Journal of Vestibular Research.* 1993; 3:383–389.

Alvord LS. Psychological status of patients undergoing electronystagmography. *Journal of the American Academy of Audiology.* 1991;2(4):261–265.

Ambekar A. The behavioural response to whiplash injury [letter]. *Journal of Bone and Joint Surgery [British].* 1998;80B(1):183.

Anonymous. Whiplash injury [letter]. *Lancet.* 1991;338:1207–1208.

Antinnes JA, Dvorak J, Hayek J, Panjabi MM, Grob D. The value of functional computed tomography in the evaluation of soft-tissue injury in the upper cervical spine. *European Spine Journal.* 1994;3:98–101.

These researchers suggest that whiplash patients may have ligament injuries in the cervical spine, as one sees by computed tomography scanning techniques. The study population is those reporting that they have chronic neck pain following an accident.

There are, however, a number of potential sources for significant bias. First, that patients attribute their neck pain to an accident does not necessarily validate that the accident is actually the cause of their symptoms. Finding a pathological lesion in those patients does not validate the idea that the lesion is from an accident injury. If one wanted to demonstrate that an injury occurred in the accident, one would do the study within days to weeks of the accident. This would ensure that other causes had not intervened and that there was a high likelihood that the accident event led to the abnormal findings. Second, the authors do not describe much about the patient study group and the control group to show that they match well, to avoid selection bias. Members of the control group (part of an earlier study) are almost 16 years younger than members of the study group, and this could affect results. Third, there is no mention of what neurological abnormalities the study patients may have. This is important, because most whiplash patients have no objective neurological findings. For one to apply the results of this study to other whiplash patients, the authors must demonstrate that the study patients are similar to most whiplash patients. Finally, the accidents were high-speed collisions (where changes in velocity of the struck vehicle were as high as 30 km/h). Most whiplash claims are from collisions of less severity in collision speed, and so these results would not be applicable to most whiplash patients.

Aplin DY, Kane JM. Personality and experimentally simulated hearing loss. *British Journal of Audiology*. 1985;19:251–255.

Aprill C, Bogduk N. Cervical zygapophyseal joint pain. *Spine*. 1990;15(6): 744–777.

Aprill C, Bogduk N. The prevalence of cervical zygapophyseal joint pain. *Spine*. 1992;17(7):744–777.

These authors suggest that neck pain commonly arises from certain joints in the cervical spine, showing that they could produce pain when injecting saline into the joints. They could relieve the pain by then injecting anesthesia into the joint. They failed to use a double-blind, placebo-controlled methodology, however, so the conclusions may not be valid.

Arnold JG Jr. The clinical manifestations of spondylochondrosis (spondylosis) of the cervical spine. *Annals of Surgery*. 1955;141(6):872–889.

Arnott DWH. Neurosis and compensation. *Medical Journal of Australia*. 1941;1:24–25.

Arntz A, De Jong P. Anxiety, attention and pain. *Journal of Psychosomatic Research*. 1993;37(4):423–432.

In this study, and others reviewed by the authors, they show that attention to pain, even when one controls for anxiety, amplifies the pain and/or lowers the pain threshold.

Aubrey JB, Dobbs AR, Rule BG. Laypersons' knowledge about the sequelae of minor head injury and whiplash. *Journal of Neurology, Neurosurgery, and Psychiatry*. 1989;52:842–846.

These authors suggest from their study that the layperson could be quite knowledgeable about what physical symptoms should arise from specific types of motor vehicle accidents. Thus, expectation may contribute to symptomatology, or at least to the tendency to attribute chronic pain symptoms to an accident event. See also W. Mittenberg et al.

Auerbach AH, Scheflen NA, Scholz CK. A questionnaire survey of the post-traumatic syndrome. *Diseases of the Nervous System.*1967;28:110–112.

Awerbuch MS. Thermography—its current diagnostic status in musculoskeletal medicine. *Medical Journal of Australia*. 1991;154:441–444.

This article lays to rest any notions that one can reliably use thermography as a diagnostic tool in evaluating patients with chronic pain.

Awerbuch MS. Thermography—wither the niche? *Medical Journal of Australia*. 1991;154:444–447.

See above.

Awerbuch MS. In reply [letter]. *Medical Journal of Australia*. 1992;157:574.

Awerbuch MS. Whiplash in Australia: illness or injury? *Medical Journal of Australia*. 1992;157:193–196.

This author offers arguments that the reporting of chronic symptoms in whiplash patients is not due to some form of chronic damage that stems from the acute injury.

Awerbuch MS. Whiplash in Australia: illness or injury? [letter]. *Medical Journal of Australia*. 1992;157:502.

Babcock JL. Cervical spine injuries. Diagnosis and classification. *Archives of Surgery*. 1976;11:646–651.

Baer N. Fraud worries insurance companies but should concern physicians too, industry says. *Canadian Medical Association Journal*. 1997;156(2):251–256.

Bailey M. Assessment of impact severity in minor motor vehicle collisions. *Journal of Musculoskeletal Pain*. 1996;4(4): 21–38.

This author reviews various experiments involving minor collisions, reaffirming that they produce only brief durations (days to weeks) of symptoms in volunteers. The author also indicates that one reaches the threshold for injury when the struck vehicle has a change in velocity of at least 8 km/h in a rear-end collision and 16 to 24 km/h in a frontal or lateral collision.

Bailey MN, Wong BC, Lawrence JM. Data and methods for estimating the severity of minor impacts. In: *Proceedings of the Thirty Ninth Stapp Car Crash Conference*. Paper #950352. Warrendale, PA: Society of Automotive Engineers; 1995:139–173.

Balla JI. The late whiplash syndrome. *Australian and New Zealand Journal of Surgery*. 1980;50(6):610–614.

This author considers how cultural and psychological factors act in leading some whiplash victims to report chronic symptoms.

Balla JI. The late whiplash syndrome: a study of an illness in Australia and Singapore. *Culture, Medicine and Psychiatry*. 1982;6:191–210.

This author draws attention to the observation that while accidents are frequent in Singapore, whiplash victims reporting chronic symptoms are not. Social and cultural phenomena apparently contribute significantly to the behavior of reporting chronic symptoms.

Balla JI. Report to the Motor Accidents Board of Victoria on Whiplash Injuries. 1984. In: Hopkins A, ed. *Headache. Problems in Diagnosis and Management*. London: WB Saunders Company; 1988:268–289.

This author reviewed the files of more than 5,000 patients (a partial review to be found in the above article), finding that outcome in whiplash is not dependent on X-ray findings. Whiplash patients are not at any greater risk of developing disc degeneration than is the general population.

Balla JI., Iansek R. Headaches arising from disorders of the cervical spine. In: Hopkins A, ed. *Headache. Problems in Diagnosis and Management*. London: WB Saunders; 1988:243–267.

These authors affirm the knowledge that a "whiplash injury" does not aggravate or lead to disc degeneration. They remind us of how common such changes are with aging.

> The relatively small number [of whiplash patients] seen in older age groups is an important finding. If the underlying degenerative disease

were a significant predisposing cause of symptoms, then one would expect to see more cases in those age groups in which cervical spondylosis is prevalent. The findings raise doubts about the importance of degenerative disease in the production of head and neck symptoms.

There is no evidence to link preexisting degenerative changes in the cervical spine to the development of chronic changes.

They also discuss Balla's study of whiplash patients in Australia.

Balla JI, Karnaghan J. Whiplash headache. In: Eadie MJ, Lander C, eds. *Proceedings of the Australian Association of Neurologists. Clinical and Experimental Neurology*. 1986:179–182.

This authors conclude that the headaches whiplash patients experience are muscle contraction headaches, likely related to anxiety. See also R. Iansek et al.

Balla JI, Moraitis S. Knights in armour. A follow-up study of injuries after legal settlement. *Medical Journal of Australia*. 1970;2:355–361.

Bankes MJK, Noble LM. The behavioural response to whiplash injury [letter]. *Journal of Bone and Joint Surgery [British]*. 1998;80-B:555–558.

Bannister G, Main C. Authors' reply [letter]. *Journal of Bone and Joint Surgery [British]*. 1998;80-B:555.

Barber HO. Head injury. Audiological and vestibular findings. *Annals of Otology, Rhinology, and Laryngology*. 1969;78:239–252.

In this study, the authors reveal that normal individuals frequently have the same findings on ocular and hearing examination as those claiming to have had injury. They could find no organic basis for the symptoms after head injury.

Barnes SM. Whiplash injury and surgically treated cervical disc disease [letter]. *Injury*. 1994;25(6):409–410.

This author renders a critique of the study by A. J. Hamer et al. See also C. L. Colton and A. D. Redmond et al.

Barnsley L, Lord SM, Bogduk N. Comparative local anaesthetic blocks in the diagnosis of cervical zygapophysial joint pain. *Pain*. 1993;55:99–106.

This is among the first of a series of exceptionally well-conducted studies that this group of authors has produced (see below). They demonstrate that specific joints in the cervical spine (zygapophysial joints) may be a source of chronic neck pain. This group of authors conducted a number of studies on patients who *claim* their neck pain is due to an accident. There are major problems, however, with the conclusion that whiplash patients suffer a zygapophysial joint injury and that is the reason why they have chronic pain. First, the patients are not consecutive whiplash patients presenting to an emergency department, for example. Also, not all the patients were in motor vehicle accidents. One of the patients (in a later study) did not have any neck pain with the accident but developed neck pain 3 months later. (That patient should not attribute the neck pain to the accident.) The major flaw, however, is that the average duration from the accident to the time of the study was 4 to 5 years. One case was 44 years after the accident! That a patient (or anyone else) attributes chronic neck pain to an accident does not validate that the *chronic* pain is due to an accident injury. Identifying the underlying pathological basis of the pain does not confirm that this pathology follows from the acute accident injury. Chronic neck pain is very frequent in the general population. Some whiplash patients may be mistakenly attributing non–accident related pain to an accident. It is interesting that these studies do not include a control group of non–traumatic neck pain patients. They may have the same prevalence of zygapophysial joint pain. This brings into question the validity of concluding that chronic neck pain is the result of zygapophysial joint injury from an accident.

To demonstrate cervical zygapophysial joint injury in whiplash patients as a cause for their pain, the study should be within at most 3 months of the accident. Then there is a reasonable probability that one can ascribe the patient's symptoms to the accident. Otherwise, these studies merely confirm the zygapophysial joint as a potential source of chronic neck pain, but do not confirm what event caused that pathology. One must also consider the possibility that chronic pain arises from the development of abnormal posture of the neck. This might generate zygapophysial joint pathology over months to years. An acute joint injury may not be necessary. One must also note that bone scans are capable of detecting joint pathology. Yet they have been routinely negative in studies of whiplash patients (see "Radiology of Whiplash" in Chapter 5). As such, these studies do not validate cervical zygapophysial joint injury as an event that occurs in most whiplash patients.

Barnsley L, Lord SM, Bogduk N. Whiplash injury. *Pain.* 1994; 58:283–307.

This is a very good review of the issues in whiplash, although the authors neglect to discuss the extensive body of literature on human whiplash experiments. Instead, they emphasize less appropriate animal studies. They also quote the Watkinson et al study, which has significant potential flaws.

Barnsley L, Lord SM, Wallis BJ, Bogduk N. False-positive rates of cervical zygapophysial joint blocks. *Clinical Journal of Pain.* 1993;9:124–130.

Barnsley L, Lord SM, Wallis BJ, Bogduk N. Lack of effect of intraarticular corticosteroids for chronic pain in the cervical zygapophysial joints. *New England Journal of Medicine.* 1994;330:1047–1050.

Barnsley L, Lord SM, Wallis BJ, Bogduk N. The prevalence of chronic cervical zygapophysial joint pain after whiplash. *Spine.* 1995;20(1):20–26.

Barry M. Whiplash injuries. *British Journal of Rheumatology.* 1992;31(9):579–581.

Barsky AJ. Amplification, somatization, and the somatoform disorders. *Psychosomatics.* 1992;33(1):28–34.

Barsky AJ, Goodson JD, Lane RS, Cleary PD. The amplification of somatic symptoms. *Psychosomatic Medicine.* 1988;50: 510–519.

Barsky AJ, Klerman GL. Overview: hypochondriasis, bodily complaints, and somatic styles. *American Journal of Psychiatry.* 1983;140(3):273–283.

Barton D, Allen M, Finlay D, Belton I. Evaluation of whiplash injuries by technetium 99m isotope scanning. *Archives of Emergency Medicine.* 1993;10: 197–202.

These researchers explain the stage that the radiologic search for whiplash injury had reached.

> The exact aetiology of the condition is unknown but many theories exist which include overstretching of soft tissues, intervertebral joints, nerve roots and peripheral nerves in the posterior cervical and lumbar spine. Radiological findings offer no characteristic or pathognomic lesion: prognostic indicators as exist are nonspecific.

> Reports on [bone scans] outline the effectiveness of this investigation in demonstrating periosteal irritation associated with ligamentous avulsion and muscle injury.

> Soft tissue trauma even in the absence of bone injury can be revealed by increased activity on a bone scan . . . and can be used to differentiate between acute muscle injury, skeletal injury, periosteal injury, or stress fracture, or an abnormality which is entirely associated with a joint or connective tissue.

In their study of 20 whiplash patients, they found that "The . . . scans were reported as normal . . . in nineteen patients with one patient demonstrating changes consistent with degenerative disease."

Thus, bone scans, which are extremely sensitive in finding significant ligament or muscle damage, are negative in typical whiplash patients. See also C. Hildingsson et al.

Beals RK. Compensation and recovery from injury. *Western Journal of Medicine.* 1984;140(2):233–237.

Becker RE. Whiplash injuries. *Academy of Applied Osteopathy—Year Book.* 1958:65–69.

Behan RC, Hirschfeld AH. The accident process II. Toward more rational treatment of industrial injuries. *Journal of the American Medical Association.* 1963;186(4):300–306.
See also A. H. Hirschfeld and R. C. Behan.

Behan RC, Hirschfeld AH. Disability without disease or accident. *Archives of Environmental Health.* 1966;12:655–659.

Bendjellal F, Tarriere C, Gillet D, et al. Head and neck responses under high G-level lateral deceleration. In: *Proceedings of the Thirty First Stapp Car Crash Conference.* Paper #872196. Warrendale, PA: Society of Automotive Engineers; 1987:29–47.

Benna P, Bergamasco B, Bianco C, et al. Brainstem auditory evoked potentials in postconcussion syndrome. *Italian Journal of Neurologic Science.* 1982;4:281–287.

Bergman H, Andersson F, Isberg A. Incidence of temporomandibularjoint changes after whiplash trauma: a prospective study using MR imaging. *American Journal of Roentgenology.* 1998;171:1237–1243.

Bernard TN Jr. Lumbar discography followed by computed tomography. *Spine.* 1990;15(7):691–707.

In this study of computed tomography scanning and discography of the lumbar spine, the author shows that a number of the abnormalities exist without causing symptoms. Only when there are specific signs of a "pinched" nerve can one link some of the abnormalities to symptoms.

Berry H. Psychological aspects of chronic neck pain following hyperextension-flexion strains of the neck. In: Morley TP, ed. *Current Controversies in Neurosurgery.* Philadelphia: WB Saunders; 1976:51–60.

Berry H. Psychological aspects of whiplash injury. In: Wilkins RH, Rengachary SS, eds. *Neurosurgery*. Vol 2. Philadelphia: McGraw-Hill; 1985:1716–1719.

Berryman JS. Diagnosis of whiplash injuries. *International Record of Medicine*. 1956;169(1):26–27.

Berton J. *Whiplash: Test of the Influential Variables*. Paper #680080. Warrendale, PA: Society of Automotive Engineers; 1968:77.

Bicik I, Radanov BP, Schäfer N, et al. PET with [18]fluorodeoxyglucose and hexamethylpropylene amine oxime SPECT in late whiplash syndrome. *Neurology*. 1998;51:345–350.

These researchers confirm that brain injury is a very unlikely event in whiplash patients and that abnormal brain scan findings have other explanations beside injury. See also M. P. Alexander and A. Otte et al.

Billig HE Jr. Traumatic neck, head, eye syndrome. *Journal of the International College of Surgeons*. 1953;20(5):558–561.

Billig HE Jr. The mechanism of whiplash injuries. *International Record of Medicine*. 1956;169(1):3–7.

Billig HE Jr. Head, neck, shoulder and arm syndrome following cervical injury. *Journal of the International College of Surgeons*. 1959;32(3):287–297.

Bjøgen IA. Late whiplash syndrome [letter]. *Lancet*. 1996;348:124.

Björnstig U, Hildingsson C, Toolanen G. Soft-tissue injury of the neck in a hospital based material. *Scandinavian Journal of Social Medicine*. 1990;18:263–267.

Blumer D, Heilbronn M. Chronic pain as a variant of depressive disease. The pain-prone disorder. *Journal of Nervous and Mental Disease*. 1982;170(7):381–406.

This article deals with the concept of a psychological basis for chronic, nonorganic pain.

Bodack MP, Tunkel RS, Marini SG, Nagler W. Spinal accessory nerve palsy as a cause of pain after whiplash injury: case report. *Journal of Pain and Symptom Management*. 1998;15:321–328.

Boden SD, Davis DO, Dina TS, Patronas NJ, Wiesel SW. Abnormal magnetic-resonance scans of the lumbar spine in asymptomatic subjects. *Journal of Bone and Joint Surgery*. 1990;72-A(3):403–408.

In this study of magnetic resonance imaging of the lumbar spine, the authors show that 20% to 57% (depending on age) of the general population have abnormalities even without symptoms. This includes patients under age 39. One cannot therefore attribute symptoms to such abnormalities since they may indeed not cause any symptoms at all. The authors also emphasize that many of the changes are part of the normal aging process.

Boden SD, McCowin PR, Davis DO, et al. Abnormal magnetic-resonance scans of the cervical spine in asymptomatic subjects. *Journal of Bone and Joint Surgery*. 1990;72-A(8):1178–1184.

These authors show that one cannot simply use the finding of disc degeneration on magnetic resonance imaging scans of the cervical spine as an explanation for neck pain, because it is so often present in asymptomatic individuals.
See also L. M. Teresi et al.

Bogduk N. In response [letter]. *Spine*. 1996;21(1):150–151.

This is a response to another author who feels that passive therapies are useful in whiplash patients.

Bogduk N, Lord SM. Cervical spine disorders. *Current Opinion in Rheumatology*. 1998;10:110–115.

This is a response to a letter by J. Y. Maigne.

Bogduk N, Lord SM, Barnsley L. In response [letter]. *Spine*. 1997;22(12): 1420–1421.

See critical reviews by R. Ferrari et al (*Journal of Rheumatology, Cephalalgia*) and O. Kwan et al (*Cephalalgia*) as well as Chapter 5.

Bohnen N, Jolles J, Verhey FRJ. Persistent neuropsychological deficits in cervical whiplash patients without direct headstrike. *Acta Neurologica Belgium*. 1993; 93:23–31.

These authors suggest that brain injury may occur in whiplash patients. Their conclusion is highly flawed as they base it on a study of only two patients, with no control group. As well, proper studies with larger numbers of patients and control groups have indicated that explanations other than brain injury are more probable for cognitive problems. See also "Disturbance of Cognition" in Chapter 7.

Boismare F, Boquet J, Moore N, Chretien P, Saligaut C, Daoust M. Hemo-dynamic, behavioural and biochemical disturbances induced by an experimen-tal cranio-cervical injury (whiplash) in rats. *Journal of the Autonomic Nervous System.* 1985;13:137–147.

While these authors report neurological injury in rats with a whiplash maneu-ver, one cannot extend this result to the human situation. The authors do not state what the exact acceleration was at the onset of the event, although they do state the deceleration. Further, the anatomy of the rat neck is quite different from that of the human neck, and the human whiplash experiments have never resulted in the injury these authors report.

Bonk A, Giebel GD, Edelmann M, Huser R. Whiplash outcome in Germany. *Journal of Rheumatology.* 1999. In press.
See also Giebel et al.

Borchgrevink GE, Kaasa A, McDonagh, et al. Acute treatment of whiplash neck sprain injuries. A randomized trial of treatment during the first 14 days follow-ing car accident. *Spine.* 1998;23(1):25–31.

In this study, the authors reveal that giving the whiplash patient advice to "act as usual" without sick leave from work significantly improves their outcome, when compared with outcomes of those given 2 weeks' sick leave and a collar. See also L. A. McKinney.

Borchgrevink GE, Lereim I, Røyneland L, Bjørndal A, Haraldseth O. National health insurance consumption and chronic symptoms following mild neck sprain injuries in car collisions. *Scandinavian Journal of Social Medicine.* 1996;24(4):264–271.

Borchgrevink G, Smevik O, Haave I, Lereim I, Haraldseth O. MRI of cerebrum and cervical column within two days after "whiplash" neck sprain injury. In: *Proceedings of the Society of Magnetic Resonance Third Scientific Meeting and Exhibition, 1995, August 19–25, Nice, France.* 1995:243.

In this study, the authors confirm that there is no evidence for nervous system injury and no evidence for any other injury than microscopic muscle or ligament tears in most whiplash patients. One can detect anything more serious than this by magnetic resonance imaging or bone scans. See also "MRI" and "Radiology of Whiplash" in Chapter 5.

Borchgrevink GE, Smevik O, Nordby A, et al. MR imaging and radiography of patients with cervical hyperextension-flexion injuries after car accidents. *Acta Radiologica.* 1995;36:425–428.

This is another study in which the authors show that the injuries others so often cite as a cause for chronic pain are absent in whiplash patients. Magnetic resonance imaging (MRI) studies find no evidence of a specific traumatic lesion. The only type of lesion these and other imaging techniques can miss is a microscopic muscle or ligament tear, that is, a minor sprain.

They also show that MRI findings do not predict symptoms or the patient's outcome.

Borchgrevink GE, Stiles TC, Borchgrevink PC, Lereim I. Personality profile among symptomatic and recovered patients with neck sprain injury, measured by MCMI-I acutely and 6 months after car accidents. *Journal of Psychosomatic Research*. 1997;42(4):357–367.

These authors report that one need not be a hypochondriac or neurotic, or have extreme personality traits, to report chronic symptoms following the acute whiplash injury. This is not to say, however, that psychological factors are unimportant in chronic symptom reporting. Psychological and cultural factors might affect so-called "normal" individuals and encourage the behavior of reporting chronic symptoms. The authors did not design the study to look for the many other psychological factors that may be acting, nor did they examine what effect life stressors after the accident had on symptom reporting. M. Karlsborg et al show, for example, that events such as birth of a baby, loss of a relative, or robbery correlate with outcome at 6 months.

Borden AGB, Rechtman AM, Gershon-Cohen J. The normal cervical lordosis. *Radiology*. 1960;74:806–809.

In this study of the normal population, the authors show that the cervical lordosis on X-ray can normally be flat or even in reverse curvature. One cannot use this as a reliable sign of whiplash injury. It occurs in individuals with no history of neck trauma. See also D. R. Gore et al, P. S. Helliwell et al, and A. M. Rechtman et al.

Bosworth DM. Whiplash—an unacceptable medical term. *Journal of Bone and Joint Surgery*. 1959;41-A:16.

Bounds JA. Chronic whiplash syndrome [letter]. *Neurology*. 1995;45:2117.

Bourbeau R, Desjardins D, Maag U, Laberge-Nadeau C. *Neck Injuries amongst Front Seat Belted and Unbelted Car Occupants (Seat Belts and Neck Injuries)*. Publication #818. Centre de recherche sur les transports; 1992.
See below.

Bourbeau R, Desjardins D, Maag U, Laberge-Nadeau C. Neck injuries among belted and unbelted occupants of the front seat of cars. *Journal of Trauma*. 1993;35(5):794–799.

In this study, the authors conclude that accident victims wearing seat belts are more likely to develop whiplash than nonbelted victims. One must note, however, that it is significant that the study does not include uninjured occupants who may have been wearing a seat belt, a fact that could dramatically alter results. See Chapter 22.

Bowman BM, Schneider LW, Lustick LS, Anderson WR, Thomas DJ. Simulation analysis of head and neck dynamic response. In: *Proceedings of the Twenty Eighth Stapp Car Crash Conference*. Paper #841668. Warrendale, PA: Society of Automotive Engineers; 1984:173–205.

Braaf MM, Rosner S. Symptomatology and treatment of injuries of the neck. *New York State Journal of Medicine*. 1955;55(1):237–242.

In this study, the authors found a high frequency of psychoneurotic symptoms in whiplash patients and found that most had social maladjustment and neurotic personalities prior to the head injury. They believed that this predicted the development of chronic symptoms after an accident.

Braaf MM, Rosner S. Whiplash injury of the neck: symptoms, diagnosis, treatment, and prognosis. *New York State Journal of Medicine*. 1958;58:1501–1507.

Braaf MM, Rosner S. Chronic headache. *New York State Journal of Medicine*. 1960;60:3987–3995.

Braaf MM, Rosner S. Meniere-like syndrome following whiplash injury of the neck. *Journal of Trauma*. 1962;2:494–501.

The authors offer a theory for the basis of vertigo in whiplash patients. One must note, however, that this remains theoretical, with the authors providing no experimental evidence.

Braaf MM, Rosner S. Headache following neck injuries. *Headache*. 1962;2: 153–159.

Braaf MM, Rosner S. Whiplash injury of neck—fact or fancy? *International Surgery*. 1966;46(2):176–182.

These authors summarize their concepts of the site of whiplash injury. One must note, however, that these authors seem to be somewhat confused and unaware of the available literature from before 1966. In this article, for instance, they state that straightening or reversal of the cervical lordosis on neck X-ray is an important radiologic sign in whiplash. Yet, A. G. B. Borden et al, J. H. Juhl et al, J. O. Lottes et al, and H. Zatzkin and F. W. Kveton had already published studies and demonstrated that there was no significance to this X-ray finding. One frequently finds it in the general population.

Braaf MM, Rosner S. Trauma of cervical spine as a cause of chronic headache. *Journal of Trauma*. 1975;15(5):441–446.

Brady C, Taylor D, O'Brien M. Whiplash and temporomandibular joint dysfunction. *Journal of the Irish Dental Association*. 1993;39(3):69–72.

These authors consider temporomandibular joint injury to occur as a result of mechanisms that have since been disproven (see R. P. Howard et al). The authors do not explain why these same symptoms do not seem to exist in whiplash patients in other countries.

Brault JR, Wheeler JB, Siegmund GP, Brault EJ. Authors' reply [letter]. *Archives of Physical Medicine and Rehabilitation*. 1998;79:722–723.

Brault JR, Wheeler JB, Siegmund GP, Brault EJ. Authors' reply [letter]. *Archives of Physical Medicine and Rehabilitation*. 1998;79:1024.

Brault JR, Wheeler JB, Siegmund GP, Brault EJ. Clinical response of human subjects to rear-end automobile collisions. *Archives of Physical Medicine and Rehabilitation*. 1998; 79:72–80.

The authors of this study give one the impression that even the most minor of rear-end collisions, being struck at 5 km/h, can cause acute whiplash symptoms. This result is contrary to all other low-velocity collision experiments, wherein a velocity of at least double is the threshold. What are the potential flaws in this study that might give such different results?

A detailed discussion of this study is in Chapter 21.

Braun BL, DiGiovanna A, Schiffman E, Bonnema J, Friction J. A cross-sectional study of temporomandibular joint dysfunction in post-cervical trauma patients. *Journal of Craniomandibular Disorders: Facial and Oral Pain*. 1992; 6:24–31.

Although these authors suggest that whiplash patients are more likely to complain of jaw pain than the general population, this in no way proves that whiplash patients have a temporomandibular joint (TMJ) injury. The whiplash patients obviously have the experience of a number of psychological factors that could be generating this reporting. The authors should have used a control group that had nontraumatic neck pain, for example, or a control group of patients with known psychological disorders. As such, this study offers no support to the theory that TMJ injury occurs in whiplash patients.

See also R. Ferrari et al, H. L. Goldberg, A. P. Heise et al, R. P. Howard et al, W. S. Kirk Jr., M. Olin, R. H. Roydhouse, E. W. Small, and D. H. West et al.

Braunstein PW, Moore JO. The fallacy of the term "whiplash injury." *American Journal of Surgery*. 1959;97:522–529.

Breck LW, Van Norman RW. Medicolegal aspects of cervical spine sprains. *Clinical Orthopaedics and Related Research*. 1971;74:124–128.

Bremner DN, Gillingham FJ. Patterns of convalescence after minor head injury. *Royal College of Surgeons of Edinburgh Journal*. 1974;19:94–97.

These authors evaluate the psychological factors responsible for delayed recovery in these patients.

Brien JA. Ototoxicity associated with salicylates. A brief review. *Drug Safety*. 1993;9(2):143–148.

Bring G, Westman G. Chronic posttraumatic syndrome after whiplash injury. *Scandinavian Journal of Primary Health Care*. 1991;9:135–141.

Brodin H. Cervical pain and mobilization. *Journal of Manual Medicine*. 1985;2:18–22.

This author discusses early mobilization techniques for the treatment of whiplash.

See also Quebec Task Force review (W. O. Spitzer et al), L. A. McKinney, K. Mealy et al, and L. Provinciali et al.

Brooke RI, Lapointe HJ. Temporomandibular joint disorders following whiplash. *Spine: State of the Art Reviews*. 1993;7(3):443–454.

This review discusses a temporomandibular joint (TMJ) injury in whiplash patients. It is largely based on theories and ignores the fact that such TMJ disorders do not exist in whiplash patients in other countries. There is also no discussion of the fact that there is a substantial body of literature showing that the very same imaging abnormalities reported to be the cause of the jaw dysfunction in a whiplash patient are commonly found in many normal (asymptomatic) subjects. R. P. Howard et al's research disproves their theories of TMJ injury. See also R. Ferrari et al.

Brooke RI, Stenn PG. Postinjury myofascial pain dysfunction syndrome: Its etiology and prognosis. *Oral Surgery, Oral Medicine, and Oral Pathology*. 1978; 45(6):846–850.

These authors discuss the psychological factors for temporomandibular joint symptoms, identifying that the difference in response to therapy of postaccident patients versus other patients lies in the psychological stressors such as the harbored resentment of a problem "someone else had caused" and the stress of litigation.

Brooks SL, Westesson P, Eriksson L, Hansson LG, Barsotti JB. Prevalence of osseous changes in the temporomandibular joint of asymptomatic persons without internal derangement. *Oral Surgery, Oral Medicine, and Oral Pathology.* 1992;73:122–126.

These authors reveal that 35% of asymptomatic subjects have abnormalities on temporomandibular joint imaging, even though they have no pain. Thus the finding of these changes in a whiplash patient with jaw pain does not identify the cause of the pain.

See also C. B. Muir and A. N. Goss, M. M. Tasaki et al, and P. Westesson et al.

Buonocore E, Hartman JT, Nelson CL. Cineradiograms of cervical spine in diagnosis of soft-tissue injuries. *Journal of the American Medical Association.* 1966;198(1):143–147.

These authors reveal that a special technique called cineradiography can find abnormalities in whiplash patients. One must note, however, that of the 57 patients (all had symptoms), only half had these abnormalities and the rest were normal. This meant that there was no correlation of symptoms to the abnormalities. As well, the study completely lacked a control population, so one does not know the prevalence of such findings in asymptomatic individuals.

Burgess J. Symptom characteristics in TMD patients reporting blunt trauma and/or whiplash injury. *Journal of Craniomandibular Disorders: Facial and Oral Pain.* 1991;5(4):251–257.

This author reviews the findings on examination of the temporomandibular joint (TMJ) in patients with blunt trauma and whiplash patients. He suggests TMJ (temporomandibular joint) pain is a consequence of injury during whiplash, but one must note that patients' symptoms, although real, may not necessarily be due to injury. The author also reports clicking as an abnormal phenomenon, which is true perhaps, but it is one frequently found in asymptomatic subjects (see R. H. Roydhouse). No one has demonstrated that rear-end collisions can produce TMJ injury. See also R. Ferrari et al, H. L. Goldberg, A. P. Heise et al, R. P. Howard et al, W. S. Kirk Jr., M. Olin, T. C. S. Probert et al, E. W. Small, and D. H. West et al.

Burgess J, Dworkin SF. Litigation and post-traumatic TMD: How patients report treatment outcome. *Journal of the American Dental Association.* 1993;124: 105–110.

These authors demonstrate that the stress of litigation worsens the treatment response of the so-called "TMJ disorders" in whiplash patients, indicating that psychological factors are indeed important in the expression of these symptoms.

Burgess JA, Kolbinson DA, Lee PT, Epstein JB. Motor vehicle accidents and TMDs: assessing the relationship. *Journal of the American Dental Association.* 1996;127:1767–1772.

Burke JP, Orton HP, West J, et al. Whiplash and its effects on the visual system. *Graefe's Archive for Clinical and Experimental Ophthalmology.* 1992;230: 335–339.

These authors suggest that whiplash has ocular complications, but they consider only a small group of patients and provide no evidence that the abnormalities were not present before the patients developed whiplash. The authors do not report a control group in the study.

Bush FM, Dolwick MF. *The Temporomanibular Joint and Related Orofacial Disorders.* Philadelphia: JB Lippincott; 1995: 72–73.

Within this text is a review of the studies dealing with the psychological factors involved in temporomandibular joint disorders, focusing on those studies chiefly after 1980.

Buskila D, Neumann L, Vaisberg G, et al. Increased rates of fibromyalgia following cervical spine injury. *Arthritis and Rheumatism.* 1997;40(3):446–452.

Although the authors of this study show that patients have a greater risk for developing fibromyalgia after neck injury than they do after leg fracture, this association does not prove that there is a causal relationship between the neck injury and fibromyalgia. The link between the two is discussed by R. Ferrari and A. S. Russell, in part, and in the section "Fibromyalgia and Motor Vehicle Accidents" of Chapter 10.

Buzzard F. Discussion on traumatic neurasthenia and the litigation neurosis. *Proceedings of the Royal Society of Medicine.* 1927;21(1):353–364.

The author discusses traumatic neurosis (neurasthenia).

Byrn C, Borenstein P, Linder LE. Treatment of neck and shoulder pain in whiplash syndrome patients with intracutaneous sterile water injections. *Acta Anaesthesiologica Scandinavica.* 1991;35:52–53.

These researchers were able to relieve patients of their symptoms of headache, neck pain, and arm pain by injecting water under the skin. The success of this therapy makes it unlikely that structures that cannot be reached or affected by water (cervical nerves, ligaments, discs, etc.) are the source of symptoms. The alternative explanation is that there is a marked placebo response in whiplash patients that explains their improvement. Otherwise, this study and that below are quite small, with an uncontrolled design, and the validity of the results is questionable. See T. Sand et al.

Byrn C, Olsson I, Falkheden L, et al. Subcutaneous sterile water injections for chronic neck and shoulder pain following whiplash injuries. *Lancet.* 1993;341:449–452.

See above.

Caldwell IW. Seat belts and head rests. *British Medical Journal.* 1972;2:163.

This author offers a passionate view that seat belts may cause serious neck injury. One must note, however, that he has no evidence to support this claim. Further criticism is offered by W. Gissane and in Chapter 22.

Caldwell JW, Crane CR, Krusen EM. Nerve conduction studies: an aid in the diagnosis of the thoracic outlet syndrome. *Southern Medical Journal.* 1971; 64(2):210–212.

Cameron BM, Cree CMN. A critique of the compression theory of whiplash. *Orthopedics.* 1960;2:127–129.

Cammack KV. Whiplash injuries to the neck. *American Journal of Surgery.* 1957; 93:663–666.

Cannistraci AJ, Fritz G. Dental applications of biofeedback. In: Basmajian JV, ed. *Biofeedback Principles and Practice for Clinicians.* 3rd ed. Baltimore: Williams & Wilkins; 1989:297–310.

Capistrant TD. Thoracic outlet syndrome in whiplash injury. *Annals of Surgery.* 1977;185:175–178.

This study attempts to prove that thoracic outlet syndrome is the cause of symptoms in patients with whiplash, and the study bases its arguments on nerve conduction studies. One must note, however, the many authors who have since made it clear that abnormalities on nerve conduction studies are in no way indicative of this rare disorder. See M. Cherington et al, A. J. Wilbourn, and J. R. Youmans.

Capistrant TD. Thoracic outlet syndrome in cervical strain injury. *Minnesota Medicine.* 1986;69:13–17.

In this article, the author admits that there are no true objective tests that confirm a true case of thoracic outlet syndrome. He also admits that he bases his diagnosis on what the patient reports or on certain physical findings (like Adson's test, which is known to be useless, as it is frequently positive in normal subjects). There has never been any scientific verification of the existence of this syndrome in whiplash patients.

See also M. Cherington et al, A. J. Wilbourn, and J. R. Youmans.

Carette S. Whiplash injury and chronic neck pain. *New England Journal of Medicine*. 1994;330(15):1083–1084.

Carlsson G, Nilsson S, Nilsson-Ehle A, et al. Neck injuries in rear end car collisions. Biomechanical considerations to improve head restraints. In: *Proceedings of the International IRCOBI/AAAM Conference on the Biomechanics of Injury*, 1985, June 24–26, Göteborg, Sweden, Bron, France. 1985:277–289.

These authors suggest that occupant height predicts neck injury and that maladjusted head restraints may account for the observed failure of head restraints to prevent whiplash injury. This study is succeeded, however, by the study of P. Lövsund et al, which is much larger and concludes the opposite.

Carnett JB, Bates W. Railway spine. *Surgical Clinics of North America*. 1932; 12:1369–1386.

These authors review railway spine. The story of railway spine is much like the story of whiplash. Many theories were offered, there were inadequate attempts to view the injury radiologically, and many authors, including this one, hoped to define the physical basis for railway spine.

Cassidy JD. Basal metabolic temperature vs. laboratory assessment in "posttraumatic hypothyroidism" [letter]. *Journal of Manipulative and Physiological Therapeutics*. 1996;19(6):425–426.

This author discusses the need for better quality of research about controversial topics such as a whiplash.

Cassidy JD, Lopes AA, Yong-Hing K. The immediate effect of manipulation versus mobilization on pain and range of motion in the cervical spine: a randomized controlled trial. *Journal of Manipulative and Physiological Therapeutics*. 1992;15(9):570–575.

The authors of this study originally reported that there was short-term benefit to chiropractic manipulation, when compared with mobilization by exercises. The authors later point out, however, that there were flaws in the study and that "the trial does not support the conclusion that manipulation provided more relief than mobilization." Thus, there are as yet no randomized studies supporting this therapy in whiplash patients. See reference below.

Cassidy JD, Lopes AA, Yong-Hing K. The immediate effect of manipulation versus mobilization on pain and range of motion in the cervical spine: a randomized controlled trial [letter]. *Journal of Manipulative and Physiological Therapeutics*. 1993; 16(4):279–280.

In this letter, the authors point out the major flaw of the study above.

Castro WHM, Schilgen M, Meyer S, et al. Do "whiplash injuries" occur in low-speed rear impacts? *European Spine Journal*. 1997;6:366–375.

In this study the authors found the threshold for whiplash injury in rear-end collision to be when the struck vehicle has a change in velocity of 10 km/h, slightly higher than the 8 km/h found by other researchers. See "Whiplash Experiments" in Chapter 5 and Chapter 20.

Cesarani A, Alpini D, Bonvier R, et al. *Whiplash Injuries. Diagnosis and Treatment*. Berlin: Springer; 1996.

The authors of this textbook present a theoretical argument for the existence of nervous system injury to explain symptoms like dizziness, visual disturbance, and hearing disturbance in whiplash patients. There are no comments, however, on the other possible causes for these symptoms, nor that simply having neck pain alone could alter these sensations by altering head movements. There is also no explanation of what type of lesion could be commonly causing these symptoms in some cultures but not in others (ie, where whiplash is rare or uncommon). There is also a lack of inclusion of much of the important whiplash literature in their considerations. When they discuss the whiplash experiments, they refer to animal and dummy studies and do not quote the human whiplash experiments.

In addition, the only psychological aspects they do consider are compensation issues. They thus ignore a large number of other psychological factors.

Finally, they state that when treatment fails, one must exhaustively search for "some lesion" but do not consider instead the much higher probability that the genuine symptoms are psychologically based or unrelated to the accident injury altogether.

Champion GD. Whiplash in Australia: illness or injury? [letter]. *Medical Journal of Australia*. 1992;157:574.

This author adds further support to M. S. Awerbuch's work.

Chappa KH, Gladstone KJ, Young RR. Brain stem auditory evoked responses. *Archives of Neurology*. 1979;36:81–87.

These authors show that what one might consider to be abnormalities, one can also find in normal individuals, thus requiring caution in interpreting abnormalities as brain damage.

Cherington M. A conservative point of view of the thoracic outlet syndrome. *American Journal of Surgery*. 1989;158: 394–395.
See below.

Cherington M, Cherington C. Thoracic outlet syndrome: reimbursement patterns and patient profiles. *Neurology*. 1992;42: 943–945.

These authors help one to understand that it is an unfounded conclusion to attribute the cause of whiplash patient's symptoms to thoracic outlet syndrome.

Cherington M, Happer I, Machanic B, Parry L. Surgery for thoracic outlet syndrome may be hazardous to your health. *Muscle and Nerve*. 1986;9:632–634.
See above.

Chester JB Jr. Whiplash, postural control, and the inner ear. *Spine*. 1991;16(7): 716–720.

The patients this author describes are a highly select group. The author examined them, in some cases, years after their accident. It may be that their symptoms at the time of the evaluation were due entirely to other disorders unrelated to the accident. There is also no mention of what medications these people were on that might contribute to findings. There is no control group.

As well, the author shows that electronystagmography was normal in more than 85% of the whiplash patients, even though those patients had symptoms, so that there was no correlation between symptoms and abnormal test findings.

Finally, authors of more recent studies of whiplash patients have not reported the abnormalities in this study.

Cholewicki J, Panjabi MM, Nibu K, et al. Head kinematics during in vitro whiplash simulation. *Accident Analysis and Prevention*. 1998;30(4):469–479.

Chrisman OD, Gervais RF. Otologic manifestations of the cervical syndrome. *Clinical Orthopedics*. 1962;24:34–39.

In this study, the authors could not find an objective cause for the symptoms of headache and hearing disturbance in whiplash patients.

Christensen LV, McKay DC. Reflex jaw motions and jaw stiffness pertaining to whiplash injury of the neck. *Journal of Craniomandibular Practice*. 1997; 15(3):242–260.

These authors conducted a detailed study of how the jaw muscles move in a neck extension (such as in whiplash injury) and discuss the physiology of jaw movements. They indicate that the touted theories of "mandibular whiplash" are scientifically unsound. See also R. Ferrari et al, H. L. Goldberg, R. P. Howard et al, R. H. Roydhouse, T. J. Szabo et al, and D. H. West et al.

Christian MS. Non-fatal injuries sustained by seatbelt wearers: a comparative study. *British Medical Journal*. 1976;2: 1310–1311.

This author concludes that seat belt wearers have a higher incidence of neck injury than do nonwearers. One must note, however, that there are potential sources of significant concern in this study. See Chapter 22 and C. P. De Fonseka.

Christie B. Appeal overturns link between multiple sclerosis and whiplash. *British Medical Journal*. 1998;316:799.

Ciccone DS, Grzesiak RC. Psychological dysfunction in chronic cervical pain. In: Tollison CD, Satterthwaite JR, eds. *Painful Cervical Trauma*. Baltimore: Williams & Wilkins; 1992:89.

These authors point out that the premorbid personality in adoption of the sick role may include individuals who appear to be leading successful, rewarding social and work lives. They too may find motivation to adopt the sick role because it relieves them of overly burdensome responsibilities without losing social approval.

Clarke TD, Gragg CD, Sprouffske JF, et al. Human head linear and angular accelerations during impact. In: *Proceedings of the Fifteenth Stapp Car Crash Conference*. Paper #710857. Warrendale, PA: Society of Automotive Engineers; 1971:269–286.

In this study, the researchers subjected 14 human volunteers to frontal collisions with head accelerations exceeding 20*g*. Six of the 14 experienced minor, temporary headache, and they reported no chronic symptoms.

Claussen CF, Claussen E. Neurootological contributions to the diagnostic followup after whiplash injuries. *Acta Otolaryngolica*. 1995;520(suppl):53–56.

Clemens HJ, Burow K. Experimental investigation on injury mechanisms of cervical spine at frontal and rear-front vehicle impacts. In: *Proceedings of the Sixteenth Stapp Car Crash Conference*. Paper #720960. Warrendale, PA: Society of Automotive Engineers; 1972:76–102.

With a cadaver experiment, these researchers show that frontal and rear-end impacts can cause serious neck damage. One must note, however, that the forces that caused injury were in some cases 10 times (see Table 20–2 in Chapter 20) those whiplash patients usually experience in rear-end collisions. Further, cadavers suffer damage more easily than do living humans (see J. R. Cromack and H. H. Ziperman). One expects that the tolerable levels for cadavers are lower than those for living humans.

Cluff LE, Trever RW, Imboden JB, Canter A. Brucellosis. *Archives of Internal Medicine.* 1959;103:398–414.

Cobb LA, Thomas GI, Dillard DH, Merendino KA, Bruce RA. An evaluation of internal-mammary-artery ligation by a double-blind technique. *New England Journal of Medicine.* 1959;260(22):1115–1118.

These authors show that even surgery can have a placebo response. That a patient's neck pain, for example, improves or resolves after surgery does not necessarily prove that one has identified the cause of the patient's symptoms. Instead of in the neck, the cause may be somewhat higher.

Coffee MS, Edwards WT, Hayes WC, White AA. Biomechanical properties and strength of the human cervical spine. *Transactions of the American Society of Mechanical Engineers (Bioengineering Division).* 1987;3:71–72.

Cohen ML, Quintner JL. Fibromyalgia syndrome, a problem of tautology. *Lancet.* 1993;342:906–909.

Cohen ML, Quintner JL. Altered nociception, but not fibromyalgia, after cervical spine injury: comment on the article by Buskila et al. *Arthritis and Rheumatism.* 1998;41(1):183–190.

Cole ES. Psychiatric aspects of compensable injury. *Medical Journal of Australia.* 1970;1:93–100.

Colton CL. Whiplash injury and surgically treated cervical disc disease [letter]. *Injury.* 1994;25(6):409–410.

This author critiques A. J. Hamer et al's study. See also S. M. Barnes and A. D. Redmond et al.

Compere WE Jr. Electronystagmographic findings in patients with "whiplash" injuries. *Laryngoscope.* 1968;78:1226–1233.

Conte A, Caruso G, Mora R. Static and dynamic posturography in prevalent laterally directed whiplash injuries. *European Archives of Otorhinolaryngology.* 1997;254:186–192.

These authors show that whiplash claimants do have problems with posture control. Others have suggested this is because neck pain influences head and neck movements. In this study, much data are missing, including how long after the accident the authors evaluated the patients. (The longer after the accident, the more likely a new condition may be producing the postural problems.) The authors do not state what medications the patients used (this could affect postural control), and they had no control group of non–traumatic neck pain patients. It may be that the control group would have had the same postural problems. This would confirm that neck pain itself, of any cause, can lead to these problems. Indeed, M. Karlberg et al have shown this to be the case.

Cook JB. The post-concussional syndrome and factors influencing recovery after minor head injury admitted to hospital. *Scandinavian Medical Journal.* 1972;4:27–30.

Coppola AR. Neck injury, a reappraisal. *International Surgery.* 1968;50(6): 510–515.

Cornes P. Return to work of road accident victims claiming compensation for personal injury. *Injury.* 1992;23(4):256–260.

Crenshaw AH. Railroad back and other compensable injuries, 1890–1894. *The Bulletin.* May 1975:25–28.

Croft P, Schollum J, Silman A. Population study of tender point counts and pain as evidence of fibromyalgia. *British Medical Journal.* 1994;309:696–699.

Cromack JR, Ziperman HH. Three-point belt induced injuries: a comparison between laboratory surrogates and real world accident victims. *Proceedings of the Nineteenth Stapp Car Crash Conference. Paper* #751141. Warrendale, PA: Society of Automotive Engineers; 1975:1–24.

This experiment compares the injury outcomes of accident victims to damage in experimental collisions using cadavers. The authors found it much easier to damage a cadaver than to injure a living human at any given severity of collision. This means that cadaver experiments underestimate the capacity of people to resist injury in collisions, and one needs to keep this in mind in reviewing cadaver experiments. (See also J. Wismans et al.)

Crowe HE. Whiplash injuries of the cervical spine. In: *Section of Insurance, Negligence, and Compensation Law, Proceedings.* American Bar Association; 1958:176–184.

The orthopaedic surgeon who coined the term "whiplash" offers a dramatic example of how a straightening of the lordotic curve of the cervical spine on X-ray can be produced by anxiety alone (or already existed).

Crowe HE. A new diagnostic sign in neck injuries. *Insurance Counsel Journal.* July 1962;463–466.

Crowe HE. A new diagnostic sign in neck injuries. *California Medicine.* 1964; 100(1):12–13.

Cuetter AC, Bartoszek DM. The thoracic outlet syndrome: controversies, over-diagnosis, overtreatment, and recommendations for management. *Muscle and Nerve.* 1989;12:410–419.

This authors dispute thoracic outlet syndrome.

Cullum DE. Whiplash in Australia: illness or injury? [letter]. *Medical Journal of Australia.* 1992;157:428–429.

Culpan R, Taylor C. Psychiatric disorders following road traffic and industrial injuries. *Australian and New Zealand Journal of Psychiatry.* 1973;7:32–39.

Culver CC, Neathery RF, Mertz HJ. Mechanical necks with humanlike responses. In: *Proceedings of the Sixteenth Stapp Car Crash Conference.* Paper #720959. Warrendale, PA: Society of Automotive Engineers; 1972:61–75.

Dansak DA. On the tertiary gain of illness. *Comprehensive Psychiatry.* 1973;14(6):523–534.

Darragh FN, O'Connor P. Whiplash injury. *Journal of Neurology, Neurosurgery, and Psychiatry.* 1991;54(3):283–284.

Daube JR. Nerve conduction studies in the thoracic outlet syndrome. *Neurology.* 1975;25:347.

This author shows how erroneous it is to use nerve conduction studies as proof of thoracic outlet syndrome, as T. D. Capistrant attempted to do. The writings of M. Cherington et al, A. J. Wilbourn, and J. R. Youmans support Daube's statements.

Davidson HA. Neurosis and malingering. *American Journal of Medical Jurisprudence.* 1939;2:94–96.

This author reviews the basis for traumatic neurosis.

Davis AG. Injuries of the cervical spine. *Journal of the American Medical Association*. 1945;127(3):149–156.

This author provides one of the earliest proposed whiplash mechanisms. Unfortunately, the mechanism he proposed was completely contrary to every mechanism others proposed thereafter, and researchers have shown the radiologic findings he quotes to be irrelevant.

Davis SJ, Teresi LM, Bradley GB Jr, Ziemba MA, Bloze AE. Cervical spine hyperextension injuries: MR findings. *Radiology*. 1991;180:245–251.

These authors show some abnormalities that one can miss on plain X-rays but detect on magnetic resonance imaging (MRI) scans. The authors indicate that the lesions they found are evidence of the chronic damage responsible for reporting of chronic symptoms by thousands of whiplash patients. The abnormalities included, however, spondylosis (which we know exists in asymptomatic individuals) and disc protrusion (L. M. Teresi et al show one commonly sees this in asymptomatic controls). The data from this study also make it clear that there is no correlation between symptoms and these MRI findings, since all patients had symptoms, but only half had abnormal MRI findings.

An additional concern with this study is that some patients were apparently also not in accidents that typically produce whiplash patients but more severe accidents. See "MRI" in Chapter 5.

Deans GT, Magalliard JN, Kerr M, Rutherford WH. Neck sprain—a major cause of disability following car accidents. *Injury*. 1987;18:10–12.

These authors suggest that seat belts may increase the risk of developing neck pain after an accident. One should, however, see Chapter 22 for a review of this study.

Deans GT, Magalliard JN, Rutherford WH. Incidence and duration of neck pain among patients injured in car accidents. *British Medical Journal*. 1986;292:94–95.

De Boever JA, Keersmaekers K. Trauma in patients with temporomandibular disorders: frequency and treatment outcome. *Journal of Oral Rehabilitation*. 1996;23:91–96.

These authors discuss what they believe may be the mechanism of temporomandibular joint injury in whiplash patients. They neglect to mention R. P. Howard et al's work, however, which shows that mandibular whiplash has been disproven.

De Fonseka CP. Neck injuries in seatbelt wearers [letter]. *British Medical Journal*. 1977;1:168.

This author offers a critique of the article by M. S. Christian, who claims neck injury to be more common in seat belt wearers. See also Chapter 22.

DeGravelles WD, Kelley JH. *Injuries Following Rear-End Automobile Collisions.* Springfield, IL: Charles C Thomas; 1969.

These authors raise the important concern that many authors discuss ideas as to what *could* happen to the spine and neck structures, but without producing the objective evidence of the actual damage that remains chronic and produces chronic symptoms: "Many of them also did excellent jobs of describing the anatomy of the neck, with varied illustrations and x-rays, and one could find suggestions of the basic pathological anatomy as involving practically any of the structures of the head and neck from the thyroid cartilage posteriorly to the tips of the spinous processes, and from the coronal suture to the gluteal folds, depending upon what article was read."

These researchers also revealed from their studies of 137 patients with whiplash that "We are not impressed with the chances of cervical osteoarthritis being a common aggravating feature of neck pain following rear-end collisions. The median age of our group of patients with neck injuries was 41.7 years, with almost half (42%) being between 30 and 49 years of age. If cervical osteoarthritis was an important cause of neck pain . . . following rear-end collision, we would have expected an older age group in our study."

Dell'Osso LF, Daroff RB, Troost BT. Nystagmus and saccadic intrusions and oscillations. In: Duane TE, Jaeger EA, eds. *Clinical Ophthalmology.* Vol 2. London: JB Lippincott Company; 1988:13, 17.

This chapter deals with some forms of nystagmus that are actually normal rather than abnormal findings. Some early authors on whiplash attributed pathology to these findings.

de Mol BA, Heijer T. Late whiplash syndrome [letter]. *Lancet.* 1996;348:124–125.

Denker PG. The prognosis of insured neurotics. *New York State Journal of Medicine.* 1939;39(1):238–247.

DePalma AF, Rothman RH, Levitt RL, Hammond NL. The natural history of severe cervical disc degeneration. *Acta Orthopaedica Scandinavica.* 1972;43:392–396.

These authors show that even in patients with severe disc degeneration, psychological factors alter the natural history of pain reporting.

DePalma AF, Subin DK. Study of the cervical syndrome. *Clinical Orthopedics.* 1965;38:135–142.

DeRoy MS. Whiplash injuries. Fact or fallacy? *Medical Times*. 1963;91(10): 976–978.

De Simoni C, Wetz HH, Zanetti M, et al. Clinical examination and magnetic resonance imaging in the assessment of ankle sprains treated with an orthosis. *Foot and Ankle International*. 1996;17(3):177–182.

De Smet AA. Magnetic resonance findings in skeletal muscle tears. *Skeletal Radiology*. 1993;22:479–484.

De Smet AA, Fisher DR, Heiner JP, Keene JS. Magnetic resonance imaging of muscle tears. *Skeletal Radiology*. 1990;19:283–286.

These authors have shown that one can find significant muscle tears, new and old, in various sites of the body by magnetic resonance imaging (MRI) scans. Yet in studies of whiplash patients with MRI, researchers have rarely found significant tears. This implies that only minor sprains occur.

See also above.

De Wijer A, Steenks MH, Bosman F, Helders PJM, Faber J. Symptoms of the stomatognathic system in temporomandibular and cervical spine disorders. *Journal of Oral Rehabilitation*. 1996;23:733–741.

De Wijer A, Steenks MH, De Leeuw JRJ, Bosman F, Helders PJM. Symptoms of the cervical spine in temporomandibular and cervical spine disorders. *Journal of Oral Rehabilitation*. 1996;23:742–750.

Dinning TAR. Whiplash in Australia: illness or injury? [letter]. *Medical Journal of Australia*. 1993;158:138, 140.

This surgeon offers some blunt reasoning why one should not expect acute soft-tissue trauma to lead to reporting of chronic pain.

Di Stefano, Radanov BP. Course of attention and memory after common whiplash: a two-year prospective study with age, education and gender pair-matched patients. *Acta Neurologica Scandinavica*. 1995;91:346–352.

These authors confirm no long-term memory deficits in whiplash patients, regardless of the presence or absence of other symptoms.

Dolinis J. Risk factors for 'whiplash' in drivers: a cohort study of rear-end traffic crashes. *Injury*. 1997;28(3):173–179.

Domer FR, King Liu Y, Chandran KB, Krieger KW. Effect of hyperextension-hyperflexion (whiplash) on the function of the blood-brain barrier of rhesus monkeys. *Experimental Neurology*. 1979;63:304–310.

These researchers experimented with monkeys and demonstrated the possibility of some injury in tissues responsible for protecting the brain. The authors leap from this observation to the conclusion that this explains a whiplash patient's symptoms. This is erroneous as the experiment is with animals only, uses 35g accelerations (much higher than many collisions producing whiplash patients). As well, there is no evidence that such changes would occur in humans or that they would lead to symptoms.

Dorman TA. Whiplash injury [letter]. *Lancet*. 1991;338:1208.

Drace JE, Enzmann DR. Defining the normal temporomandibular joint: closed-, partially open-, and open-mouth MR imaging of asymptomatic subjects. *Radiology*. 1990;177:67–71.

Drottning M, Staff PH, Levin L, Malt UF. Acute emotional response to common whiplash predicts subsequent pain complaints. A prospective study of 107 subjects sustaining whiplash injury. *Nordic Journal of Psychiatry*. 1995;49: 293–299.

These authors indicate potential flaws with B. P. Radanov et al's research (see also O. Kwan and J. Friel). Their own research indicates that emotional factors predict symptom reporting at 4 weeks after the accident.

DuBois RA, McNally BF, DiGregorio JS, Phillips GJ. Low velocity car-to-bus test impacts. *Accident Reconstruction Journal*. 1996;8(5):44–51.

Dunn EJ, Blazar S. Soft-tissue injuries of the lower cervical spine. In: Griffin PP, ed. *Instructional Course Lectures*. American Academy of Orthopaedic Surgeons; 1987:499–512.

These authors give a general overview of whiplash, but many statements are potentially erroneous. For instance, the statement that "experimental and pathologic evidence and the mechanism and types of injuries have been delineated" is not valid. There is great doubt that most whiplash patients receive anything more than a minor muscle or ligament sprain (microscopic tears).

Dunsker SB. Hyperextension and hyperflexion injuries of the cervical spine. In: SB Dunsker, ed. *Seminars in Neurological Surgery: Cervical Spondylosis*. New York: Raven Press; 1981:135–143.

This author states that the pathology seen in the animal whiplash experiments is "impressive." That the author finds fracturing monkey and rabbit spines "impressive" does not mean that such pathology occurs in typical whiplash claimants.

Du Toit GT. The post-traumatic painful neck. *Forensic Science*. 1974;3:1–18.

Dvorák J. Soft-tissue injuries of the cervical spine (whiplash injuries): classification and diagnosis. In: Gunzburg R, Szpalski M, eds. *Whiplash Injuries. Current Concepts in Prevention, Diagnosis, and Treatment of the Cervical Whiplash Syndrome*. Philadelphia: Lippincott-Raven; 1998:53–60.

This author appears to misinterpret the findings of A. Otte et al with brain scan of whiplash patients. The author appears to believe that these scans might show evidence of brain injury in whiplash patients. In actuality, Otte et al found abnormal brain scans in posttraumatic and non–traumatic neck pain groups. Thus, trauma is not the cause of the findings. Instead, Otte et al explain that simply having neck pain (of any cause) will generate these abnormalities. There is no evidence of brain injury in whiplash patients.

Otherwise, the author is correct in suggesting that other psychological factors are responsible for cognitive symptoms in whiplash patients.

Dvorák J, Herdmann J, Janssen B, Theiler R, Grob D. Motor-evoked potentials in patients with cervical spine disorders. *Spine*. 1990;15(10):1013–1016.

These authors reveal abnormalities of a specific neurological test in whiplash patients as well as control populations of patients with disc degeneration and rheumatoid arthritis. There is no control population, however, of asymptomatic subjects from the general population, who may also happen to have these abnormalities, indicating there may actually be little correlation between abnormalities and symptoms. The study in no way confirms a specific nervous system injury in whiplash patients. Moreover, the patients are a referral group, and this may greatly affect the results.

Dvorák J, Valach L, Schmid S. Cervical spine injuries in Switzerland. *Journal of Manual Medicine*. 1989;4:7–16.

Eck DB. Flexion-extension injury of the cervical spine. *Journal of the Medical Society of New Jersey*. 1960;57:300–306.

Editorial. Are the 1956 cars safer? Consumers' *Research Bulletin*. 1956;37:16–19.

Editorial. Crashes cause most neck pain. *AMA News*. December 5, 1956:7.

Editorial. Neck injury and the mind. *Lancet*. 1991;338: 728–729.

This article (anonymous) deals with the argument that the neck pain of patients with whiplash is not at all psychological. The argument is made on the basis of MacNab's monkey-dropping experiments. One must note, however, the many flaws of MacNab's experiments and animal experiments in general (see "Whiplash Experiments" in Chapter 5), and this editorial author misinterprets Radanov et al's work to mean that psychological factors are not at all involved in reporting chronic pain.

Editorial. Railway spine. *Boston Medical and Surgical Journal*. 1883;109(17): 400.

Editorial. Therapy for whiplash: leave alone. *Medical World News*. 1962;3:69.

Elias F. Roentgen findings in the asymptomatic cervical spine. *New York State Journal of Medicine*. 1958;58:3300–3303.

This author shows that signs of disc degeneration on neck X-ray are common, and one should not attribute them to injury or symptoms since they are common in asymptomatic individuals.

Ellard J. Psychological reactions to compensable injury. *Medical Journal of Australia*. 1970;2:349–355.

Ellard J. Being sick and getting better. *Medical Journal of Australia*. 1974;1: 867–872.

This author offers a brief discussion of the sick role.

Ellerbroek WC. Whiplash injuries and cervical pain. *Headache*. 1966;6(2): 73–77.

Ellertsson AB, Sigurjonsson K, Thorsteinsson T. Clinical and radiographic study of 100 cases of whiplash injury. *Proceedings of the 22nd Scandinavian Congress of Neurology. Acta Neurologica Scandinavica Supplementum*. 1978; 67:269.

Ellis SJ. Tremor and other movement disorders after whiplash type injuries. *Journal of Neurology, Neurosurgery, and Psychiatry*. 1997;63:110–112.

The author considers the possibility that patients who report tremor after an accident might have some nervous system injury as the cause. The author does not consider, however, that the fact that a number of the patients developed their symptoms months later might mean they are completely unrelated to the accident. The author does not consider that they may be related to hysteria or anxiety (it still does occur, although this reaction was more fitting for the nineteenth century). As regards the possibility of secondary gain, the author appears to rule this out by stating that there did not appear to be motivation for monetary gain. He does not point out that there are many other forms of secondary gain.

Epstein JB. Temporomandibular disorders, facial pain and headache following motor vehicle accidents. *Canadian Dental Association Journal.* 1992;58(6): 488–495.

This article deals with jaw pain and whiplash, but such discussion of any possible mechanisms is theoretical. There are others who criticize these theories. See R. Ferrari et al, H. L. Goldberg, A. P. Heise et al, R. P. Howard et al, W. S. Kirk Jr, M. Olin, R. H. Roydhouse, E. W. Small, and D. H. West et al.

As well, the author states that temporomandibular joint injuries may accelerate degenerative changes in the osseous components of the joint, a phenomenon that researchers have never closely studied in whiplash patients and that remains unproven. See also Chapter 6.

Erichsen JE. *Railway and Other Injuries.* Philadelphia: Henry C Lea; 1867.

The book that started it all.

Erichsen JE. *Concussion of the Spine.* New York: William Wood and Company; 1886.

The book that kept the *train* rolling.

Erlandsson SI, Rubinstein B, Axelsson A, Carlsson SG. Psychological dimensions in patients with disabling tinnitus and craniomandibular disorders. *British Journal of Audiology.* 1991; 25:15–24.

Ernest EA III. The orthopedic influence of the TMJ apparatus in whiplash: report of a case. *General Dentistry.* 1979;27(2):62–64.

Ettlin TM, Kischka U, Reichmann S, et al. Cerebral symptoms after whiplash injury of the neck: a prospective clinical and neuropsychological study of whiplash injury. *Journal of Neurology, Neurosurgery, and Psychiatry.* 1992; 55:943–948.

These authors show the negative results of some objective tests and argue that many of the symptoms (like decrease in attention and concentration) that whiplash patients complain of could be due to pain itself and to depression.

These authors suggest that there may be an organic basis for whiplash symptoms as well. One must note, however, that researchers have shown brainstem auditory evoked potentials, which are an extremely sensitive tool for detecting the damage, to either be normal in whiplash patients or have the same changes as asymptomatic controls. See J. H. Noseworthy et al, J. M. S. Pearce, M. J. Rowe et al, J. J. Stockard et al, and P. R. Yarnell and G. V. Rossie.

Evans RW. Some observations on whiplash injuries. *Neurologic Clinics.* 1992;10(4):975–997.

This author provides a useful review of the history of whiplash.

Evans RW. Chronic whiplash syndrome [letter]. *Neurology.* 1995;45:2117.

Evans RW. Whiplash around the world. *Headache.* 1995;35:262–263.

Evans RW, Evans RI, Sharp MJ. The physician survey on the post-concussion and whiplash syndromes. *Headache.* 1994;34(5):268–274.

Ewing CL. Injury criteria and human tolerance for the neck. In: Saczalski K, ed. *Aircraft Crashworthiness.* Charlottesville, VA: University Press of Virginia; 1975:141–151.

Ewing CL, Thomas DJ. Torque versus angular displacement response of human head to −Gx impact acceleration. *Proceedings of the Seventeenth Stapp Car Crash Conference.* Paper #730976. Warrendale, PA: Society of Automotive Engineers; 1973:309–342.

Twelve volunteers tolerated head and neck hyperflexion forces of 320 newtons and hyperextension forces of 605 newtons with no symptoms. These forces may be higher than those experienced in some collisions producing whiplash patients.

Ewing CL, Thomas DJ, Beeler GW Jr, et al. Dynamic response of the head and neck of the living human to −Gx impact acceleration. *Proceedings of the Twelfth Stapp Car Crash Conference.* Paper #680792. Warrendale, PA: Society of Automotive Engineers; 1968:424–439.

These researchers studied volunteers in experimental rear-end collisions without head restraints and found that the volunteers tolerated peak head accelerations of greater than 47g. They also found that it did not matter at what height above the seat the head rested, since the amount of extension of the neck did not vary with sitting height. Further, there was no evidence of any electroencephalogram abnormalities in the subjects in almost 200 test runs.

Ewing CL, Thomas DJ, Beeler GW Jr, et al. Living human dynamic response to −Gx impact acceleration. *Proceedings of the Thirteenth Stapp Car Crash Con-*

ference. Paper #690817. Warrendale, PA: Society of Automotive Engineers; 1969:400–415.

See above.

Ewing CL, Thomas DJ, Lustik L. Multiaxis dynamic response of the human head and neck to impact acceleration. In: *Proceedings of the AGARD Conference 253, November 1978, France.* 1979:1–27.

Ewing CL, Thomas DJ, Lustick L, et al. The effect of the initial position of the head and neck on the dynamic response of the human head and neck to $-Gx$ impact acceleration. *Proceedings of the Nineteenth Stapp Car Crash Conference.* Paper #751157. Warrendale, PA: Society of Automotive Engineers; 1975:487–512.

These authors (see also below) demonstrate that nothing more than minor injury occurs in volunteers subjected to hyperflexion with accelerations similar to that in typical collisions producing whiplash patients.

Ewing CL, Thomas DJ, Lustick L, et al. The effect of duration, rate of onset, and peak sled acceleration on the dynamic response of the human head and neck. *Proceedings of the Twentieth Stapp Car Crash Conference.* Paper #760800. Warrendale, PA: Society of Automotive Engineers; 1976:3–41.

See above.

Ewing CL, Thomas DJ, Lustik L, et al. Dynamic response of the human head and neck to +Gy impact acceleration. *Proceedings of the Twenty First Stapp Car Crash Conference.* Paper #770928. Warrendale, PA: Society of Automotive Engineers; 1977:549–586.

These authors examine the effects of forces of collision that cause the neck to bend laterally (ear toward shoulder). They review similar previous experiments and show that even though the forces used in these experiments are 10 times that occurring in typical rear-end collisions producing whiplash patients, no significant injury occurs. See "Whiplash Experiments" in Chapter 5.

Ewing CL, Thomas DJ, Lustik L, et al. Effect of initial position on the human head and neck response to +Gy impact acceleration. *Proceedings of the Twenty Second Stapp Car Crash Conference.* Paper #780888. Warrendale, PA: Society of Automotive Engineers; 1978.

See above.

Ewing CL, Thomas DJ, Majewski PL, et al. Measurement of head, T1, and pelvic response to $-Gx$ impact acceleration. *Proceedings of the Twenty First Stapp*

Car Crash Conference. Paper #770927. Warrendale, PA: Society of Automotive Engineers; 1977:509–545.

See above.

Fagerlund M, Björnebrink J, Pettersson K, Hildingsson C. MRI in acute phase of whiplash injury. *European Radiology*. 1995;5:297–301.

These authors studied 39 whiplash patients 4 to 15 days after their accidents. One patient was actually found to have a muscle sprain on magnetic resonance imaging, as the imaging was done early enough. They found no evidence of acute trauma to the discs, bones, or joints. They were able to find evidence of minor ligament and muscle sprains in 3 cases.

Otherwise, all the other abnormalities are found in the same frequency as for asymptomatic controls. At most, these patients had minor sprains.

Farbman AA. Neck sprain. Associated factors. *Journal of the American Medical Association*. 1973;223(9):1010–1015.

This author noted that emotional and psychological factors are the ones most closely associated with an increased duration of symptoms after whiplash.

Farquhar D. Misconceived ideas [letter]. *Canadian Family Physician*. 1995; 41:563.

Fattori B, Borsari C, Vannucci G, et al. Acupuncture treatment for balance disorders following whiplash injury. *Acupuncture & Electro-Therapeutics Research International Journal*. 1996; 21:207–217.

Although the authors suggest acupuncture is effective in treating the chronic symptoms of whiplash patients, there are several potential flaws with the study. First, there is a small number of patients. Second, there may very well be a placebo effect. Third, the researchers have not demonstrated that the symptoms are actually a result of the accident and do not explain how long after the accident the symptoms had been present. (It may be that the patients think they are currently whiplash patients but actually are not.) Fourth, there is very short follow-up, and the authors do not indicate whether there was any measure of pain relief. The study falls far short of the type one needs before one could routinely recommend acupuncture over active treatments.

Faverjon G, Henry C, Thomas C, Tarriere C. Head and neck injuries for belted front occupants in real frontal crashes: patterns and risks. In: *Proceedings of the International IRCOBI Conference on the Biomechanics of Impacts, September 14–16, 1988, Bergisch, Gladbach, Germany. Bron, France*. 301–317.

Ferrari R. Rear-end auto collisions [letter]. *Archives of Physical Medicine and Rehabilitation.* 1998;79:721.

This is a commentary on Brault et al 1998. See Appendix 10.

Ferrari R. Whiplash-associated headache [letter]. *Cephalalgia.* 1998;18(8): 585–586.

Ferrari R. Comment on Polatin et al, Predictive value of Waddell's signs [letter]. *Spine.* 1999;24(3):306.

A discussion of the clinical application and meaning of Waddell's signs.

Ferrari R, Kwan O. Perceived physical and emotional trauma as precipitating events in fibromyalgia: Comment on article by Aaron et al [letter]. *Arthritis and Rheumatism.* April 1999. In press.

Ferrari R, Kwan O, Friel J. Illness behaviour and adoption of the sick role in whiplash claimants. *Forensics* [serial online]. 1999. In press. Available from http://www.acfe.com.

Ferrari R, Kwan O, Russell AS, Schrader H. The best approach to the problem of whiplash? One ticket to Lithuania, please. *Clinical and Experimental Rheumatology.* 1999. In press.

Ferrari R, Leonard M. Whiplash and temporomandibular disorders. *Journal of the American Dental Association.* 1998;129: 1739–1745.

Ferrari R, Russell AS. The whiplash syndrome—common sense revisited. *Journal of Rheumatology.* 1997;24(4):618–623.

Ferrari R, Russell AS. Authors' reply [letter]. *Journal of Rheumatology.* 1998;25(7):1438–1440.

Ferrari R, Russell AS. Neck injury and chronic pain syndromes: comment on article by Buskila et al [letter]. *Arthritis and Rheumatism.* 1998;41(4):758–759.

Ferrari R, Russell AS. A rheumatologist's pain in the neck. *Scandinavian Journal of Rheumatology.* 1998. In press.

Ferrari R, Russell AS. Development of persistent neurological symptoms in patients with simple neck sprain. *Arthritis Care & Research.* 1999;12(1): 70–75.

Ferrari R, Russell AS. Epidemiology of whiplash—an international dilemma. *Annals of Rheumatic Diseases.* 1999;58:1–5.

A review of the cultural variances in the epidemiology of whiplash—why some cultures are whiplash cultures while others are not.

Ferrari R, Russell AS. Whiplash—heading for higher ground. A point of view. *Spine.* 1999;24(1):97–98.

Ferrari R, Schrader H, Obelieniene D. Prevalence of temporomandibular disorders associated with whiplash injury in Lithuania. *Oral Surgery, Oral Medicine, Oral Pathology.* 1999. In press.

Field H. Post-traumatic syndrome [letter]. *Journal of the Royal Society of Medicine.* 1981;74:630.

This author disputes the conclusions of R. Kelly's writings on this subject.

Fields A. The autonomic nervous system in whiplash injuries. *International Record of Medicine.* 1956;169(1):8–10.

Fineman S, Borrelli FJ, Rubinstein BM, Epstein H, Jacobson HG. The cervical spine: transformation of the normal lordotic pattern into a linear pattern in the neutral posture. *Journal of Bone and Joint Surgery.* 1963;45-A(6):1179–1206.

These authors show that a straight or even kyphotic cervical spine on X-ray can be entirely normal, regardless of the view one uses for the X-ray. They also show that slight variations in technique can change the shape of the cervical curve on X-ray. Thus, one cannot consider these X-ray changes as evidence for the existence of chronic neck damage from an acute injury.

Fischer AJEM, Huygen PLM, Folgering HT, Verhagen WIM, Theunissen EJJM. Hyperactive VOR and hyperventilation after whiplash injury. *Acta Otolaryngolica (Stockholm).* 1995;520 (suppl):49–52.

These authors confirm the view that one can link visual and balance disturbances to neck pain as the probable cause rather than a nervous system injury.

Fischer AJEM, Verhagen WIM, Huygen PLM. Whiplash injury. A clinical review with emphasis on neuro-otological aspects. *Clinical Otolaryngology.* 1997; 22:192–201.

These authors review all of the studies considering why whiplash patients report symptoms such as dizziness, vertigo, or hearing disturbances. The authors point out that many studies have several major flaws or biases. They add that there is yet no evidence that actual nervous system injury occurs in whiplash patients to cause such symptom reporting. They also point to evidence that considers that emotional distress is likely to be acting in some cases of reporting of these symptoms.

See also "Disturbances of Balance and Hearing" in Chapter 7.

Fishbain DA. Secondary gain concept. Definition problems and its abuse in medical practice. *American Pain Society Journal.* 1994;3(4):264–273.

Fite JD. Neuro-ophthalmologic syndromes in automobile accidents. *Southern Medical Journal.* 1970;63:567–570.

Fitzgerald DC. Head trauma: hearing loss and dizziness. *Journal of Trauma.* 1996;40(3):488–496.

This is a good general review, but the author has made some possible errors in a brief discussion of some engineering aspects of whiplash injury. He quotes a 5g acceleration as being capable of causing injury. In actuality, it is the same acceleration experienced in sneezing (see M. E. Allen et al). A review of the entire literature on whiplash experiments (see "Whiplash Experiments" in Chapter 5) shows that such a head acceleration in a volunteer does not cause injury. It is also interesting that none of the volunteer experiments have resulted in an individual reporting chronic symptoms, even though it is relatively easy to reproduce acute symptoms.

Finally, the symptom of dizziness in whiplash patients is unlikely to be due to a nervous system injury. See also "Disturbances of Balance and Hearing" in Chapter 7.

Fitz-Ritzon D. Assessment of cervicogenic vertigo. *Journal of Manipulative and Phsyiological Therapeutics.* 1991;14(3): 193–198.

The author of this study suggests that chiropractic treatment can relieve the sensations of vertigo seen in some accident victims. There is no control group, however, so there is no accounting for the natural resolution over time, and of course no accounting for placebo effect (ie, the author could have had a group where a "sham" chiropractic adjustment or manipulation was done).

Flax HJ, Fernández B, Rodríguez-Ramón A. The "whiplash" injury. *Boletin Asociacion medica de Puerto Rico.* 1971;63(6): 161–165.

Fleming JFR. The neurosurgeon's responsibility in "whiplash" injuries. *Clinical Neurosurgery.* 1973;20:242–252.

The author points out that the severe and often traumatic handling of soft tissues of the neck during neurosurgical procedures does not result in any chronic symptoms. This raises the question of why patients with whiplash and minor trauma should report chronic symptoms.

Foley-Nolan D, Moore K, Codd M, et al. Low energy high frequency pulsed electromagnetic therapy for acute whiplash injury. *Scandinavian Journal of Rehabilitation Medicine.* 1992;24:51–59.

In this study, the authors confirm that laser therapy is no better than placebo at 12 weeks follow-up in whiplash patients. See Quebec Task Force on Whiplash-Associated Disorders (W. O. Spitzer et al).

Foley-Nolan D, O'Connor P. Whiplash injury [letter]. *Journal of Neurology, Neurosurgery, and Psychiatry.* 1991;54(3):283–284.

Ford CV. *The Somatizing Disorders. Illness as a Way of Life.* New York: Elsevier Biomedical; 1983.

This text deals with the concepts behind illness behavior. It also addresses the effects of the individual's personality, societal views on illness, and patient–physician interaction in contributing to and modifying illness behavior.

Foreman SM, Croft AC. *Whiplash Injuries. The Cervical Acceleration/Deceleration Syndrome.* Baltimore: Williams & Wilkins; 1988.

This text includes a very good, thorough discussion on many aspects of accident injury. However, there are a number of aspects missing from the text, namely a discussion of the large body of literature surrounding the psychological aspects of whiplash and a thorough review of the human volunteer experiments.

Foreman SM, Croft AC. *Whiplash Injuries. The Cervical Acceleration/Deceleration Syndrome.* Baltimore: Williams & Wilkins; 1995.

See above.

Foret-Bruno JY, Tarriere C, Le Coz JY, et al. Risk of cervical lesions in real-world and simulated collisions. In: *Proceedings of the Thirty Fourth Conference of the American Association of Automotive Medicine, Scottsdale, Arizona.* 1990:373–389.

Forsyth HF. Extension injuries of the cervical spine. *Journal of Bone and Joint Surgery.* 1964;46-A(8):1792–1797.

Foster LJ. Traumatic neurosis. *American Journal of Roentgenology.* 1933;30(1): 44–50.

Foust DR, Chaffin DB, Snyder RG, Baum JK. Cervical range of motion and dynamic response and strength of cervical muscles. In: *Proceedings of the Seventeenth Stapp Car Crash Conference*. Paper #730975. Warrendale, PA: Society
of Automotive Engineers; 1973:285–308.

In this study of human neck muscle reflexes in response to extension or flexion, the authors suggest that at high velocity rear-end collisions, muscle reflexes
may not be protective. That is, the higher the velocity of collision, the less likely
the muscle reflex will act in time to protect the neck. One must note, however,
that they determined this for collision velocities of 30 mph only and that many
whiplash patients are in collisions of much lower velocities. If one needs such
high velocities to negate the protective muscular reflex, then it is quite likely that
at lower velocities of collision (which produce most whiplash patients) the reflexes are likely protective.

Frankel CJ. Medical-legal aspect of injuries to the neck. *Journal of the American
Medical Association*. 1959;169(3):216–223.

Frankel VH. Temporomandibular joint pain syndrome following deceleration injury to the cervical spine. *Bulletin of the Hospital for Joint Diseases*. 1965;26:
47–51.

This author gives one of the earliest descriptions of a theory of temporomandibular joint injury in whiplash patients. One must note, however, that
the statement "when an automobile is struck from behind . . . the mouth flies open
. . . [and then] the jaw snaps shut" was without data to support it. Since then, R. P.
Howard et al and D. H. West et al have shown that this theory is not valid. See
also R. Ferrari et al, H. L. Goldberg, A. P. Heise et al, W. S. Kirk Jr, M. Olin,
R. H. Roydhouse, and E. W. Small.

Frankel VH. Whiplash injuries to the neck. In: Hirsch C, Zotterman Y, eds. *Cervical Pain*. Oxford, England: Pergamon Press; 1971:97–112.

Frankel VH. Pathomechanics of whiplash injuries to the neck. In: Morley TP, ed.
Current Controversies in Neurosurgery. Philadelphia: WB Saunders; 1976:
39–50.

Frankel VH. Comments on soft tissue injuries of the neck. In: *Head and Neck Injury Criteria. A Consensus Workshop. National Highway Traffic Safety Administration*, 1981, March 26–27, Washington, DC. 1981:121–122.

Frankel summarizes his ideas on whiplash over the years, packing the discussion with theory and conjecture.

Fredin Y, Elert J, Britschgi N, et al. A decreased ability to relax between repetitive muscle contractions in patients with chronic symptoms after whiplash trauma of the neck. *Journal of Musculoskeletal Pain*. 1997;5(2):55–70.

These authors found more muscle tension in whiplash claimants as compared to controls, but they could not determine whether this was due to neck damage, psychological factors, abnormal posture, or combinations of these. To do so, they would need control groups such as chronic neck pain patients who are not whiplash victims and patients with psychological distress who are not complaining of neck pain. They would also need to correct abnormal posture. As well, many of the claimants had their accidents years before the study. That they yet attribute their pain to the accident does not make this attribution valid. Neck pain exists in the general population, and there could be many reasons for these patients to have neck pain that have nothing to do with whiplash injury. It is important to conduct such studies within weeks of the accident.

Freed S, Fishman Hellerstein L. Visual electrodiagnostic findings in mild traumatic brain injury. *Brain Injury*. 1997;11(1):25–36.

These authors conducted a study of 50 patients with so-called mild traumatic brain injury to see if visual complaints were related to any nervous system or eye damage. Using specialized techniques, the authors found that indeed some patients had abnormalities of eye function. What this means, in terms of the whiplash claimant reporting these symptoms, is not clear. They do not state how long after the accident they evaluated the patients (ie, if it was weeks, months, or years after the accident, there is the opportunity for new events to have led to these abnormal findings). They do not state if they checked the patients' records for any preaccident complaints, and they do not state how often these abnormalities are found in a control group (the general population) complaining of similar visual symptoms. It may be that the accident is not the risk factor for developing such complaints.

As such, this study does not prove that whiplash claimants actually suffer any eye or brain injury.

Freeman MD, Croft AC. Late whiplash syndrome [letter]. *Lancet*. 1996;348:125.

Freeman MD, Croft AC, Rossignol AM. "Whiplash associated disorders: redefining whiplash and its management" by the Quebec Task Force. A critical evaluation. *Spine*. 1998;23:1043–1049.

A fair, albeit sometimes irrelevant, critique of the methodology of the Quebec Task Force. The authors' key point is that the Quebec Task Force underestimates how severe whiplash injury really is and how poor the outcome is. This may be true. It draws attention, even more, however, to how disparate the outcomes are between North America and Germany, Greece, and Lithuania. These differences are important and require an explanation.

Friedenberg ZB, Broder HA, Edeiken JE, Spencer HN. Degenerative disk disease of cervical spine. *Journal of the American Medical Association.* 1960;174(4): 375–380.

The authors examined a group of patients with cervical spondylosis to determine any correlation between the clinical course and to note any correlation between the clinical and the X-ray findings. They found that "there was . . . no correlation between the intensity of pain and the degree of [radiographically] visible changes at the involved cervical disk level."

Friedenberg ZB, Miller WT. Degenerative disc disease of the cervical spine. A comparative study of asymptomatic and symptomatic patients. *Journal of Bone and Joint Surgery.* 1963;45-A(6):1171–1178.

The authors compared 160 asymptomatic individuals with an equal number of symptomatic individuals between age 30 and 70. They found that:

> In each group, the highest incidence of change [on X-ray] was between the fifth and sixth and sixth and seventh vertebral bodies.
>
> No significant difference was apparent either in the incidence or in the severity of these degenerative changes.
>
> It was our hope that some roentgen findings could be designated as a probable cause of symptoms. However, comparing the symptomatic with the asymptomatic individuals, there was essentially no difference between them in our series. . . .
>
> Our findings cast doubt on the relative value of roentgenograms in determining the clinical significance of degenerative disease of the cervical spine.

There is, therefore, no difference between patients with neck pain and those without in the X-ray findings of the neck. Thus, X-ray findings do not provide a basis for the symptoms.

Friedman AP, Ransohoff J. Post-traumatic headache. *Trauma.* 1964;5:33–61.

This article reviews the concepts that theories of the anatomical basis for post-traumatic headache have no basis in fact, that posttraumatic headache seldom occurs after recreational activities, and that individuals who were neurotic prior to the accident have the highest incidence of headaches.

Frost FA, Jessen B, Siggaard-Andersen J. A control, double-blind comparison of mepivacaine injection versus saline injection for myofascial pain. *Lancet.* March 1980:499–500.

Furman JM, Jacob RG. Psychiatric dizziness. *Neurology.* 1997;48:1161–1166.

Gadd CW, Culver CC. A study of responses and tolerances of the neck. In: *Proceedings of the Fifteenth Stapp Car Crash Conference.* Warrendale, PA: Society of Automotive Engineers; 1971:256.

In lateral flexion studies, the researchers subjected cadavers to head and neck forces up to 290 newtons without damage to the cadavers. Although these forces are near those one encounters in typical collisions producing whiplash patients, this particular study was able to produce injury above 290 newtons only by fixing the neck in a position in which it was bent more than 20° toward the left ear. Since most people do not drive in this position, the results would not be applicable to whiplash patients in any case. As well, cadaver experiments underestimate resistance to injury because the tissues have lost the properties of living tissue, and supportive tissues are lacking (see J. R. Cromack and H. H. Ziperman and J. Wismans et al).

Galasko CSB, Murray PM, Pitcher M, et al. Neck sprains after road traffic accidents: a modern epidemic. *Injury.* 1993;24(3): 155–157.

Garcia R Jr, Arrington JA. The relationship between cervical whiplash and temporomandibular joint injuries: an MRI study. *Journal of Craniomandibular Practice.* 1996;14(3):233–239.

Although these authors find a high incidence of abnormalities on temporomandibular joint (TMJ) imaging in whiplash patients compared to controls, there are a number of concerns in the study. First, the patients are part of a referral group, with the potential for selection bias and concentration of abnormal findings. More important, however, identifying an imaging abnormality does not immediately prove that the abnormality is due to an injury, or that it is the cause of pain. Indeed, the epidemiological literature is replete with associations researchers find in retrospective studies like this one, which, when one does proper prospective studies, disappear. Moreover, demonstrating an association is not the same as demonstrating a causal relationship.

As well, the authors of the study do not state how long after the accident the symptoms of so-called "TMJ dysfunction" actually began. It may be that the symptoms and signs do not relate to any accident event, especially if the symptoms arose months later.

The authors do not consider that an alteration in jaw muscle activity may create abnormalities over time (see B. A. Loughner et al 1996). If the imaging abnormalities occur often in individuals with no symptoms, why conclude that an alteration in jaw muscle activity is the cause of symptoms in whiplash patients?

The authors also appear to assume that if patients state that they had no preaccident symptoms, then they did not have any preaccident symptoms. Insurance fraud does exist, and it is also possible that patients do not recall preaccident symptoms that are now amplified as the patients have become hypervigilant since the accident. There exists a high frequency of TMJ symptoms in the general population, many cases not having a history of trauma. These whiplash claimants were once part of the general population. How did they all just happen to be the members of the general population that had no TMJ symptoms before the accident?

Finally, the authors present a theory of TMJ injury that R. P. Howard et al have since disproved. See also R. Ferrari et al, H. L. Goldberg, A. P. Heise et al, W. S. Kirk Jr, M. Olin, R. H. Roydhouse, E. W. Small, and D. H. West et al.

Gargan MF. What is the evidence for an organic lesion in whiplash injury? *Journal of Psychosomatic Research*. 1995; 39(6):777–781.

The author states that there is indirect evidence for a physical lesion in whiplash, from studies that show an acceleration of disc degeneration in whiplash patients. The author, however, may not realize that one study he references (A. Watkinson et al) has a number of potential flaws, and the other reference (turns out to be a reference to a book that referenced another article), when one actually pursues it, makes no such claim.

Moreover, the author has not examined the other numerous studies that have conclusions opposite those of Watkinson et al. (See "Radiology of Whiplash" in Chapter 5.)

Gargan MF, Bannister GC. Long-term prognosis of soft-tissue injuries of the neck. *Journal of Bone and Joint Surgery*. 1990;72-B:901–903.

Gargan MF, Bannister GC. Soft tissue injuries to the neck [letter]. *British Medical Journal*. 1991;303:786.

Gargan MF, Bannister GC. The rate of recovery following whiplash injury. *European Spine Journal*. 1994;3:162–164.

Gargan MF, Bannister GC, Main C, Hollis S. The behavioural response to whiplash injury. *Journal of Bone and Joint Surgery [British]*. 1997;79-B: 523–526.

This article deals with a study that demonstrated that many whiplash patients become psychologically distressed within the first 3 months of their accident. The authors do not discuss, however, the many psychological factors that might be involved but focus chiefly on litigation and monetary issues. The authors do not state whether the reporting of chronic pain is due to ongoing physical damage from the acute injury or due to a variety of other factors (including, for example, the tendency to amplify and misattribute pain to the accident). They also do not state whether the psychological distress itself can alter pain reporting.

As well, they do not consider whether individuals who have just been in an accident (like many individuals, even those not in a car accident) might underreport psychological distress from their life, but later admit to it, this time because they have a socially acceptable reason (distress due to chronic pain) upon which they can deposit all their preaccident miseries.

Garmoe W. Rear-end collisions [letter]. *Archives of Physical Medicine and Rehabilitation*. 1998;79:1024.

Gates EM, Cento D. Studies in cervical trauma. Part 1. *International Surgery*. 1966;46(3):218–222.

Gay JR, Abbott KH. Common whiplash injuries of the neck. *Journal of the American Medical Association*. 1953;152(18):1698–1704.

These authors give one of the earlier descriptions of whiplash symptoms. This article is also a very good example of how conjecture can lead one astray. These authors thought hyperflexion was the first event after a rear-end collision, that cars hit in rear-end collisions were traveling several hundred feet, and that the human head and neck could oscillate back and forth. J. H. Schaefer would later comment on how incorrect their ideas were.

Gebhard JS, Donaldson DH, Brown CW. Soft-tissue injuries of the cervical spine. *Orthopaedic Review*. May 1994;(suppl):9–17.

Geigl BC, Steffan H, Leinzinger P, Roll, Mühlbauer M, Bauer G. The movement of head and cervical spine during rearend impact. In: *Proceedings of the International IRCOBI Conference on the Biomechanics of Impact, 1994, Lyon, France*. 127–137.

Gelber LJ. Medico-legal aspects of whiplash injuries. *Mississippi Valley Medical Journal*. 1956;78:215–216.

Gelber LJ. Medico-legal aspects of whiplash injuries. *Nassau Medical News*. 1956;28(8):1–6.

Gennarelli TA, Segawa H, Wald U, et al. Physiological response to angular acceleration of the head. In: Grossman RG, Gildenberg PL, eds. *Head Injury: Basic and Clinical Aspects*. New York: Raven Press, 1982:128–140.

This chapter deals with animal experiments producing head acceleration to assess the threshold for brain injury. The authors indicate that one has to exceed accelerations of more than 45*g* to cause detectable brain injury. This greatly exceeds the acceleration that whiplash patients usually experience. Moreover, the duration of the acceleration was longer than one expects in whiplash patients, and the range of head movement (60° rotation) far exceeds that in volunteer experiments. Thus, there is no experimental evidence that the types of collisions producing whiplash patients are capable of producing brain injury.

B. P. Radanov et al (1996) have explained that the symptoms others sometimes attribute to brain injury in whiplash patients are not due to physical injury but to noninjurious factors. See "Disturbance of Cognition" in Chapter 7.

Gennis P, Miller L, Gallagher EJ, et al. The effect of soft cervical collars on persistent neck pain in patients with whiplash injury. *Academic Emergency Medicine*. 1996;3(6):568–573.

The authors of this study compare treatment with rest, analgesia, and collar to rest and analgesia alone. They found that collar use offered no advantage.

Gibbs FA. Objective evidence of brain disorder in cases of whiplash injury. *Clinical Electroencephalography*. 1971;2(2):107–110.

These authors suggest that electroencephalogram studies might prove the basis for some whiplash symptoms to be organic. The works of T. M. Ettlin et al, E. S. Gurdjian and L. M. Thomas, and D. E. Jacome and M. Risko dispute this notion altogether.

Gibson WJ. The eye and whiplash injuries. *Journal of the Florida State Medical Association*. 1968;55(10):917–918.

This author reports 3 cases of abnormalities on eye examination of patients complaining of whiplash. He presents a theoretical basis for the cause of ocular injury from whiplash. One must note, however, that there were no preaccident examinations and no discussion of the incidence of these abnormalities in asymptomatic individuals. The conclusions are therefore doubtful.

Gillies GT. Temporomandibular joint injury potential imposed by the low-velocity extension-flexion maneuver [letter]. *Journal of Oral and Maxillofacial Surgery*. 1995;53:263.

Gimse R, Bjørgen IA, Straume A. Driving skills after whiplash. *Scandinavian Journal of Psychology*. 1997;38:165–170.

The difficulties in driving are likely due to difficulties with neck movements and perhaps the effects of having pain. One could also modify these skills, however, by intentional lack of effort or drugs (stopping drug use on the day of the test does not necessarily remove the effects of the drug). It is also difficult to prove or disprove the reported difficulties.

Gimse R, Bjørgen IA, Tjell C, Tyssedal JS, Bø K. Reduced cognitive functions in a group of whiplash patients with demonstrated disturbances in the posture control system. *Journal of Clinical and Experimental Neuropsychology*. 1997;19(6):838–849.

These authors suggest that the abnormal posture control of the neck influences reading technique, partly as a distractor, or interfering with the automation of reading. They plan to study whiplash patients without postural control problems, however, to see if this connection is valid. In either case, they are indicating that there is no evidence of brain damage as a cause for cognitive dysfunction in whiplash patients. They also indicate that pain, depression, and medications may be important factors generating these symptoms.

Gimse R, Tjell C, Bjørgen IA, Saunte C. Disturbed eye movements after whiplash due to injuries to the posture control system. *Journal of Clinical and Experimental Neuropsychology*. 1996;18(2):178–186.

These authors confirm the possibility that neck pain, in affecting neck posture and movements, may be responsible for dizziness and reading problems in whiplash patients. There is no evidence of a nervous system injury as the reason for these symptoms in whiplash patients. See also "Disturbance of Vision" in Chapter 7.

Girling WNM. Whiplash injuries. Their effect on accommodation convergence, peripheral and central field together with treatment used. Concilium Ophthalmologicum (Belgium). 1958;18(2):1550–1557.

The author claims to have identified a nervous system injury responsible for visual symptoms in whiplash patients. One must note, however, that there are many potential flaws with this study and studies like it, as pointed out in "Radiology of Whiplash" in Chapter 5.

Gissane W. The causes and the prevention of neck injuries to car occupants. *Annals of the Royal College of Surgeons of England*. 1966;39:161–163.

Gissane W. Seat belts and head rests [letter]. *British Medical Journal*. 1972;2:288.
This letter to the editor criticizes the article by I. W. Caldwell.

Gissane W, Bull JP. A seat belt syndrome? [letter]. *British Medical Journal*. 1974;1:394.

Giebel GD, Edelmann M, Huser R. Neck sprain: physiotherapy versus collar treatment. *Zentralblatt fur Chirurgie*. 1997;122(7):517–521.

Goff CW, Alden JO. *Traumatic Cervical Syndrome and Whiplash*. Philadelphia: JB Lippincott Company; 1964.
These authors review some of the topics concerning whiplash. Research had (even by 1964), however, shown some of their statements regarding the radiology of whiplash to be incorrect.

Goldberg AL, Rothfus WE, Deeb ZL, et al. The impact of magnetic resonance imaging on the diagnostic evaluation of acute cervicothoracic spinal trauma. *Skeletal Radiology*. 1988;17:89–95.
See below.

Goldberg AL, Rothfus WE, Deeb ZL, et al. Hyperextension injuries of the cervical spine. *Skeletal Radiology*. 1989;18:283–288.
This study of 11 patients, some of whom had falls rather than motor vehicle accidents, shows that hyperextension can lead to fractures and spinal cord injury that one can detect by magnetic resonance imaging. This does not, however, verify that whiplash patients have some form of this type of injury.

Goldberg HL. Trauma and the improbable anterior displacement. *Journal of Craniomandibular Disorders: Facial and Oral Pain*. 1990;4(2):131–134.
This author refutes the theories of S. Weinberg and others of temporomandibular joint injury in rear-end collisions. See also the work of R. Ferrari et al, A. P. Heise et al, R. P. Howard et al, W. S. Kirk Jr, M. Olin, R. H. Roydhouse, E. W. Small, T. J. Szabo et al, and D. H. West et al.

Goldberg MB, Mock D, Ichise M, et al. Neuropsychologic deficits and clinical features of posttraumatic temporomandibular disorders. *Journal of Orofacial Pain*. 1996;10:126–140.
This study is of limited use because the total number of patients is only 27, divided into two groups. Such small numbers, unless they definitely represent the larger population of patients, are unreliable.

Golding DN. Whiplash injuries. *British Journal of Rheumatology*. 1992;32(2): 174.

This author offers another theory regarding neck pain in whiplash, although it is not a concept with support elsewhere.

Goldney RD. "Not cured by verdict": A re-evaluation of the literature. *Australian Journal of Forensic Science*. 1989;20:295–300.

This author reviews previous studies that examine the effects of settlement on recovery from whiplash symptoms. Goldney reminds readers that one cannot generalize about such issues, in that clearly there are some individuals in which settlement improves their symptoms and others in which settlement has no impact. There are many other psychological factors besides the secondary gains of compensation that could potentially perpetuate the illness in those patients not improving with settlement.

Gordon DA. The rheumatologist and chronic whiplash syndrome. *Journal of Rheumatology*. 1997;24(4):617–618.

Gore DR, Sepic SB, Gardner GM. Roentgenographic findings of the cervical spine in asymptomatic people. *Spine*. 1986;11(6):521–524.

In this study, the authors show that changes in cervical lordosis or even kyphosis of the cervical spine do not correlate with symptoms and that one often finds these in asymptomatic individuals. Also see article below.

Gore DR, Sepic SB, Gardner GM, Murray MP. Neck pain: a long-term follow-up of 205 patients. *Spine*. 1987;12(1):1–5.

These researchers followed 205 patients for durations varying from 10 to 25 years. Half of them were patients who had claimed some form of neck injury, and the others had spontaneous neck pain without any history of trauma. The researchers had several important findings. First, they looked at patients (from both groups) who had normal X-rays at the beginning of the study, and the researchers checked their X-rays years later. They found no difference in the number of patients who went on to develop degenerative changes in each group. Thus, whiplash patients developed the same X-ray changes as they grew older as did non–whiplash patients. A prior study by these authors and others noted that most people develop degenerative changes in their neck at a rate similar to that of whiplash patients and other patients with neck pain.

Second, they found that whiplash patients with abnormal X-rays at the beginning of the study developed further changes at no greater rate than patients without injury.

Finally, they found absolutely no difference in the prognosis for patients with abnormal X-rays and for those with normal X-rays. Each group had the same incidence of symptoms and outcome. Thus, an abnormal X-ray at the onset or the development of an abnormal X-ray later has no effect on prognosis. This study suggests, then, that one cannot predict a worse prognosis because of an abnormal X-ray. The X-ray findings are irrelevant to outcome.

This means that there is no basis for claiming a greater degree of disability or worse long-term prognosis on the basis of X-ray findings.

Gorman WF. The alleged whiplash "injury." *Arizona Medicine*. 1974;31(6):411–413.

Gorman WF. "Whiplash": fictive or factual? *Bulletin of the American Academy of Psychiatry and Law*. 1979;7:245–248.

Gorman W. Whiplash—a neuropsychiatric injury. *Arizona Medicine*. 1974;31(6): 414–416.

Gosch HH, Gooding E, Schneider RC. An experimental study of cervical spine and cord injuries. *Journal of Trauma*. 1972;12(2):570–576.

These authors show that if you ram a monkey's head into a steel plate hard enough, you can cause injury.

Gotten N. Survey of one hundred cases of whiplash injury after settlement of litigation. *Journal of the American Medical Association*. 1956;162(9):865–867.

This represents one of the early articles dealing with psychological factors affecting whiplash patients.

Gough JP. Human occupant dynamics in low-speed rear end collisions: an engineering perspective. *Journal of Musculoskeletal Pain*. 1996;4(4):11–19.

This is an excellent review of the literature on low-velocity collisions. One does not expect physical injury in most of them. If physical injury does occur, symptoms last for just hours to days.

Grader JN, Panjabi MM, Cholewicki J, Nibu K, Dvorak J. Whiplash produces an S-shaped curvature of the neck with hyperextension at lower levels. *Spine*. 1997;22:2489–2494.

Graham GJ, Butler DS. Whiplash in Australia: illness or injury? [letter]. *Medical Journal of Australia*. 1992;157:429.

Greco CM, Rudy TE, Turk DC, Herlich A, Zaki HH. Traumatic onset of temporomandibular disorders: positive effects of a standardized conservative treatment program. *Clinical Journal of Pain*. 1997;13:337–347.

This study examines an interesting group of patients, all nonlitigants, noncompensated patients. With this group of patients, the authors found no difference in response to treatment between those with temporomandibular disorder (TMD) following trauma and those with TMD not following trauma.

Greenfield J, Ilfeld FW. Acute cervical strain. *Clinical Orthopedics and Related Research.* 1977;122:196–200.

Gregory GF, Crockett DJ. Chronic benign pain syndrome: A legal and psychological overview. *Advocate.* 1988;46(3):369–378.

These authors discuss illness behavior and adoption of the sick role in whiplash patients as well as issues of compensability.

Griffiths HJ, Olson PN, Everson LI, Winemiller BA. Hyperextension strain or "whiplash" injuries to the cervical spine. *Skeletal Radiology.* 1995;24: 263–266.

In this study, the authors suggest methods by which one can detect ligamentous tears in whiplash patients. However, they do not use an objective technique to determine if they are correct, such as verifying the existence of a tear in whiplash patients by magnetic resonance imaging (MRI) or bone scan. Also, they conducted a retrospective study on a selected group of whiplash patients, which raises significant concerns.

There is no clear proof that significant ligamentous tears are occurring in most whiplash patients, and human and animal experiments do not find evidence of significant ligamentous tears but rather minor tears in experimental collisions using forces whiplash patients typically experience. See Tables 20–1 to 20–4 in Chapter 20.

Also, the numerous MRI studies on whiplash patients reveal that such significant tears seldom occur. See "MRI" in Chapter 5.

Gross A, Gale EN. A prevalence study of the clinical signs associated with mandibular dysfunction. *Journal of the American Dental Association.* 1983; 107:932–936.

This study of the general population indicates that a number of the symptoms or signs of so-called "temporomandibular joint disorders," especially joint clicking, are common in the general population and should thus not necessarily be attributed to disease or injury.

Grunsten RC, Gilbert NS, Mawn SV. The mechanical effects of impact acceleration on the unconstrained human head and neck complex. *Contemporary Orthopaedics.* 1989;18(2):199–202.

Grzesiak RC. Psychologic considerations in temporomandibular dysfunction. *Dental Clinics of North America*. 1991;35(1): 209–226.

Grzesiak RC, Ciccone DS. *Psychological Vulnerability to Chronic Pain*. New York: Springer Publishing; 1994.

Gukelberger M. The uncomplicated post-traumatic cervical syndrome. *Scandinavian Journal of Rehabilitation Medicine*. 1972;4:150–153.

Gundrum LK. Whiplash injuries to the ear. *International Record of Medicine*. 1956;169(1):21–25.

Gundry CR, Fritts HM. Magnetic resonance imaging of the musculoskeletal system. Part 8. The spine, section 2. *Clinical Orthopaedics and Related Research*. 1997;343:260–271.

These authors review the exceptional capacity of magnetic resonance imaging (MRI) scans to detect all but the most minor of abnormalities. Yet when MRI studies with whiplash are done, no acute trauma is found. The only injuries to be missed are the minor muscle or ligament sprains.

Gunzburg R, Szpalski M. *Whiplash Injuries. Current Concepts in Prevention, Diagnosis, and Treatment of the Cervical Whiplash Syndrome*. Philadelphia: Lippincott-Raven; 1998.

This is a relatively pleasant, easy-to-read book. It is mostly a collection of articles or studies, some of which are years out of date now but of interest nevertheless.

Some of the chapters (or the authors' work) are elsewhere in this bibliography. See the bibliographic entries under the lead authors' names: S. Meyer, M. M. Panjabi, B. P. Radanov, W. Rauschning, M. Y. Svensson, and P. F. van Akkerveeken for more comments.

There are some obvious deficiencies, but still it is a useful and balanced discussion of a few aspects of the whiplash controversy, which is not an easy task. The editors of the text did not apparently intend to review all the important or current literature.

There is a lack of discussion in this text of the numerous current magnetic resonance imaging (MRI) studies of whiplash patients. In these studies, researchers fail to find evidence of significant muscle tears, ligament tears, and other injuries that MRI scans are capable of detecting. There is a failure to discuss how bone scans are capable of detecting the types of injuries that MRI scans do not detect. Studies of whiplash patients with bone scans have not detected injuries even though experts know that bone scans can detect numerous types of injuries to bone and joints, and even significant injuries to ligaments or muscles.

Animal and cadaver data contribute to some degree to our understanding of whiplash but do not much advance the understanding of why whiplash claimants report chronic symptoms. Current emphasis is being placed on subjecting living humans to collisions and monitoring the clinical short-term and long-term effects.

There is a limited discussion of the current engineering literature with human volunteers. There appears to be a belief that animal experiments are somehow more relevant. There is also a lack of discussion of what it means that a human volunteer has never reported chronic symptoms after whiplash injury. Has anyone wondered why? There is a limited but very important discussion of low-velocity collisions. The authors make no statement, however, why there are so many claims after low-velocity collisions. Meyer et al do a good job of saying why one does not expect this but do not point out why it occurs nevertheless. Current efforts are being made to introduce more of the engineering literature into the medical literature.

There are the obvious flaws with the conclusions regarding cervical zygapophysial joint injuries supposedly occurring in whiplash patients. See the articles of L. Barnsley et al as well as the articles by R. Ferrari and A. S. Russell (*Journal of Rheumatology,* 1998), Ferrari (*Cephalalgia,* 1998), and O. Kwan and J. Friel (*Cephalalgia,* 1998).

While the authors cite some cultural epidemiological differences, they make little attempt to explain those differences. Others are currently making efforts to do so.

This text on current concepts includes data from Radanov et al that is now about 7 years out of date. M. Karlsborg et al reveal current data (1997) and show that psychosocial factors predict symptom reporting in whiplash patients. (See O. Kwan and J. Friel for criticisms of the Radanov et al studies.)

Surprisingly, although temporomandibular disorders and whiplash are such a current topic of interest, there is little mention of them.

Gurdjian ES, Thomas LM, eds. *Neckache and Backache.* Springfield, IL: Charles C Thomas; 1970.

This text deals with many aspects of whiplash. It includes effects of psychological factors and information about early experimental work with human volunteers.

Gurdjian and L. M. Thomas also studied the electroencephalograms (EEGs) of whiplash patients and found that "the EEG in the majority were normal, with a few showing [mild abnormalities]."

Gurumoorthy D, Twomey L. The Quebec task force on whiplash-associated disorders [letter]. *Spine.* 1996;21(7):897–899.

Guy JE. The whiplash: tiny impact, tremendous injury. *Industrial Medicine and Surgery.* 1968;37:688–691.

Haas DC. Chronic posttraumatic headache. In: Olesen J, Tfelt-Hansen P, Welch KMA, eds. *The Headaches*. New York: Raven Press; 1993:629–637.

This author provides a useful review on the relationship of posttraumatic headaches to psychological factors and the lack of organic basis for the headaches in most cases.

Haas DC. Chronic post-traumatic headaches classified and compared with natural headaches. *Cephalalgia*. 1996;16:486–493.

The author confirms that these posttraumatic headaches are really no different than tension-type headaches in the general population.

Hachinski V. The thoracic outlet syndrome. *Archives of Neurology*. 1990;47:330.

A reminder of the lack of evidence for this proposed disorder and, therefore, the caution to all who claim it to be the source of symptoms in whiplash patients. See also M. Cherington et al, A. J. Wilbourn, and J. R. Youmans.

Hackett GS. Whiplash injury. *American Practitioner*. 1959;10(8):1333–1336.

Hadley LA. Roentgenographic studies of the cervical spine. *American Journal of Roentgenology*. 1944;52(2):173–195.

Hadley LA. *Anatomico-Roentgenographic Studies of the Cervical Spine*. Springfield, IL: Charles C Thomas; 1956:119–128.

Hagberg M. ABC of work related disorders. Neck and arm disorders. *British Medical Journal*. 1996;313(7054):419–422.

Hagström Y, Carlsson J. Prolonged functional impairments after whiplash injury. *Scandinavian Journal of Rehabilitation Medicine*. 1996;28:139–146.

These authors are correct in identifying that there are many psychological factors other than monetary compensation that promote chronic pain in whiplash patients. The authors neglect, however, to point out that one need not ascribe cognitive difficulties to a brain injury, but rather to the effects of pain and other psychological factors, as B. P. Radanov et al (1996) and A. E. Taylor et al point out. See also "Disturbance of Cognition" in Chapter 7.

Halliday JL. Psychoneurosis as a cause of incapacity among insured persons. *British Medical Journal*. March 1935(suppl): 85–88.

Halliday JL. *Psychosocial Medicine. A Study of the Sick Society*. New York: WW Norton and Company; 1948.

This text deals with the relationship between individuals' psychological characteristics and their response to disease or likelihood of developing symptoms of an illness.

Hamel HA, James OE Jr. Acute traumatic cervical syndrome (whiplash injury). *Southern Medical Journal*. 1962;55:1171–1177.

Hamer AJ. Reply from the authors [letter]. *Injury*. 1994;25(6):410.

Hamer AJ, Gargan MF, Bannister GC, Nelson RJ. Whiplash injury and surgically treated cervical disc disease. *Injury*. 1993;24(8):549–550.

These authors argue that disc degeneration occurs earlier in whiplash patients than in non–whiplash patients. One must note, however, that there are many significant concerns with this *retrospective* study, particularly that there is a highly select group of patients. Also, many studies have shown that having a whiplash injury does not accelerate disc degeneration. "Radiology of Whiplash" in Chapter 5 deals with this further.

See also S. M. Barnes, C. L. Colton, and A. D. Redmond et al for more criticisms.

Hammacher ER, van der Werken C. Acute neck sprain: 'whiplash' reappraised. *Injury*. 1996;27(7):463–466.

In this article, the authors state that chronic pain may follow ankle sprain, and so it is possible that ongoing physical damage from the accident injury may be causing chronic pain in whiplash patients. They neglect to point out that the sprains they are discussing are severe ankle sprains with complete tears of ligaments and tendons, a phenomenon rarely seen in whiplash patients. Minor ankle sprains have an excellent prognosis, and there is no evidence to suggest that most whiplash patients receive anything more than a minor neck sprain. Both sites of minor sprain should have similar outcomes. In addition, one of the studies they quote (P. Gebuhr et al) actually demonstrates that even for severe ankle sprains, return to normal activities (like sports) occurs within several weeks. So even severe ankle sprains appear to have a quicker recovery than most whiplash patients.

Hancock J. Comments on Barnsley et al [letter]. *Pain*. 1995;61:487–495.

Harder S, Veilleux M, Suissa S. The effect of socio-demographic and crash-related factors on the prognosis of whiplash. *Journal of Clinical Epidemiology*. 1998;51(5):377–384.

Hardesty WH, Whitcare WB, Toole JF, Randall P, Royster HP. Studies on vertebral artery blood flow in man. *Surgery, Gynecology, and Obstetrics*. 1963; 116:662–664.

These authors show that healthy individuals frequently have abnormalities in blood flow through the vertebral arteries of the neck. For this reason it is important to have a control group when studying whiplash patients, because any abnormalities one finds may be just as a common in the healthy control group. The lack of such a control group hampers the study by M. Yagi in which he attempts to explain whiplash symptoms by finding abnormalities of the vertebral artery. Yagi did not take into consideration that the abnormalities he found in whiplash patients with symptoms are also frequently found in the general population, and so their causal link to symptoms is doubtful.

Harms-Ringdahl K, Ekholm J. Intensity and character of pain and muscular activity levels elicited by maintained extreme flexion position of the lower-cervical-upper thoracic spine. *Scandinavian Journal of Rehabilitation Medicine.* 1986;18: 117–126.

Harris JH, Yeakley JW. Hyperextension-dislocation of the cervical spine. Ligament injuries demonstrated by magnetic resonance imaging. *Journal of Bone and Joint Surgery.* 1992;74(4)-B:567–570.

These authors show that some patients with apparent hyperextension injuries demonstrate ligament injuries on magnetic resonance imaging (MRI). One must note, however, that the patients in this study are completely different from whiplash patients in that the study patients had obvious spinal cord damage. Also, studies with bone scans and MRI scans, which are extremely efficient at detecting significant ligament injuries, do not find such injuries exist in virtually all whiplash patients. See D. Barton et al and C. Hildingsson et al as well as "Radiology of Whiplash" in Chapter 5.

Harriton MB. *The Whiplash Handbook.* Springfield, IL: Charles C Thomas; 1989.

This text is a general review. Although published in 1989, the discussion of whiplash is largely on animal or dummy experiments.

Harth M, Teasell RW. Chronic whiplash re-revisited [letter]. *Journal of Rheumatology.* 1998;25(7):1437–1438.

Hartigan C, Miller L, Liewehr SC. Rehabilitation of acute and subacute low back and neck pain in the work-injured patient. *Orthopedic Clinics of North America.* 1996;27(4):841–860.

Hartley J. Modern concepts of whiplash injury. *New York State Journal of Medicine.* 1958;58(2):3306–3310.

Haslett RS, Duvall-Young J, McGalliard JN. Traumatic retinal angiopathy and seat belts: pathogenesis of whiplash injury. *Eye*. 1994;8:615–617.

This articles includes discussion on 3 cases of visual disturbances patients reported following supposed whiplash injury. One must consider, however, that (1) the patients may have had symptoms before the accident but are claiming them as part of their personal injury, (2) the authors do not state exactly how long after the accident the symptoms started (just because a symptom occurs after an accident does not mean it is due to an injury during the accident), and (3) patients become hypervigilant for bodily symptoms after an accident, especially if they are involved in a claim. As such, they may have had some minor symptoms prior to the accident that they largely ignored but are now registering at a different level since the accident.

Hawkes CD. Whiplash injuries of the head and neck. *Archives of Surgery*. 1957; 75:828–833.

Hawkins GW. Flexion and extension injuries of the cervico-capital joints. *Clinical Orthopedics*. 1962;24:22–33.

Hayes JG. Whiplash in Australia: illness or injury? [letter]. *Medical Journal of Australia*. 1992;157:429.

Hayes PE, Kristoff CA. Adverse reactions to five new antidepressants. *Clinical Pharmacy*. 1986;5(6):471–480.

Hedman TP, Fernie GR. Mechanical response of the lumbar spine to seated postural loads. *Spine*. 1997;22(7):734–743.

Heilig D. "Whiplash" mechanics of injury: management of cervical and dorsal involvement. *Journal of the American Osteopathic Association*. 1963;63: 113–120.

Heikkilä H, Aström PG. Cervicocephalic kinesthetic sensibility in patients with whiplash injury. *Scandinavian Journal of Rehabilitation Medicine*. 1996;28: 133–138.

In this small study, the authors demonstrate that neck pain may cause abnormal postural dynamics and lead to symptoms such as dizziness. Thus, it is not necessary to suspect a nervous system lesion in whiplash patients as the cause of these symptoms. See also "Disturbances of Balance and Hearing" in Chapter 7.

Surprisingly, the authors also do go on to suggest that reporting of chronic symptoms by whiplash patients may be due to some chronic damage from the acute injury. They do not explain the evidence for such a conclusion.

Heikkilä H, Wenngren BI. Cervicocephalic kinesthetic sensibility, active range of cervical motion, and oculomotor function in patients with whiplash injury. *Archives of Physical Medicine and Rehabilitation.* 1998;79:1089–1094.

Including patients who have both Grade 2 and Grade 3 whiplash-associated disorders, these authors once again found that limited neck range of motion influences and correlates with eye function. This may account for dizziness and visual complaints in some whiplash patients. See also "Disturbances of Balance and Hearing" in Chapter 7.

In this case, the authors suggest a muscular source for this phenomenon rather than a nervous system injury.

Heise AP, Laskin DM, Gervin AS. Incidence of temporomandibular joint symptoms following whiplash injury. *Journal of Oral and Maxillofacial Surgery.* 1992;50:825–828.

These authors offer arguments against the concept of temporomandibular joint injury in rear-end collisions. See also R. Ferrari et al, H. L. Goldberg, R. P. Howard et al, W. S. Kirk Jr, M. Olin, R. H. Roydhouse, E. W. Small, and D. H. West et al.

Helliwell PS, Evans PF, Wrigth V. The straight cervical spine: Does it indicate muscle spasm? *Journal of Bone and Joint Surgery [British].* 1994;76-B:103–106.

These authors confirm that a straightening of the cervical lordosis is just as common in the general population as it is in whiplash patients. It is not a sign of injury or a perhaps not even a sign of muscle spasm.

Hendler N, Bergson C, Morrison C. Overlooked physical diagnoses in chronic pain patients involved in litigation, part 2. The addition of MRI, nerve blocks, 3-D CT, and qualitative flow meter. *Psychosomatics.* 1996;37:509–517.

These authors believe they are able to find a "diagnosis" in many chronic pain claimants. They seem to confuse abnormalities on test results with an actual explanation for the patient's symptom reporting. They cite various imaging abnormalities, for example, but do not point out that the abnormalities found (and the frequency in their study) are all commonly seen in the general healthy population with no symptoms at all. The authors do not have a control population, so they cannot appreciate that there actually is no difference in unselected populations of accident victims and the general population in this regard. Finding a bulging disc or other abnormalities on a magnetic resonance imaging scan does not confirm an explanation for the patient's symptoms. Moreover, the authors use "diagnoses" like "temporomandibular joint pain," "myofascial disease," and "rib tip syndrome." None of these have been validated as actually reflecting specific pathology causing chronic pain. The authors also appear to diagnose thoracic outlet syndrome frequently, even though experts regard it as a rare condition. No doubt they made use of physical examination signs that are also found in most of the normal population.

This study illustrates how important it is to have control populations (because so many abnormal test results exist in healthy individuals), how one must not associate a given finding with symptoms and then immediately conclude causation, and how one should not be duped into believing that because a "scientific" sounding term has been used, that there actually is a disease associated with that term. "Myofascial," for instance, simply means that the patient reports pain and no one has explained why.

Readers are referred to "Radiology of Whiplash" in Chapter 5. Compare the studies showing how many asymptomatic subjects have abnormalities with various imaging techniques to the frequency of abnormalities in this study. They are the same. The reader is also referred to the text addressing thoracic outlet syndrome in Chapter 7.

Hendler NH, Kozikowski JG. Overlooked physical diagnoses in chronic pain patients with litigation. *Psychosomatics.* 1993;34:494–501.

See above.

Hildingsson C, Hietala SO, Toolanen G. Scintigraphic findings in acute whiplash injury of the cervical spine. *Injury.* 1989; 20:265–266.

In this study, the authors evaluated bone scans, which are sensitive to any bony or significant ligamentous pathology, in whiplash patients. The authors found that "skeletal and ligamentous injuries are rare after whiplash injury. . . . Somewhat surprisingly the current scintigraphic study could not verify the earlier reported damage to the anterior longitudinal ligaments and the separation of the discs from associated vertebrae after whiplash injury."

Hildingsson C, Toolanen G. Outcome after soft-tissue injury of the cervical spine. *Acta Orthopaedica Scandinavica.* 1990; 61(4): 357–359.

These researchers studied 93 patients and noted that "our radiographic findings . . . do not support the theory that . . . the presence of degenerative spondylosis is prognostically unfavourable."

They revealed that finding changes in cervical lordosis on X-ray and the presence of disc degeneration on X-ray do not worsen the prognosis. See also J. Greenfield and F. W. Ilfeld and M. Hohl.

Hildingsson C, Wenngren BI, Bring G, Toolanen G. Oculomotor problems after cervical spine injury. *Acta Orthopaedica Scandinavica.* 1989;60(5):513–516.

These authors suggest that there may be a nervous system injury responsible for some of the visual (ocular) symptoms of whiplash patients. Note, however, that the study is of a small number of patients and that patients who were asymptomatic had abnormalities similar to those who were symptomatic, making it difficult to correlate findings to symptoms. Also, there were no preaccident examinations in these patients, and the control group was too small to rule out finding these abnormalities in the general population.

The other suggestion the authors make is that the neck pain alters the way the head moves and therefore interferes with ocular function. This seems a more probable explanation given the recent work of M. Karlberg et al.

Hildingsson C, Wenngren BI, Toolanen G. Eye motility dysfunction after soft-tissue injury of the cervical spine. *Acta Orthopedica Scandinavica.* 1993; 64(2):129–132.

See above.

Hinoki M. Vertigo due to whiplash injury: a neurotological approach. *Acta Otolaryngologica (Stockholm).* 1985;419(suppl):9–29.

These authors review theories and animal experiments that support the view of vertigo (a type of dizziness) in whiplash patients as being due to a nervous system injury. Note, however, that the discussion is largely theoretical and that one cannot so readily apply animal experiments to the human situation. See also "Disturbances of Balance and Hearing" in Chapter 7.

Hirsch SA, Hirsch PJ, Hiramoto H, Weiss A. Whiplash syndrome: fact or fiction? *Orthopedic Clinics of North America.* 1988;19(4):791–795.

The authors base this article on their own anecdotal experience.

Hirschfeld AH, Behan RC. The accident process I. Etiological considerations of industrial injuries. *Journal of the American Medical Association.* 1963;186(3): 193–199.

Hirschfeld AH, Behan RC. The accident process III. Disability: acceptable and unacceptable. *Journal of the American Medical Association.* 1966;197(2): 85–89.

These authors deal with how an accident, rather than being the cause of disability, is instead an opportunity for socially acceptable disability.

Hitselberger WE, Witten RM. Abnormal myelograms in asymptomatic patients. *Journal of Neurosurgery.* 1968;28:204–206.

These authors discuss the utility of myelography in the evaluation of neck, arm, and leg pain. Some people believed at the time that the abnormalities on myelogram would show the injury responsible for the patient's symptoms. On the contrary, the authors of this study revealed that "myelographic defects occurred in 37% of 300 asymptomatic patients."

This casts doubt on the significance of findings on a myelogram in relation to pain symptoms alone.

Hodge JR. The whiplash injury. A discussion of this phenomenon as a psychosomatic illness. *Ohio State Medical Journal.* 1964;60:762–766.

This author offers further discussion on the psychological aspects of whiplash. Also see below.

Hodge JR. The whiplash neurosis. *Psychosomatics.* 1971;12: 245–249.

Hodgson SP, Grundy M. Neck sprains after car accidents [letter]. *British Medical Journal.* 1989;298:1452.

Hodgson VR. Tolerance of the neck to impact acceleration. In: *Technical Report 9.* Contract no. N00014-75-C-1015. Washington, DC: Department of Navy; 1979.

Hoffman BF. The demographic and psychiatric characteristics of 110 personal injury litigants. *Bulletin for the American Academy of Psychiatry and the Law.* 1991;19(3):227–236.

This author discusses the emotional state of accident victims from a variety of accident types. The author apparently concludes that much of the psychological suffering is due to the accident and does not believe that secondary gain is an issue. The author fails to describe that secondary gain is more than monetary. Recall that A. J. Barsky and G. L. Klerman (1983) have defined secondary gain as:

> the acceptable and "legitimate" interpersonal advantages that result when one has the symptoms of a physical disease. The somatically distressed individual is excused from certain responsibilities and obligations and can avoid challenges and duties. The physically symptomatic person also garners sympathy, attention, support, and many types of concrete assistance. . . . All of this occurs without a loss of pride or self-esteem and without a sense of failure, fault, or defeat. This is because the patient cannot be blamed for his or her inability and is not held responsible or culpable.

Recall also that D. S. Ciccone and R. C. Grzesiak (1992) point out that:

> Many patients who go on to develop chronic pain following an acute injury or illness report a premorbid pattern of excessive self-sacrifice,

hyperactivity, or overachievement. They often have a history of going to work at an early age, putting in frequent overtime hours, and holding more than one job at a time. They may have permitted or encouraged others to rely upon them excessively and, as a result, were routinely called upon and expected to perform special tasks or favors. These tasks were often burdensome in nature or at least not intrinsically rewarding for the patient. Following the onset of pain, this pattern of unrelenting self-sacrifice and overachievement typically comes to an abrupt halt with the patient becoming the recipient of special care instead of the provider. . . . The onset of physical injury or illness apparently offers these patients an opportunity to relieve themselves of their occupational and social obligations without any need for self-reproach and without any loss of social approval.

Hoffman also states that plaintiff lawyers referred all these patients to him and does not state whether he has seen an equal number of patients from defense lawyers. This review of patients is thus a very highly select group, and the discussion might be entirely different from a psychiatrist who has seen 110 patients from defense lawyers.

Hohl M. Soft-tissue injuries of the neck in automobiles accidents. Factors influencing prognosis. *Journal of Bone and Joint Surgery*. 1974;56-A(8):1675–1682.

Some quote this study to indicate that whiplash patients have a high incidence of developing disc degeneration. Wrong choice. M. Hohl attempted to determine whether whiplash patients who had no evidence of disc degeneration at the time of an accident would develop such changes later. He had 534 patients with normal X-rays initially but could follow up on only 146 patients 5 years later. Hohl admits, "It was not possible to establish whether or not these 146 patients were a valid sample of the total pool."

Indeed, when the number of patients missing in follow-up is greater than the number one includes in the study, the study results become highly suspect. Did the process somehow concentrate patients who had abnormal changes on X-ray? Do patients who know they have abnormal X-rays remain in litigation or attend physicians more often? Who knows? That is why it is essential to have had as many of the 534 patients as possible. One can make assumptions about the missing patients, but this does not make study conclusions any more valid.

Hohl did find that 39% (57 patients) of the 146 had changes on their X-rays later. What does this mean in terms of the likelihood that whiplash patients get disc degeneration more readily than a control group? It is difficult to know because he could not account for 388 patients, and it would require only 10% of them to alter the results dramatically.

Hohl did not have a control group, which is not acceptable. He used the data from other studies of asymptomatic people to state that a control group would have had an incidence of disc degeneration of 6%. It is true that 39% is greater than 6%, but because there is a lack of 388 patients in the follow-up study, one cannot validate the conclusion that whiplash patients get disc degeneration more often than those not in collisions.

Some have quoted the figure of 63% in this study, to indicate that this is the incidence of whiplash patients developing disc degeneration. This number in Hohl's article is derived from 7 patients out of 11 with restricted motion at one intervertebral joint, out of 47 patients who had flexion-extension X-rays, out of 146 followed up 5 years after, out of 534 patients with no disc degeneration at the time of the accident!

This may obviously mislead the reader into believing that whiplash patients have a 63% chance of developing disc degeneration. They do not. The value of 34% is the only one that can be interpreted in this way, but unfortunately even that value may not be valid because of the study's poor quality.

Nevertheless, Hohl reported that "the occurrence of new degenerative changes did not affect recovery."

The author also adds proof that neck X-ray changes have little to do with symptoms. The study found that 58% of patients with abnormal X-rays became asymptomatic in time, while 44% of those with normal X-rays remained symptomatic!

Hohl M. Soft tissue injuries of the neck. *Clinical Orthopedics*. 1975;109:42–49.

This author suggests that one can find the source of the symptoms of whiplash in radiologic studies. One must note, however, that this has been completely disproved. See also "Disturbances of Balance and Hearing" in Chapter 7.

Hohl M. Soft-tissue neck injuries. In: *The Cervical Spine*, H.H. Sherk et al, eds. Philadelphia: JB Lippincott Company; 1989:436–441.

This author reviews whiplash, explaining the mechanism of injury and the experiments to reproduce the injury, but one must note that the experiments he cites are either outdated (McKenzie 1971, D. M. Severy et al 1955) or of animals (I. MacNab 1964, A. K. Ommaya et al 1968, J. Wickstrom et al 1968). More recent studies supersede these earlier, inadequate studies.

Hohl M. Soft tissue injuries—a review. *Revue de Chirurgie Orthopedique et Reparatrice de L'appareil Mateur (Paris)*. 1990;76(suppl 1):15–25.

See above.

Hohl M, Hopp E. Soft tissue injuries of the neck—II: Factors influencing prognosis. *Orthopedic Transactions*. 1978;2:29.

These authors show that the appearance of new degenerative changes on cervical X-ray after whiplash does not affect prognosis. See "Radiology of Whiplash" in Chapter 5.

Holt EP Jr. Fallacy of cervical discography. *Journal of the American Medical Association*. 1964;188(9):799–801.

This author addresses the question of whether discograms are helpful in finding the cause of chronic whiplash symptoms. He examined 50 asymptomatic individuals ages 21 to 50 with no history of prior neck injury, neck pain, or arm pain, and no physician records of such complaints. Each underwent discography. He found that practically 100% of the discograms show so-called abnormalities. He concluded that "the results of discography in 148 spaces of 50 symptom-free, uninjured cervical spines indicated that the test, so far as extravasation of contrast media is concerned, is without diagnostic value. The claim of reproduction of discogenic pain by injection of the responsible disk space seems likely to be equally fallacious. Injection into any cervical disk causes great pain and brings on tonic neck muscle contracture."
See below and also the work of S. E. Sneider et al.

Holt EP Jr. Further reflections on cervical discography. *Journal of the American Medical Association*. 1975;231(6):613–614.

This author makes it clear that discography is of little value in assessing the cause of neck pain.

Hone MR. What's in a name? [letter]. *Medical Journal of Australia*. 1997;167:175.

Horwich H. The ocular effects of whiplash injury. *Transactions of the Section of Ophthalmology of the American Medical Association*. 1956:86–90.
See below.

Horwich H, Kasner D. The effect of whiplash injuries on ocular functions. *Southern Medical Journal*. 1962;55:69–71.

These authors make the statement that the whiplash mechanism can cause eye injury. One must note, however, that the authors admit "we are at the mercy of the patient's volition and motivation" because the symptoms are subjective (not objective) and dependent on patient reporting. The one objective finding they note (differences in pupillary size from one side to the other) is found frequently in the normal population. (See T. L. Slamovits and J. S. Glaser.)

Howard RP, Benedict JV, Raddin JH, Smith HL. Assessing neck extension-flexion as a basis for temporomandibular joint dysfunction. *Journal of Oral and Maxillofacial Surgery*. 1991; 49:1210–1213.

This is an important article in that it casts serious doubt on the theories of jaw pain or dysfunction coming from temporomandibular joint injury in whiplash patients. It is particularly critical of Weenberg's work. See also R. Ferrari et al, H. L. Goldberg, A. P. Heise et al, W. S. Kirk Jr, M. Olin, R. H. Roydhouse, E. W. Small, and D. H. West et al.

Howard RP, Bowles AP, Guzman HM, Krenrich SW. Head, neck, and mandible dynamics generated by "whiplash." *Accident Prevention and Analysis*. 1998; 30(4):525–534.

These authors extend their studies further, with dual plates for the upper and lower jaw, surface monitoring of muscle contraction and relaxation, and detailed analyses of data about rear-end collisions. They show why one does not expect rear-end collisions without jaw impact to produce any forces on the joint or supporting structure that one does not routinely encounter in daily jaw activities.

Howard RP, Hatsell CP, Guzman HM. Temporomandibular joint injury potential imposed by the low-velocity extension-flexion maneuver. *Journal of Oral and Maxillofacial Surgery*. 1995; 53:256–262.

These authors report the first detailed analysis of the temporomandibular joint forces occurring in low-velocity rear-end collisions. They demonstrate that these forces are within the range of normal jaw activities such as chewing and yawning. This further refutes theories of mandibular whiplash. See also R. Ferrari et al, H. L. Goldberg, A. P. Heise et al, W. S. Kirk Jr, M. Olin, R. H. Roydhouse, E. W. Small, and D. H. West et al.

Hu AS, Bean SP, Zimmerman RM. Response of belted dummy and cadaver to rear impact. In: *Proceedings of the Twenty First Stapp Car Crash Conference*. Paper #770929. Warrendale, PA: Society of Automotive Engineers; 1977: 589–625.

Huddleston OL. Whiplash injuries. Diagnosis and treatment. *California Medicine*. 1958;89(5):318–321.

Hudson AJ. Chronic whiplash [letter]. *Neurology*. 1996; 47:615–616.

Hundley JM. "Whiplash" injuries of the cervical spine. *Journal of the Arkansas Medical Society*. 1961;57(12):499–502.

Iansek R, Heywood J, Kornaghan J, Balla JJ. Cervical Spondylosis and Headaches. *Clinical and Experimental Neurology*. 1986;23:175–178.

These authors reveal that cervical spondylosis is not likely to be a cause for headache, but rather posterior (occipital) headaches may be due to anxiety or at least a muscular source of pain.

Imboden JB, Canter A, Cluff LE. Convalescence from influenza. *Archives of Internal Medicine.* 1961;108:115–121.

This is an interesting demonstration that the outcome from an infection depends on the preinfection psychosocial status, indicating that our station in life and our personality have the potential to influence the outcome of illness.

Imboden JB, Canter A, Cluff LE. Symptomatic recovery from medical disorders. *Journal of the American Medical Association.* 1961;178(13):1182–1184.

Immega G. Whiplash injuries increase with seat belt use. *Canadian Family Physician.* 1995;41:203–204.

Irvine DH, Foster JB, Newell DJ, Klukvin BN. Prevalence of cervical spondylosis in a general practice. *Lancet.* 1965;1: 1089–1092.

Jaanus SD. Ocular side effects of selected systemic drugs. *Optometry Clinics.* 1992;2(4):73–96.

Jackson R. *The Cervical Syndrome.* 3rd ed. Springfield, IL: Charles C Thomas; 1966.

Jacobs H. Whiplash legitimized by clinical support [letter]. *Canadian Family Physician.* 1995;41:202–203.

Jacome DE. EEG in whiplash: a reappraisal. *Clinical Electroencephalography.* 1987;18(1):41–45.

In this study, this author lays to rest the notion that one can use electroencephalograms to prove chronic brain damage as the basis for the chronic symptoms in whiplash patients.

Jacome DE, Risko M. EEG features in post-traumatic syndrome. *Clinical Electroencephalography.* 1984;15(4):214–221.

These authors studied posttraumatic syndrome and electroencephalogram (EEG) findings, noting that "we conclude that the great majority of patients with post-traumatic syndrome due to minor head trauma . . . had normal standard and 24-hour EEG ambulatory recordings. The symptoms . . . were not accompanied with any EEG abnormality."

Conducting further studies in 1987, they added:

> Torres and Shapiro performed clinical standard EEGs on . . . patients [who] had a multiplicity of abnormalities in their clinical examinations

which included . . . [objective neurologic abnormalities]. . . . Radiographic data was not described in their study and the investigation was performed in the pre-CT (computer tomography) scan era.

The divergence of [our] results and those of Torres and Shapiro is attributed to probable differences in the degree of severity of trauma, since their patients often showed abnormalities in their clinical examination. The unavailability of CT made it impossible for them to detect and discard those patients with intracranial structural lesions.

Jaeschke R, Guyatt GH, Sackett DL. Users' guides to the medical literature. III. How to use an article about a diagnostic test. *Journal of the American Medical Association*. 1993;271(5):389–391.

These authors provide a useful methodology for critically reviewing the medical literature. Their article is worth reviewing.

James OE Jr, Hamel HA. Whiplash injuries of the neck. *Missouri Medicine*. 1955;52(6):423–426.

Janecki CJ Jr, Lipke JM. Whiplash syndrome. *American Family Physician*. 1978; 17(4):144–151.

Janes JM, Hooshmand H. Extension-flexion injury of the neck. *Modern Medicine (Review Edition)*. 1965;33:894–895.

Janes JM, Hooshmand H. Extension-flexion injury of the neck. *Modern Medicine*. August 1965:128–129.

Jayson MI. ABC of work related disorders. Back pain. *British Medical Journal*. 1996;313(7053):355–358.

Jensen MC, Brant-Zawadzki MN, Obuchowski N, et al. Magnetic resonance imaging of the lumbar spine in people without back pain. *New England Journal of Medicine*. 1994;331:69–73.

These authors show that healthy subjects frequently have abnormalities of the spine with no symptoms at all.

Jensen OK, Justesen T, Nielsen FF, Brixen K. Functional radiographic examination of the cervical spine in patients with post-traumatic headache. *Cephalalgia*. 1990;10:295–303.

These authors conclude that changes in the cervical curve on X-ray are due to muscle spasm rather than any underlying disorder in the cervical spine itself.

Jensen OK, Nielsen FF. The influence of sex and pre-traumatic headache on the incidence and severity of headache after head injury. *Cephalalgia*. 1990;10: 285–293.

Johnson G. Hyperextension soft tissue injuries of the cervical spine—a review. *Journal of Accident and Emergency Medicine*. 1996;13:3–8.

Although providing a good general review, the author does not note the thousands of human whiplash experiments and the failure of those experiments to produce an individual with chronic symptoms. The author also does not quote the many magnetic resonance imaging studies of whiplash patients failing to show any of the injuries others so often quote as being possible explanations for chronic pain. Finally, R. P. Howard et al have shown that there is no temporomandibular joint injury in rear-end collisions.

Jónsson H Jr, Bring G, Rauschning W, Sahlstedt B. Hidden cervical spine injuries in traffic accident victims with skull fractures. *Journal of Spinal Disorders*. 1991;4(3):251–263.

These authors provide autopsy data of the structures that may undergo injury in accidents, albeit of a different accident type than most whiplash patients experience. All of the injuries they cite would be identifiable by magnetic resonance imaging (MRI) or bone scans. If these lesions were commonly occurring in whiplash patients, studies of whiplash patients using MRI and bone scans would find the lesions. Yet the many MRI studies of whiplash patients and the bone scan studies do not find such lesions even though the patients are reporting chronic pain. See also "Disturbances of Balance and Hearing" in Chapter 5.

Jónsson H Jr, Cesarini K, Sahlstedt B, Rauschning W. Findings and outcome in whiplash-type neck distortions. *Spine*. 1994; 19(24):2733–2743.

These authors confirm that the outcome in accident victims with neck pain but no identifiable neck injury (ie, whiplash) varies from full recovery in 6 weeks to pain for 5 years. This suggests that noninjurious mechanisms are responsible for the outcome in whiplash patients.

The authors also confirm that whiplash patients are not at any increased risk for disc degeneration.

Juhl JH, Miller SM, Roberts GW. Roentgenographic variations in the normal cervical spine. *Radiology*. 1962;78:591–597.

These authors show that there is little correlation between a patient's symptoms and the severity of changes on neck X-ray.

Juhl M, Kjærgaard-Seerup K. Cervical spine epidemiological investigation. Medical and social consequences. In: *Proceedings of the International IRCOBI*

Conference on the Biomechanics of Impacts, 1981, Salonde-Provence. 1981: 49–58.

Jung TT, Rhee CK, Lee CS, Park YS, Choi DC. Ototoxicity of salicylate, nonsteroidal antiinflammatory drugs, and quinine. *Otolaryngologic Clinics of North America.* 1993;26(5):791–810.

Kahane CJ. *Evaluation of Head Restraints: Federal Motor Vehicle Safety Standard 202.* Washington, DC: National Highway Traffic Safety Administration (NHTSA), Office of Program Evaluation; 1982.

In this in-depth study, the author shows that head restraints appear to result in only a 10% to 15% reduction in whiplash patients. He also points out, however, that head restraints should be effective even if they are in the "down" position because they are high enough for most people even then.

Head restraints in the down position would be high enough for most women, as they are designed for men. Yet women get whiplash more than men. Further, no one has shown that tall occupants in rear-end collisions develop whiplash symptoms more frequently than short occupants.

Maladjusted head restraints cannot explain increasing claims of whiplash injury.

See Chapter 22 and also R. C. Grunsten et al, W. E. McConnell et al, D. B. Olney and A. K. Marsden, B. O'Neill et al, C. Thomas et al, and D. H. West et al.

Kallieris D, Mattern R, Miltner E, Schmidt G, Stein K. Considerations for a neck injury criterion. In: *Proceedings of the Thirty Fifth Stapp Car Crash Conference.* Paper #912916. Warrendale, PA: Society of Automotive Engineers; 1991:401–417.

See below and legend for Tables 20–1 to 20–4 in Chapter 20.

Kallieris D, Schmidt G. Neck response and injury assessment using cadavers and the US-SID for far-side lateral impacts of rear seat occupants with inboard-anchored shoulder belts. In: *Proceedings of the Thirty Fourth Stapp Car Crash Conference.* Paper #902313. Warrendale, PA: Society of Automotive Engineers; 1990:93–99.

These authors show that the lateral forces (like those from a side collision) necessary to cause significant muscle damage in cadavers are higher than those most whiplash patients experience. This suggests that the injury in most whiplash patients in side-impact collisions is relatively minor.

Kamman GR. Traumatic neurosis, compensation neurosis or attitudinal pathosis? *Archives of Neurology and Psychiatry.* 1951;65:593–603.

Karlberg M, Johansson R, Magnusson M, Fransson PA. Dizziness of suspected cervical origin distinguished by posturographic assessment of human postural dynamics. *Journal of Vestibular Research.* 1996;6(1):37–47.

See below.

Karlberg M, Magnusson M, Malmström EM, Melander A, Moritz U. Postural and symptomatic improvement after physiotherapy in patients with dizziness of suspected cervical origin. *Archives of Physical Medicine and Rehabilitation.* 1996; 77:874–882.

In this study of patients with neck pain (but not whiplash patients), the authors confirm that neck pain alone generates postural abnormalities of the head. This may lead to dizziness. A nervous system injury is not necessary, and this study confirms that the dizziness goes away when one treats the neck pain. See also "Disturbances of Balance and Hearing" in Chapter 7.

Karlsborg M, Smed A, Jespersen H, et al. A prospective study of 39 patients with whiplash injury. *Acta Neurologica Scandinavica.* 1997;95:65–72.

These authors attempt to determine factors that predict outcome in whiplash patients. Although the study has potential problems in that the study group is small, it is interesting that the authors conclude that one can best predict long-lasting distress and poor outcome by the occurrence of non–accident-related stressful life events. This is contrary to the conclusions of B. P. Radanov et al. O. Kwan and J. Friel, however, have pointed out at least a dozen major flaws with Radanov et al's work.

The authors also show that magnetic resonance imaging scans do not detect any evidence of chronic damage stemming from an acute injury and that there is no evidence of brain injury in whiplash patients. See also "Disturbances of Balance and Hearing" in Chapter 7.

Kassirer MR, Manon N. Head banger's whiplash. *Clinical Journal of Pain.* 1993; 9:138–141.

These authors show that even the extreme, repetitive hyperflexion and hyperextension of "head bangers" results in reporting only mild, short-lived pain, suggesting that most collisions producing whiplash patients should do the same.

Katon W, Kleinman A, Rosen G. Depression and somatization: a review. *American Journal of Medicine.* 1982;72:127–135, 241–247.

Katsarkas A. Postural stability following mild head or whiplash injuries [letter]. *American Journal of Otology.* 1996;17:172–175.

This author deals with some concerns with the conclusions of A. M. Rubin et al.

Katzberg RW, Westesson PL, Tallents R, Drake CM. Orthodontics and temporomandibular joint derangement. *American Journal of Orthodontics and Dentofacial Orthopedics*. 1996; 109:515–520.

These authors find no relationship between prior orthodontic treatment and temporomandibular joint disc displacement.

They also point out that there is a high prevalence of disc displacement in asymptomatic volunteers (around 30%), which would presumably be the case in 30% of whiplash patients before their accident as well.

Kay DWK, Kerr TA, Lassman LP. Brain trauma and the postconcussional syndrome. *Lancet*. 1971;2:1052–1055.

This study shows the importance of psychological factors in producing the symptoms and affecting the recovery from concussion.

Keats TE. *An Atlas of Normal Roentgen Variants That May Simulate Disease*. 2nd ed. Chicago: Year Book Medical Publishers Inc; 1980.

This author gives numerous examples, especially of the cervical spine, where apparent abnormalities are actually normal findings and can be mistaken for injury or disease.

Keiser L. *The Traumatic Neurosis*. Philadelphia: JB Lippincott Company; 1968.

This author summarizes the concepts of traumatic neurosis in the first part of the twentieth century.

Kelley JS, Hoover RE, George T. Whiplash maculopathy. *Archives of Ophthalmology*. 1978;96:834–835.

Kellner R. *Psychosomatic Syndromes and Somatic Symptoms*. Washington, DC: American Psychiatric Press; 1991.

Kelly M. Whiplash syndrome. *Irish Medical Journal*. 1992; 85(3):85–87.

This is a good review of the major issues in whiplash, although the author still perpetuates some myths. He refers to the forces and acceleration of the human head and neck complex, for example, as being "quite considerable" but does not define them.

Kelly R. The post-traumatic syndrome. *Pahlavi Medical Journal*. 1972;3: 530–547.

See below.

Kelly R. The post-traumatic syndrome: an iatrogenic disease. *Forensic Science.* 1975;6:17–24.

This author makes a plea for the argument that the symptoms of posttraumatic syndrome are organic (physical) and not psychological. The argument is faulty, as it ignores many of the psychological factors that can contribute to symptom reporting. See below for further criticisms.

Kelly R. The post-traumatic syndrome [letter]. *Journal of the Royal Society of Medicine.* 1981;74:242–245.

See article below.

Kelly R, Smith BN. Post-traumatic syndrome: another myth discredited. *Journal of the Royal Society of Medicine.* 1981;74:275–277.

These authors show that not all patients return to work after claim settlements. The authors believe they thus discredit the myth that posttraumatic syndrome is nonorganic by this fact alone. That patients do not return to work after settlement does not, however, immediately lead one to conclude patients' symptoms are organic. There are many other reasons for an individual to maintain an illness (see Chapter 10).

What the authors are really demonstrating is that chronic symptoms do not exist for monetary reasons, and that is certainly reasonable.

Kenna CJ. The whiplash syndrome. A general practitioner's viewpoint. *Australian Family Physician.* 1984;13(4):256–257.

Kennedy F. Neuroses following accident. *Bulletin of the New York Academy of Medicine.* 1930;6(1):1–17.

This early twentieth century author explains that individuals, preconsciously or consciously, may use a traumatic event to cope with their preaccident difficulties.

Kent DL, Haynor DR, Larson EB, Deyo RA. Diagnosis of lumbar spinal stenosis in adults: A metaanalysis of the accuracy of CT, MR, and myelography. *American Journal of Roentgenography.* 1992;158:1135–1144.

This review of the literature reveals that computed tomography scans and magnetic resonance imaging scans frequently show abnormalities in normal people. These authors (and many others) show that asymptomatic individuals can have the very same abnormalities some claim to be the source of pain in whiplash patients. The conclusion that those abnormalities are the site of origin of symptoms is erroneous.

Kent H. BC tackles whiplash-injury problem. *Canadian Medical Association Journal.* 1998;158(8):1003–1005.

Kessels RPC, Keyser A, Verhagen WIM, van Luitelaar ELJM. The whiplash syndrome: a psychophysiological and neuropsychological study towards attention. *Acta Neurologica Scandinavica.* 1998;97:188–193.

Khan H, McCormack D, Burke J, McManus F. Incidental neck symptoms in high energy trauma victims. *Irish Medical Journal.* 1997;90(4):143.

In this study, the authors found that accident victims in more severe collisions who have limb fractures did not report neck or back pain. There could be many reasons for this. It may be that in Ireland acute whiplash injury occurs. The presence of a more significant injury (and more pain) from the fracture, with one's attention focused on the therapy for that fracture, may lead to the minimal awareness of the initial neck or back pain. If the neck and back pain only lasts for days to weeks, then at 6 weeks, when the authors questioned the patients again, they should have little or no neck or back pain.

On the other hand, the number of patients (30) may have simply been too few. Even with this number, one would expect at least 10 to 15 patients to have neck or back pain.

Kihlberg JK. Flexion-torsion neck injury in rear impacts. In: *Proceedings of the Thirteenth Annual Meeting of the American Association of Automotive Medicine.* 1969:1–16.

This author found no relationship between vehicle occupant height and the incidence of whiplash. This further confounds the theory that inadequately adjusted head restraints contribute to whiplash injury. The height of the occupant does not appear to modify risk of becoming a whiplash patient.

Kikuchi S, MacNab I, Moreau P. Localisation of the level of symptomatic cervical disc degeneration. *Journal of Bone and Joint Surgery.* 1981;63-B(2): 272–277.

In this study of discography of the cervical spine, the authors show that 23% to 50% of the abnormalities cause no symptoms. One cannot therefore always attribute symptoms to such abnormalities.

King AB, Oberc E. Instability of the neck due to trauma. *Guthrie Clinic Bulletin.* 1955;24:191–200.

Kinloch BM. Whiplash in Australia: illness or injury? [letter]. *Medical Journal of Australia*. 1993;158:70–71.

This author adds further comment to F. T. McDermott's arguments regarding the effects of legislative changes on whiplash claims.

Kinsey FR. Pain in the neck. *Pennsylvania Medical Journal*. 1958;61:1628–1631.

Kircos LT, Ortendahl DA, Mark AS, Arakawa M. Magnetic resonance imaging of the TMJ disc in asymptomatic volunteers. *Journal of Oral and Maxillofacial Surgery*. 1987;45:852–854.

These authors confirm that up to 30% of asymptomatic subjects have internal temporomandibular joint derangements on magnetic resonance imaging. Thus, finding this in a whiplash patient does not necessarily mean it is responsible for their symptoms.

Kirk WS Jr. Whiplash as a basis for TMJ dysfunction. *Journal of Oral and Maxillofacial Surgery*. 1992;50:427–428.

This author points out the lack of experimental evidence supporting the concept of jaw pain arising from a temporomandibular joint injury in whiplash patients. See also R. Ferrari et al, H. L. Goldberg, A. P. Heise et al, R. P. Howard et al, M. Olin, R. H. Roydhouse, E. W. Small, and D. H. West et al.

Kischka U, Ettlin T, Heim S, Schmid G. Cerebral symptoms following whiplash injury. *European Neurology*. 1991;31: 136–140.

These authors suggest that some of the cognitive symptoms whiplash patients complain of may be of physical origin (eg, brain injury). One must note, however, that the population they studied was extremely select (even the authors of the article admit this) and that in a later article (see T. M. Ettlin et al) the authors state that pain and underlying depression could also be possible explanations. B. P. Radanov et al (1996) and A. E. Taylor et al confirmed this. See also "Disturbances of Balance and Hearing" in Chapter 7.

Kischka U, Ettlin T, Plohmann A, Stahl H. SPECT findings in patients with whiplash injury of the neck. *Neurology*. 1994; 44(suppl 2):763P.

See A. Otte et al.

Knapp PC. Traumatic neurasthenia and hysteria. *Brain*. 1897; 20:385–406.

Knibestöl M, Hildingsson C, Toolanen G. Trigeminal sensory impairment after soft-tissue injury of the cervical spine. *Acta Neurologica Scandinavica*. 1990;82:271–276.

Knight G. Post-traumatic occipital headache. *Lancet.* 1963;1:6–8.

This author suggests that damage to a specific nerve is the cause of chronic head and neck pain after minor trauma. He bases his argument, in part, on the success of a surgical procedure that severs a certain nerve to provide pain relief. One must note, however, that the work of L. M. Weinberger completely denounces this theory.

Knight PO, Wheat JD. The whiplash injury—clinical and medico-legal aspects. *Bulletin of the Tulane University Medical Facility.* 1959;18(4):199–214.

Kolbinson DA, Epstein JB, Burgess JA. Temporomandibular disorders, headaches, and neck pain following motor vehicle accidents and the effects of litigation: review of the literature. *Journal of Orofacial Pain.* 1996;10:101–125.

This is a good general review of this literature, but the authors do not discuss issues of secondary gain in attempting to understand why symptoms may be chronic. Such issues may help to understand why there might not be much difference between litigants and nonlitigants (other secondary gains exist for members of both groups), and particularly why symptoms may not resolve after litigation settles (there are gains other than monetary ones from the illness).

Kolbinson DA, Epstein JB, Burgess JA, Senthilselvan A. Temporomandibular disorders, headaches, and neck pain following motor vehicle accidents: a pilot investigation of persistence and litigation effects. *Journal of Prosthetic Dentistry.* 1997;77(1): 46–53.

See above.

Kolbinson DA, Epstein JB, Senthilselvan A, Burgess JA. A comparison of TMD patients with or without prior motor vehicle accident involvement: initial signs, symptoms, and diagnostic characteristics. *Journal of Orofacial Pain.* 1997;11:206–214.

See below.

Kolbinson DA, Epstein JB, Senthilselvan A, Burgess JA. A comparison of TMD patients with or without prior motor vehicle accident involvement: treatment and outcomes. *Journal of Orofacial Pain.* 1997;11:337–345.

These authors look back on 50 charts of patients reporting temporomandibular disorder (TMD) symptoms either without a recent accident or with one. They find that members of the group reporting symptoms after an accident are reporting far more severe symptoms, with a lesser response to therapy, as well as other disturbances such as more sleep disturbance. The authors admit that the study design has many limitations or potential biases, but the results are interesting.

Their conclusion that trauma may be an important etiologic event in some TMD may be overstated. More exactly, being an accident victim may be an important event in some TMD. There is much more to being an accident victim than just physical injury.

One merely has to ask what factors exist in the accident victim (or someone who believes his or her pain is someone else's fault) that do not exist in the non–accident victim.

Kolbinson DA, Epstein JB, Senthilselvan A, Burgess JA. Effect of impact and injury characteristics on post-motor vehicle accident temporomandibular disorders. *Oral Surgery, Oral Medicine, Oral Pathology, Oral Radiology, and Endodontics*. 1998; 85(6):665–673.

The most interesting finding in this study is that patients in the most minor of accidents requested more therapy than those who had actually hit their face in the collision. This is out of keeping with an "injury model" for temporomandibular disorder following accident.

Kozol HL. Pretraumatic personality and psychiatric sequelae of head injury. *Archives of Neurology and Psychiatry*. 1945; 33:358–364.

This author explains that the pretraumatic personality is not the only factor that leads to posttraumatic symptoms, as other factors (battles with insurance companies, fear of disability, litigation, compensation, and posttraumatic anxieties) could contribute to these symptoms.

Krogstad BS, Jokstad A, Dahl BL, Soboleva U. Somatic complaints, psychologic distress, and treatment outcome in two groups of TMD patients, one previously subjected to whiplash injury. *Journal of Orofacial Pain*. 1998;12:136–144.

This study reveals how rare temporomandibular disorder (TMD) following whiplash is in Norway compared to in, say, North America. These researchers advertised (although it is not stated for how long) for whiplash claimants with symptoms of TMD. In a large (capital) city filled with huge numbers of whiplash claimants, the authors came up with 16.

Kronn E. The incidence of TMJ dysfunction in patients who have suffered a cervical whiplash injury following a traffic accident. *Journal of Orofacial Pain*. 1993;7:209–213.

This author finds that temporomandibular disorder (TMD) symptoms are more common in whiplash patients than in normal subjects. This does not, of course, mean that the accident is the cause of those symptoms, as there may be other explanations for why accident victims complain of such symptoms. That whiplash claimants report such symptoms so commonly in Ireland and not so commonly in

Lithuania, for example, does raise important questions about the cause of such symptom reporting.

The researcher used healthy subjects as a control group. In reality, a better control group is subjects with anxiety, as whiplash patients have a great deal of psychological distress (see M. Gargan et al 1997). Given that psychological factors play a role in such TMD symptoms, having a control group with measures of psychological distress would be more appropriate.

Krusen EM Jr. Acute injuries to the neck. *Modern Medicine (Review Edition).* 1960;20:29–38.

Krusen EM Jr, Krusen UL. Cervical syndrome especially the tension-neck problem: clinical study of 800 cases. *Archives of Physical Medicine and Rehabilitation.* 1955;36:518–523.

Kulowski J. Auto crash injury research. *Canadian Services Medical Journal.* 1955;11:761–775.

Kulowski J. Residual spinal injuries from automotive crashes: biomechanical considerations of pre-impact, impact, and post-impact factors involved in their production. *Southern Medical Journal.* 1958;51:367–372.

Kupperman A. Whiplash and disc derangement [letter]. *Journal of Oral and Maxillofacial Surgery.* 1988;46(6):519.

This author points out the potential flaws with S. Weinberg and H. LaPointe's theory of temporomandibular joint (TMJ) injury in whiplash patients. The author also reminds readers that the radiological abnormalities said to represent TMJ injury in whiplash patients are commonly found in normal subjects. See Chapter 6.

Kwan O. Rear-end auto collisions. Another view [letter]. *Archives of Physical Medicine and Rehabilitation.* 1998;79:721–722.

A commentary on Brault et al. See Chapter 21.

Kwan O, Friel J. The dilemma of whiplash [letter]. *Cephalalgia.* 1998;18(8): 586–587.

The authors explain the results of a recent study on the etiology of headache in whiplash patients by Wallis et al 1998.

Kwan O, Friel J. Comment on Radanov et al [letter]. *Journal of Rheumatology.* 1999. In press.

In this article, the authors point out the necessary methodology for an appropriate study of psychosocial factors in whiplash patients. They indicate that none of these criteria were met by Radanov et al in their Swiss study.

Lader E. Cervical trauma as a factor in the development of TMJ dysfunction and facial pain. *Journal of Craniomandibular Disorders.* 1983;1(2):85–90.

In this article, a theoretical explanation for temporomandibular joint injury in whiplash is given, but one must note the potential flaws in the reasoning. See R. Ferrari et al, H. L. Goldberg, A. P. Heise et al, R. P. Howard et al, W. S. Kirk Jr, M. Olin, R. H. Roydhouse, E. W. Small, and D. H. West et al.

Lader MH. Tolerability and safety: essentials in antidepressant pharmacotherapy. *Journal of Clinical Psychiatry.* 1996;57 (suppl 2):39–44.

Lalli JJ. Cervical vertebral syndromes. *Journal of the American Osteopathic Association.* 1972;72:121–128.

Landy PJB. Neurological sequelae of minor head and neck injuries. *Injury.* 1998;29(3):199–206.

Lange W. Mechanical and physiological response of the human cervical vertebral column to severe impacts applied to the torso. In: *Symposium on Biodynamic Models and Their Applications, Wright-Patterson Air Force Base, Ohio.* 1970: 141.

Using hyperextension studies with cadavers, the author shows that one must use head and neck forces greater than 2,700 newtons to cause significant ligament injury without head restraints.

Langwieder K, Backaitis SH, Fan W, Partyka S, Ommaya A. Comparative studies of neck injuries of car occupants in frontal collisions in the United States and in the Federal Republic of Germany. In: *Proceedings of the Twenty Fifth Stapp Car Crash Conference.* Paper #811030. Warrendale, PA: Society of Automotive Engineers; 1981:71–127.

La Rocca H. Cervical sprain syndrome. In: Frymoyer JW, Ducker TB, Hadler NM, Kostuik JP, Weinstein JN, Whitcloud III TS, eds. *The Adult Spine.* Vol 2. New York: Raven Press; 1991:1051–1061.

This author reviews some of the studies examining the cause of chronic symptoms in whiplash. The discussion has a few deficiencies. First, the author states that certain findings, other than fracture, are evidence of whiplash injury (which many studies have shown not to be true). Second, the author refers to the theoretical explanations of temporomandibular joint (TMJ) injury in whiplash as if they were factual and points out that arthrograms of the TMJ show injury. (Such findings are common in asymptomatic individuals.) Third, the author discusses a magnetic resonance scan with a herniated disc and assumes this was due to whiplash (even though studies have shown that at least 20% to 30% of the general population can have such findings on (magnetic resonance imaging) scan. (See, for example, L. M. Teresi et al and S. D. Boden et al.) Finally, the author refers to experiments done in 1955 and experiments done with animals, but not otherwise to human whiplash experiments.

Lavin RA. Cervical pain: a comparison of three pillows. *Archives of Physical Medicine and Rehabilitation.* 1997;78:193–198.

Some pillows are better than others. The study population includes a variety of causes of neck pains, only some of which are posttraumatic.

Lawrence JS. Disc degeneration. Its frequency and relationship to symptoms. *Annals of Rheumatic Diseases.* 1969;28:121–137.

Lawton F. A judicial view of traumatic neurosis. *Medicolegal Journal.* 1979;47: 6–17.

Lee F, Turner JWA. Natural history and prognosis of cervical spondylosis. *British Medical Journal.* 1963;2:1607–1610.

Lee J, Giles K, Drummond PD. Psychological disturbances and an exaggerated response to pain in patients with whiplash injury. *Journal of Psychosomatic Research.* 1993;37(2):105–110.

Lees-Haley PR, Brown RS. Neuropsychological complaint base rates of 170 personal injury claimants. *Archives of Clinical Neuropsychology.* 1993;8: 203–209.

These authors demonstrate that any litigating injury claimants, even those not claiming head injury, have a high rate of cognitive complaints. When compared to litigants without head injury, those litigants claiming head injury have the same frequency of these complaints. A brain injury thus account for symptoms that would be present in any litigant.

The authors explain that psychologically significant complaints may arise from preexisting conditions, the stress of litigation, emotional distress associated with pain, unrelated illnesses, malingering, medications, inspiration of hysteria by prior medical and legal evaluations, or influence of third parties. Thus, there remains no evidence that these complaints are due to brain injury in whiplash claimants.

Leopold RL, Dillon H. Psychiatric considerations in whiplash injuries of the neck. *Pennsylvania Medical Journal.* 1960;63(3):385–389.

Lesoin F, Thomas CE, Lozes G, Villette L, Jomin M. Has the safety-belt replaced the hangman's noose? [letter]. *Lancet.* 1985;1:1341.
Letter to the Editor. New Zealand Medical Journal. 1989;102:264.
Further comments to add to the article by K. M. Porter.

Levandoski RR. Mandibular whiplash. Part 1, An extension-flexion injury of the temporomandibular joints. *Functional Orthodontist.* January/February 1993: 26–29, 32–33.
This two-part (see below) article discusses the concept of mandibular whiplash, but one must note that the discussion is largely theoretical and that others have disproved theories of mandibular whiplash.
There are many authors who dispute the existence of mandibular or temporomandibular joint whiplash. See R. Ferrari et al, H. L. Goldberg, A. P. Heise et al, R. P. Howard et al, W. S. Kirk Jr, M. Olin, R. H. Roydhouse, E. W. Small, and D. H. West et al.

Levandoski RR. Mandibular whiplash. Part 2, An extension-flexion injury of the temporomandibular joints. *Functional Orthodontist.* January/February 1993: 45–51.
See above.

Levitt MA. Research can be a pain in the neck. *Academic Emergency Medicine.* 1996;3(6):563–564.
This author reviews the collar study by P. Gennis et al.

Lewy E. Contribution to the problem of compensation neurosis. *Bulletin of the Menninger Clinic.* 1940;4:88–92.

Liguori G, Cioffi M, Sebastiani A. Letter to the Editor. *Eye II* (part 1):139–140, 1997.

Lind JE. Traumatic neurasthenia, especially "railway spine." *Medical Record.* 1937;146:65–71.

Linson MA, Crowe CH. Comparison of magnetic resonance imaging and lumbar discography in the diagnosis of disc degeneration. *Clinical Orthopedics and Related Research.* 1990;250:160–163.

These authors use discography and magnetic resonance imaging of the lumbar spine and show that a number of the abnormalities actually caused no symptoms. One cannot therefore always attribute symptoms to such abnormalities since they may indeed not cause any symptoms at all.

Lipman FD. Malingering in personal injury cases. *Temple Law Quarterly.* 1962;35:141–162.

Lipow EG. Whiplash injuries. *Southern Medical Journal.* 1955;48:1304–1311.

Lipowski ZJ. Somatization: the concept and its clinical application. *American Journal of Psychiatry.* 1988;145(11):1358–1368.

This is a review of the concept of somatization.

Lipowksi ZJ. Somatization and depression. *Psychosomatics.* 1990;31(1):13–21.

Liu YK, Chandran KB, Heath RG, Unterharnscheidts F. Subcortical EEG changes in rhesus monkeys following experimental hyperextension-hyperflexion (whiplash). *Spine.* 1984;9(4):329–338.

In this study, the authors show that EEG abnormalities occur in monkeys they subjected to hyperextension injuries. One must note, however, that the accelerations they used were far greater than those whiplash patients typically experience, and that even then only 33% of the monkeys had EEG changes, all minor.

Liu YK, Wickstrom JK, Saltzberg B, et al. Subcortical EEG changes in rhesus monkeys following experimental whiplash. *26th Annual Conference on Engineering in Medicine and Biology (ACEMB).* 1973;15:404.

See above.

Livingston M. Neck and back sprains from MVAs: a retrospective study. *British Columbia Medical Journal.* 1991;33(12): 654–656.

Livingston M. Whiplash injury [letter]. *Lancet.* 1991;338:1208.

Livingston M. Whiplash injury: misconceptions and remedies. *Australian Family Physician.* 1992;21(11):1642–1644.

This author reveals the interesting observation that the British medical literature did not report on whiplash until many years after the American literature did. Medical literature regarding new diseases or injuries spreads rather quickly but had not in this case. The author argues that if the reporting of chronic symptoms in accident victims were due to some form of chronic neck damage that proceeds from the acute injury, it should have been occurring in the United Kingdom for as many years as in the United States. The literature in the United Kingdom should have had reports of it then but did not, until recently. Why? Collisions have been present in the United Kingdom for as long as in the United States.

Livingston M. Whiplash injury and peer copying. *Journal of the Royal Society of Medicine.* 1993;86:535–536.

This author reviews the concept of cultural information and the effect of the therapeutic community in generating illness. He also emphasizes the need for a more comprehensive and careful review of the scientific literature on whiplash—just like the review provided in this book.

Livingston M. Whiplash injury: some continuing problems. *Humane Medicine.* 1993;9(4):274–281.

See above.

Livingston M. Wise words of Malleson accordant. *Canadian Family Physician.* 1995;41:204.

Lord SM, Barnsley L, Bogduk N. The utility of comparative local anaesthetic blocks versus placebo-controlled blocks for the diagnosis of cervical zygapophysial joint pain. *Clinical Journal of Pain.* 1995;11:208–213.

See the articles by L. Barnsley et al.

Lord SM, Barnsley L, Wallis BJ, Bogduk N. Chronic cervical zygapophysial joint pain after whiplash. *Spine.* 1996;21: 1737–1745.

See the articles by L. Barnsley et al.

Lord SM, Barnsley L, Wallis BJ, McDonald GJ, Bogduk N. Percutaneous radio frequency neurotomy for chronic cervical zygapophyseal joint pain. *New England Journal of Medicine.* 1996;335:1721–1726.

These authors demonstrate that in a very small percentage of what they label as whiplash patients, there may be an identifiable joint injury as a cause of their pain. There is effective therapy for this source of pain. The authors discuss some of the problems with this study and state clearly that one should not generalize that this is the site of pain in all whiplash patients. This study provokes the same concern that other L. Barnsley et al studies provoke. Just because patients believe their pain several months or years after an accident is actually due to the accident does not mean that it is the source of the pain. The Lithuanian data (see H. Schrader et al) indicate that chronic neck pain is common in the general population and may arise spontaneously in many individuals who might in other settings attribute their pain to an accident. See the articles by L. Barnsley et al.

What is also apparent from the study is that the control group had 10 of 12 in litigation and the treatment group had only 4 of 12 in litigation. Clearly, being in litigation can prevent an individual from reporting improvement, no matter what treatment occurs. The control group is not a control group when this major confounding variable exists. No amount of statistics removes this obvious and important difference between the two groups.

Lottes JO, Luh AM, Leydig SM, Fries JW, Burst DO. Whiplash injuries of the neck. *Missouri Medicine*. 1959;56(6):645–650.

Loudon JK, Ruhl M, Field E. Ability to reproduce head position after whiplash injury. *Spine*. 1997;22(8):865–868.

In this study, the authors confirm that neck pain impairs whiplash patients' ability to use their neck muscles as part of the normal system by which people maintain equilibrium and balance. This may result in dizziness in whiplash patients. The need not be a nervous system injury. See also the "Disturbances of Balance and Hearing" in Chapter 7.

Loughner BA, Gremillion HA, Larkin LH, Mahan PE, Watson RE. Muscle attachment to the lateral aspect of the articular disk of human temporomandibular joint. *Oral Surgery, Oral Medicine, and Oral Pathology*. 1996;82:139–144.

This study deals with the possibility that abnormal muscle activity, rather than a temporomandibular joint injury, may be responsible for disk displacement.

Lövsund P, Nygren A, Salen B, Tingvall C. Neck injuries in rear end collisions among front and rear seat occupants. In: *Proceedings of the International IRCOBI Conference on the Biomechanics of Impacts, 1988, September 14–16, Bergisch, Gladbach, Germany, Bron, France*. 1988:319–325.

In this study, the authors found that occupant height bore no relationship to risk of neck injury. Thus, maladjustment of head restraints cannot explain their failure to reduce whiplash injury claims. The study is superior to others particularly because of the large sample size. See also C. J. Kahane and Chapter 22.

Lubin S, Sehmer J. Are automobile head restraints used effectively? *Canadian Family Physician*. 1993;39:1584–1588.

In this survey, the authors found that women more often have their head restraints adjusted properly than do men. Yet women are more often whiplash claimants. Adding to this is the fact that head restraints, even in the down position, are adequate for most women. See Chapter 22 for more discussion.

Lupton DE. Psychological aspects of temporomandibular joint dysfunction. *Journal of the American Dental Association*. 1969;79:131–136.

This author reviews the psychological factors responsible for the so-called "temporomandibular joint disorders" and the history of studies on this subject from 1955 to 1969.

See also R. Ferrari et al, and F. M. Bush and M. F. Dolwick.

Maag U, Desjardins D, Bourbeau R, Laberge-Nadeau C. Seat belts and neck injuries. In: *Proceedings of the International Research Council on the Biomechanics of Impacts (IRCOBI) Conference,1990, Bron, France*. 1990:1–13.

These authors conclude that accident victims wearing seat belts are more likely to develop whiplash than nonbelted victims. One must note, however, that this study does not include uninjured occupants who may have been wearing a seat belt (and therefore would alter the analysis conclusions). See Chapter 22.

Maag U, Laberge-Nadeau C, Xiang-Tong T. Neck sprains in car crashes: incidence, associations, length of compensation and costs to the insurer. In: *Proceedings of the 37th Annual Conference of the Association for the Advancement of Automotive Medicine, 1993, November 4–6, San Antonio, Texas, Des Plaines, Illinois*. 1993:15–26.

MacNab I. Acceleration injuries of the cervical spine. *Journal of Bone and Joint Surgery*. 1964;46-A(8):1797–1799.

This is MacNab's original description of monkey-dropping experiments. Many have criticized it and other animal experiments. See below and J. P. Gough for further criticisms.

MacNab I. Whiplash. *Modern Medicine of Canada*. 1966;21:43–55.

This article offers a repeat of MacNab's previous article above.

MacNab I. Whiplash injuries of the neck. *Manitoba Medical Review*. 1966;46: 172–174.

MacNab I. The "whiplash syndrome." *Orthopedic Clinics of North America*. 1971;2(2):389–403.

The author reviews the various issues regarding whiplash. One must note the many potential flaws of MacNab's work, however, and its limited applicability to humans (see "Whiplash Experiments" in Chapter 5).

MacNab I. The whiplash syndrome. *Clinical Neurosurgery*. 1973;20:232–241.

This article offers no new data. MacNab focuses on only one psychological aspect of whiplash patients (monetary compensation) and ignores the rest. He bases his discussion of pathology on monkey-dropping experiments that are not appropriate to most whiplash patients. See "Whiplash Experiments" in Chapter 5 for more criticism.

MacNab I. Acceleration extension injuries of the cervical spine. *Advocates' Quarterly*. 1979–1981;2:77–93.

This author reviews the topic in general, and essentially this is a repeat of his 1971 and 1973 articles. "Whiplash Experiments" in Chapter 5 for more criticism.

MacNab I. Acceleration extension injuries of the cervical spine. In: Rothman RH, Simeone FA, eds. *The Spine*. Philadelphia: WB Saunders; 1982:647–660.

This offers no new information and is based on MacNab's experiments before 1970. It has statements such as "when the head rotates backward the mouth is flung open" that many have now shown to be false.

Magnusson ML, Aleksiev A, Wilder DG, et al. Unexpected load and asymmetric posture as etiologic factors in low back pain. *European Spine Journal*. 1996; 5(1):23–35.

Magnússon T. Extracervical symptoms after whiplash trauma. *Cephalalgia*. 1994;14:223–227.

This author attempts a theory that the chronic pain of whiplash patients must be due to some form of chronic damage arising from the acute injury. The author bases this on the argument that such patients' diagnoses may also include fibromyalgia, low back pain, and oromandibular dysfunction. The author considers these diagnoses to be based in some form of physical pathology.

Many view fibromyalgia as nonorganic, and back pain is a symptom, not a disease. Many experts consider chronic back pain to be primarily dependent on psychological factors. And many consider oromandibular dysfunction to be dependent on psychological factors. By demonstrating that these diagnoses often occur in whiplash patients, this author has actually confirmed significant psychological mechanisms may be influencing whiplash patients.

Magnússon T, Ragnarsson T, Björnsson A. Occipital nerve release in patients with whiplash trauma and occipital neuralgia. *Headache*. 1996;36:32–36.

Magoun HI. Whiplash injury: a greater lesion complex. *Journal of the American Osteopathic Association*. 1964;63:524–535.

Maguire WB. Whiplash in Australia: illness or injury? [letter]. *Medical Journal of Australia*. 1993;158:138.

Maigne JY. Letter to editor. *Spine*. 1997;22(12):1420.

Maimaris C. Neck sprains after car accidents [letter]. *British Medical Journal*. 1989;299:123.

This author explains that there is no evidence of a form of chronic damage that arises from the acute injury, as one judges by studies with magnetic resonance imaging.

Maimaris C, Barnes M, Allen M. Whiplash injuries of the neck: a retrospective study. *Injury*. 1988;19:393–396.

See above.

Malleson A. Whiplash: folly and fakery. *Humane Medicine*. 1990;6(3):193–196.

Malleson A. Chronic whiplash syndrome. Psychosocial epidemic. *Canadian Family Physician*. 1994;40:1906–1909.

Malleson A. Response [letter]. *Canadian Family Physician*. 1995;41:204–206.

Malleson A. Response [letter]. *Canadian Family Physician*. 1995;41:563, 565.

Malt UF. Coping with accidental injury. *Psychiatric Medicine*. 1992;10(3):135–147.

This continues discussions started in the below study, focusing on the importance of coping skills and psychosocial variables in outcome.

Malt UF, Olafsen OM. Psychological appraisal and emotional response to physical injury: a clinical, phenomenological study of 109 adults. *Psychiatric Medicine*. 1992;10(3):117–134.

In this study of accident victims in general, these authors conclude that the accident or injury is only a provoking agent. The short- and long-term effect is to a large extent predicted by predisposing (vulnerability) and symptom formation (pathoplastic) variables. Issues such as attribution, learned illness behavior and operant conditioning and reinforcing variables related to the society, including its lawyers and doctors, are all important factors in the etiology of posttraumatic suffering.

Mannheimer J, Attanasio R, Cinotti WR, Pertes R. Cervical strain and mandibular whiplash: Effects upon the craniomandibular apparatus. *Clinical Preventative Dentistry*. 1989;11(1):29–32.

These authors build upon a theory of temporomandibular joint injury that R. P. Howard et al have since disproved. As well, the signs of "joint injuries" the authors cite as possibilities in whiplash patients are common in asymptomatic individuals. Finally, the authors attempt to impress the reader by citing many severe injuries that are completely irrelevant to typical whiplash patients, who by definition are almost exclusively a population without these injuries.

See also R. Ferrari et al, H. L. Goldberg, A. P. Heise et al, W. S. Kirk Jr, R. H. Roydhouse, E. W. Small, and D. H. West et al.

Marchiori DM, Henderson CNR. A cross-sectional study correlating cervical radiographic degenerative findings to pain and disability. *Spine*. 1997;21(23): 2747–2752.

These authors appear to reveal an association between severity of neck pain and severity of degenerative changes seen on neck X-ray. The study, however, does not have a control group. If it did, it might show that many people in the general population have severe degenerative changes and are not complaining of symptoms. If that is so, then this study's results do not demonstrate a cause and effect relationship, merely that an association exists in this particular study group. A reviewer of this article, P. Shekelle (p 2753 of the journal), states, "The epidemiologic literature is replete with associations observed in cross-sectional studies that later were shown to be spurious."

Marshall HW. Neck injuries. *Boston Medical and Surgical Journal*. 1919;158(4): 93–98.

Marshall PD, O'Connor M, Hodgkinson JP. The perceived relationship between neck symptoms and precedent injury. *Injury*. 1995;26:17–19.

In this study, these authors indicate that accident victims may be underreporting preaccident histories of neck pain. To appreciate the background prevalence of neck pain in the general population, the authors asked a group of individuals who had not been in an accident about neck pain. They then asked a group of accident victims if they had preaccident neck pain, and these patients reported a lower incidence of preaccident neck pain than one expects for their age. They are part of the general population as well and should have a similar background prevalence of preaccident neck pain. That they do not means that they are either intentionally underreporting preaccident neck pain or forgetting their preaccident pain for other reasons.

Martin GM. Sprains, strains, and whiplash injuries. *Physical Therapy Review.* 1959;39(12):808–817.

Matsushita T, Sato TB, Hirabayashi K, et al. X-ray study of the human neck motion due to head inertia loading. In: *Proceedings of the Thirty Eighth Stapp Car Crash Conference.* Paper #942208. Warrendale, PA: Society of Automotive Engineers; 1994:55–64.

Mayfield FH, Griffith JC. Whiplash injuries. *Journal of the Michigan State Medical Society.* 1957;56:1142–1146, 1161.

Mayou R. Somatization. *Psychotherapy and Psychosomatics.* 1993;59:69–83.

Mayou R. Medico-legal aspects of road traffic accidents. *Journal of Psychosomatic Research.* 1995;39(6):789–798.

Mayou R, Bryant B. Outcome of 'whiplash' neck injury. *Injury.* 1996;27(9): 617–623.

In this study of 63 whiplash patients, the authors conclude that psychological and social variables at the time of the accident do not correlate with outcome. This study has some of the same problems as the studies of B. P. Radanov et al (see O. Kwan and J. Friel). There is a rather simple attempt to uncover the psychosocial history and verify that the individuals are representing themselves accurately. The determination of an individual's psychosocial status as it may relate to illness outcome requires far more in-depth psychosocial data, with an analysis of family dynamics, job satisfaction, and life events.

Interestingly, the M. Karlsborg et al study concludes the exact opposite of the study by these authors.

Mayou R, Bryant B, Duthie R. Psychiatric consequences of road traffic accidents. *British Medical Journal.* 1993;307:647–651.

These authors consider that fright at the time of the accident and other psychological factors that act after the accident may lead to reporting of chronic symptoms.

Mayou R, Radanov BP. Whiplash neck injury. *Journal of Psychosomatic Research.* 1996;40(5):461–474.

This article reviews the need for more systematic and standard evaluation of the psychological and social variables affecting outcome in whiplash patients.

McConnell WE, Howard RP, Guzman HM, et al. Analysis of human test subject kinematic responses to low speed rear end impacts. In: *Proceedings of the Thirty Seventh Stapp Car Crash Conference*. Paper #930889. Warrendale, PA: Society of Automotive Engineers; 1993:21–30.

These authors show that in human experiments with rear-end collisions, there is usually (at the typical velocities of most such collisions) very little neck extension, with or without head restraints, and that the body does not slide up the seat at all. This work clearly denounces the theory of B. R. Selecki that a low head restraint will cause more neck hyperextension. Also, C. J. Kahane states that most head restraints, even in the down position, should prevent whiplash by a hyperextension mechanism.

Even in the down position, head restraints would be high enough for most women, as the design is for men. Yet women appear to get whiplash more than men. Further, no one has shown that tall occupants develop whiplash symptoms more frequently than shorter occupants.

That head restraints do not appear to reduce the incidence of whiplash patients to any great degree suggests other factors must be involved.

McConnell WE, Howard RP, Van Poppel J, et al. Human head and neck kinematics after low velocity rear-end impacts—understanding "whiplash." In: *Proceedings of the Thirty Ninth Stapp Car Crash Conference*. Paper #952724. Warrendale, PA: Society of Automotive Engineers; 1995:215–238.

McDermott FT. Reduction in cervical "whiplash" after new motor vehicle accident legislation in Victoria. *Medical Journal of Australia*. 1993;158: 720–721.

This author considers how simply changing legislation for whiplash claims causes a major decrease in claims for chronic "injury." One should not interpret this to mean that whiplash patients are malingering but perhaps that the process of dealing with insurance companies, therapists, and lawyers may itself contribute to symptoms.

McElhaney JH, Doherty BJ, Paver JG, et al. Combined bending and axial loading responses of the human cervical spine. In: *Proceedings of the Thirty Second Stapp Car Crash Conference*. Paper #881709. Warrendale, PA: Society of Automotive Engineers; 1998:21–28.

McElhaney JH, Myers BS. Biomechanical aspects of cervical trauma. In: Nahum AM, Melvin JW, eds. *Accidental Injury. Biomechanics and Prevention*. New York: Springer-Verlag; 1993:323–325.

This text deals with experiments measuring forces the cervical spine tolerates. These forces are often greater than those that occur in typical collisions producing whiplash patients.

McElhaney JH, Paver JG, McCrackin JH, Maxwell GM. Cervical spine compression responses. In: *Proceedings of the Twenty Seventh Stapp Car Crash Conference*. Warrendale, PA: Society of Automotive Engineers; 1983:163–178.

McGee FO. Whiplash injury of the cervical spine. *Orthopedics*. 1959;1:105–108, 115–116.

McIntire RT. Whiplash injuries. *Journal of the Medical Association of Alabama*. 1959;29:170.

McIntire RT, Compere EL, Watts JW, Abbott KH. Whiplash injuries: a panel discussion. *Journal of the International College of Surgeons*. 1957;28(1):54–63.

McKay DC, Christensen LV. Whiplash injuries of the temporomandibular joint in motor vehicle accidents: speculations and facts. *Journal of Oral Rehabilitation*. 1998;25(10):731–746.
See L. V. Christensen and D. C. McKay, and Chapter 6.

McKeever DC. The mechanics of the so-called whiplash injury. *Orthopedics*. 1960;2:3–6.

McKellar CC. "Whiplash"—should we discard the name? Medical *Journal of Australia*. 1979;2:494.

McKenzie RA. *The Cervical and Thoracic Spine*. New Zealand: Spinal Publications Ltd; 1990.

McKinney LA. Early mobilisation and outcome in acute sprains of the neck. *British Medical Journal*. 1989;299:1000–1008.
This is one of the few controlled trials of therapy in whiplash. The authors demonstrate that independent therapy with postural advice and neck stretches is superior to rest and to local physiotherapy with modalities such as heat, diathermy, hydrotherapy, traction, and manipulation.
See also G. E. Borchgrevink et al, K. Mealy et al, L. Provinciali et al, and Quebec Task Force (W. O. Spitzer et al).

McNeal HJ. "Whiplash"—an unrealistic psychological word. *Insurance Counsel Journal*. April 1963:275–278.

McOsker TC. Neck injury and rear-end collision. *Rhode Island Medical Journal.* 1962;45:252–257.

Mealy K, Brennan H, Fenelon GC. Early mobilization of acute whiplash injuries. *British Medical Journal.* 1986;6:27–33.

Another study dealing with the benefits of exercises and stretches versus rest in whiplash patients. See also G. E. Borchgrevink et al, H. Brodin, L. A. McKinney, and L. Provinciali et al.

Mechanic D. The concept of illness behavior. *Journal of Chronic Diseases.* 1961;15:189–194.

Mechanic D. Response factors in illness: the study of illness behavior. *Social Psychiatry.* 1966;1(1):11–20.

Mechanic D, Volkart EH. Illness behavior and medical diagnoses. *Journal of Health and Human Behavior.* 1960;1:86–94.

This article deals with the concept of illness behavior.

Mechanic D, Volkart EH. Stress, illness behavior, and the sick role. *American Sociological Review.* 1961;26:51–58.

This article deals with the psychological variables in illness, and the authors further elaborate on these concepts in the other Mechanic articles.

Melville PH. "Research" in car crashes [letter]. *Canadian Medical Association Journal.* 1963;89:275.

This author offers the interesting observation that in car-crashing contests, the occupants frequently experience collisions but do not appear to report chronic pain.

Melvin JW, McElhaney JH, Roberts VL. Evaluation of dummy neck performance. In: King WF, Mertz HJ, eds. *Human Impact Response.* New York: Plenum Press; 1973:247–261.

Mendelson G. Not "cured by a verdict." Effect of legal settlement on compensation claimants. *Medical Journal of Australia.* 1982;2:132–134.

This is a review of previous studies on this subject.

Mendelson G. Follow-up studies of personal injury litigants. International *Journal of Law and Psychiatry.* 1984;7:179–188.

This author concludes that the desire for compensation has little to do with the outcome of personal injury patients. One must note, however, R. D. Goldney's work that reminds us that one cannot generalize about such issues. Clearly, there are some individuals whose symptoms are improved after settlement and others for whom settlement has no impact. There are many other secondary gains besides monetary compensation to consider. See D. A. Fishbain.

Mendelson G. Measurement of conscious symptom exaggeration by questionnaire: a clinical study. *Journal of Psychosomatic Research*. 1987;31(6): 703–711.

Merskey H. Psychiatry and the cervical sprain syndrome. *Canadian Medical Association Journal*. 1984;130:1119–1121.

Merskey H. The importance of hysteria. *British Journal of Psychiatry*. 1986; 149:23–28.

Merskey H. Psychological consequences of whiplash. *Spine: State of the Art Reviews*. 1993;7(3):471–480.

This author quite correctly points out that many of the psychological factors responsible for chronic pain follow the accident and do not simply come from the patient's preaccident history or personality. This does not rule out the relevance of the personality and preaccident psychosocial history but simply affirms that the individual need not be neurotic or a hypochondriac. What he neglects to address, however, is a simple question: At, say, 6 months after an accident, does a whiplash patient reporting chronic pain actually have physical damage that yet remains from the acute injury? Is this author saying that psychological factors maintain the chronic pain reporting or that both physical damage and psychological factors are acting? If so, what is the damage and how does it become chronic after the acute injury?

Merskey H. Chronic whiplash syndrome [letter]. *Neurology*. 1995;45:2116.

Merskey H, Woodforde JM. Psychiatric sequelae of minor head injury. *Brain*. 1972;95:521–528.

These authors make the argument, as does R. Kelly, that there is probably an organic (physical) basis for chronic symptoms after minor head injury or whiplash because financial gain cannot fully explain the patient's chronic symptoms. One must note, however, that there are many other secondary gains. See D. A. Fishbain.

Mertz HJ, Patrick LM. Investigation of the kinematics of whiplash. In: *Proceedings of the Eleventh Stapp Car Crash Conference*. Paper #670919. Warrendale, PA: Society of Automotive Engineers; 1967:175–206.

These authors reveal that human volunteers experience only minor symptoms (no chronic symptoms) with the same magnitude of forces most whiplash patients experience. See also L. M. Patrick.

Mertz HJ, Patrick LM. Strength and response of the human neck. *Proceedings of the Fifteenth Stapp Car Crash Conference*. Paper #710855. Warrendale, PA: Society of Automotive Engineers; 1971:2903–2928.

In this study, the authors show that humans can tolerate (without any significant symptoms) often much higher forces to the head and neck than occur in most rear-end collisions.

Meyer S, Weber M, Castro W, Schilgen M, Peuker C. The minimal collision velocity for whiplash. In: Gunzburg R, Szpalski M, eds. *Whiplash Injuries. Current Concepts in Prevention, Diagnosis, and Treatment of the Cervical Whiplash Syndrome*. Philadelphia: Lippincott-Raven; 1998:95–115.

In this study the authors found the threshold for whiplash injury in rear-end collision to be when the struck vehicle has a change in velocity of 10 km/h, slightly higher than the 8 km/h found by other researchers. See "Whiplash Experiments" in Chapter 5 and Chapter 20. See also under W. H. M. Castro et al.

Michael M, Boyce WT, Wilcox AJ. *Biomedical Bestiary*. Boston: Little, Brown, and Company; 1984.

This is an amusing discussion about the flaws that may occur in medical research.

Middaugh S, Kee W, Nicholson J. Muscle overuse and posture as factors in the development and maintenance of chronic musculoskeletal pain. In: Grzesiak R, Ciccone D, eds. *Psychological Vulnerability to Chronic Pain*. New York: Springer; 1994: 55–89.

Middleton JM. Ophthalmic aspects of whiplash injuries. *International Record of Medicine*. 1956;169(1):19–20.

Miles KA, Maimaris C, Finlay D, Barnes MR. The incidence and prognostic significance of radiological abnormalities in soft tissue injuries to the cervical spine. *Skeletal Radiology*. 1988; 17:493–496.

These authors reveal important findings regarding radiologic abnormalities in whiplash patients. They show that angular deformities on X-ray are of no significance with regard to prognosis, nor is prevertebral soft tissue swelling. The authors state that this may be important in cases involving litigation.

They conclude that:

The presence of an angular deformity is certainly not associated with a poor outcome and hence no special treatment or follow-up of these patients is required. This may also be of relevance in cases of litigation.

In the absence of bony injury or clinical evidence of spinal cord injury, an increased prevertebral soft tissue space appears to be of little clinical importance.

Milette PC, Raymond J, Fontaine S. Comparison of high-resolution computed tomography with discography in the evaluation of lumbar disc herniations. *Spine*. 1990;15(6):525–533.

In this study of computed tomography scanning of the lumbar spine, the authors show that 23% to 50% of the abnormalities cause no symptoms. One cannot, therefore, always attribute symptoms to such abnormalities since they may indeed not cause any symptoms at all.

Miller H. Accident neurosis. *British Medical Journal*. April 1961:919–925.

This study shows that clearly some personal injury litigants are motivated, preconsciously or consciously, by the prospect of financial gain. Other patients' symptoms may not improve after financial settlement because other factors maintain them.

Miller H. Accident neurosis. Lecture II. *British Medical Journal*. April 1961: 992–998.

Miller H. Posttraumatic headache. In: Vinken PJ, Bruyn GW, eds. *Handbook of Clinical Neurology*. Vol 24. Amsterdam, the Netherlands: North-Holland Publishing Company; 1977: 178–184.

This chapter addresses many of the psychological factors responsible for posttraumatic headache. The author has had a great deal of experience with such patients.

Miller H, Brain R, Russell WR, O'Connell JEA. Discussion on cervical spondylosis. *Proceedings of the Royal Society of Medicine*. 1955;49:197–208.

This discussion reminds us that one cannot always ascribe symptoms to cervical spondylosis (disc degeneration) as seen on X-ray because there is a poor correlation between symptoms and X-ray changes.

Mills H, Horne G. Whiplash—manmade disease. *New Zealand Medical Journal*. 1986;99:373–374.

These authors note that differences in legislation and claims procedures between New Zealand and Australia have led to a dramatic difference in the number of whiplash claims (there are fewer in New Zealand). This does not mean that patients were malingering but rather that the process of dealing with insurance companies, therapists, and lawyers may itself contribute to symptoms.

Minc S. Psychological aspects of backache. *Medical Journal of Australia*. 1968;1:964–965.

Mittenberg W, DiGiulio DV, Perrin S, Bass AE. Symptoms following mild head injury: expectation as aetiology. *Journal of Neurology, Neurosurgery, and Psychiatry*. 1992;55:200–204.

These authors show that society in general is so aware of what symptoms whiplash and head injury should produce that individuals can produce a stereotypical syndrome based in part on expectation itself.

Modic MT, Pavlicek W, Weinstein MA. Magnetic resonance imaging of intervertebral disk disease. *Radiology*. 1984;152:103–111.

Modlin HC. The postaccident anxiety syndrome: psychosocial aspects. *American Journal of Psychiatry*. 1967;123(8):1008–1012.

Moffat M. Letter to editor. Spine. 1996;21(1):150.

Moldofsky H, Wong MTH, Lue FA. Litigation, sleep symptoms and disabilities in postaccident pain (fibromyalgia). *Journal of Rheumatology*. 1993;20:1935–1940.

The authors conducted this study to examine the sleep and symptoms of those patients with postaccident pain with litigation settlement and with outstanding litigation. They found that the claim status did not influence these outcomes. That is not surprising. There are many reasons some patients do not improve after settlement. Those who have adopted the sick role find the illness affords them secondary gains perhaps far beyond any monetary gains. Chronic pain patients may persist in that illness behavior for so long that they develop a "pain identity," which means that even after settlement, to stop having pain is to lose their identity. Some may harbor resentment that their settlement was too little and somatize this distress by complaining of ongoing suffering.

The study did demonstrate that delaying compensation is unjustified, since the outcome is much the same for early or late settlement. Those who are adopting the sick role, for example, will do so regardless of when they receive their settlement, because the sick role has other potential gains.

Moody PM, Kemper JT, Okesen JP, et al. Recent life changes and myofascial pain syndrome. *Journal of Prosthetic Dentistry*. 1982;48(3):328–330.

The authors consider that patients complaining of temporomandibular joint symptoms often have a high incidence of psychologically distressing events prior to the onset of their symptoms.

Moorhead JJ. Traumatic neuroses. *Postgraduate Medicine*. 1947;2:184–187.

Morehouse LE. Body functions and controls in whiplash injuries. *International Record of Medicine*. 1956;169(1):11–13.

Morris F. Do head-restraints protect the neck from whiplash injuries? *Archives of Emergency Medicine*. 1989;6:17–21.

Morrow J. Surgical anatomy of whiplash injuries. *International Record of Medicine*. 1956;169(1):14–18.

Muir CB, Goss AN. The radiologic morphology of asymptomatic temporomandibular joints. *Oral Surgery, Oral Medicine, and Oral Pathology*. 1990;70:349–354.

In this study of asymptomatic subjects with temporomandibular joint (TMJ) tomograms, the authors reveal that many of the radiological abnormalities on TMJ imaging are found in subjects with no pain, yet many claim these to be the cause of pain in whiplash patients.

See also S. L. Brooks et al and P. Westesson et al.

Muir CB, Goss AN. The radiologic morphology of painful temporomandibular joints. *Oral Surgery, Oral Medicine, Oral Pathology*. 1990;70:355–359.

See above.

Munro D. Relation between spondylosis cervicalis and injury of the cervical spine and its contents. *New England Journal of Medicine*. 1960;262(17):839–846.

This author states that previous injury cannot be seen as the cause of disc degeneration or as a factor that aggravates disc degeneration.

Muzzy WH, Lustick L. Comparison of kinematic parameters between hybrid II head and neck system with human volunteers for -Gx acceleration profiles. In: *Proceedings of the Twentieth Stapp Car Crash Conference*. Paper #760801. Warrendale, PA: Society of Automotive Engineers; 1976:45–74.

Myers A. Degeneration of cervical intervertebral discs following whiplash injury. *Bulletin of the Hospital for Joint Diseases*. 1953;14:74–85.

This author suggests that previous neck trauma is the cause of the X-ray changes seen as disc degeneration. The author has, however, disregarded the need for control populations in reaching such conclusions. See "Radiology of Whiplash" in Chapter 5.

Myers BS, McElhaney JH, Doherty BJ, et al. Responses of the human cervical spine to torsion. In: *Proceedings of the Thirty Third Stapp Car Crash Conference*. Paper #892437. Warrendale, PA: Society of Automotive Engineers; 1989:215–222.

Nagle DB. Whiplash of the cervical spine. Radiology. 1957; 69:823–827.

Napier M, Wheat K. *Recovering Damages for Psychiatric Injury*. London: Blackstone Press Ltd.; 1995.

Navin FDP, Macnabb MJ, Romilly DP, Thomson RW. An investigation into vehicle and occupant response subjected to low-velocity rear impacts. In: *Proceedings of the Multidisciplinary Road Safety Conference VI*. 1989:159–169.

In this study, the authors show that in a rear-end collision, a dummy's head will move backward. They use this as evidence to prove the mechanism of whiplash. One must note, however, that dummies seldom complain of whiplash (not having a mouth or a desire for litigation). There are even more differences between the dummy and human head and neck complex than there are between that of a human and a monkey.

Neal LA. The pitfalls of making a categorical diagnosis of post-traumatic stress disorder in personal injury litigation. *Medical Sciences and the Law*. 1994; 34(2):117–122.

Nelson DA. Thoracic outlet syndrome and dysfunction of the temporomandibular joint: proved pathology or pseudosyndromes? *Perspectives in Biology and Medicine*. 1990;33(4): 567–576.

This author disputes thoracic outlet syndrome.

Newman PK. Author's reply [letter]. *British Medical Journal*. 1990;301:610.

Newman PK. Whiplash injury [letter]. *British Medical Journal*. 1990;301: 395–396.

Nicholson MW. Whiplash: fact, fantasy or fakery. *Hawaii Medical Journal*. 1974;33(5):168–170.

Nick J, Sicard-Nick C. Chronic post-traumatic headache. In: Friedman AP, ed. *Research and Clinical Studies in Headache*. Vol 2. New York: S. Karger; 1969:116–168.

In this study, the authors conclude that psychological factors are an important aspect of causation of chronic posttraumatic headaches.

Nielsen GP, Gough JP, Little DM, West DH, Baker VT. Human subject responses to repeated low speed impacts using utility vehicles. *Proceedings of the Forty First Stapp Car Crash Conference*. Paper #970394. Warrendale, PA: Society of Automotive Engineers; 1997:189–212.

Nielsen JM. Whiplash injury with amnesia for life experiences. *Bulletin of Los Angeles Neurological Society*. 1959;24:27–30.

Norris JW. Whiplash injury [letter]. *Lancet*. 1991;338:1207–1208.

Norris SH, Watt I. The prognosis of neck injuries resulting from rear-end vehicle collisions. *Journal of Bone and Joint Surgery*. 1983;65-B(5):608–611.

Some quote this study to indicate that whiplash patients have a high incidence of developing disc degeneration.

These authors conclude that patients with more abnormal X-rays at the time of rear-end collision have a worse outcome. One must note, however, that they had only 8 patients in the worse outcome group, far too small a number to make such conclusions. These authors also include patients with neck fractures in the study. Clearly the outcome of patients with neck fractures and the factors that affect that outcome may be very different from those of whiplash patients without neck fractures. It is inappropriate to include patients with neck fracture in this outcome study. See "Radiology of Whiplash" in Chapter 5.

Noseworthy JH, Miller J, Murray TJ, Regan D. Auditory brainstem response in postconcussion syndrome. *Archives of Neurology*. 1981;38:275–278.

In this study, the authors show that auditory brainstem responses in postconcussion patients are not indicative of brain damage.

Nygren A. Injuries to car occupants—some aspects of the interior safety of cars. *Acta Otolaryngologica*. 1984;395(suppl):1–164.

This author suggests that neck injuries occur more often in occupants wearing seat belts than in occupants who are not wearing seat belts. One should, however, refer to Chapter 22 to note the potential flaws with this conclusion.

Nygren A, Gustafsson H, Tingvall C. Effects of different types of headrests in rear-end collisions. In: *Proceedings of the Tenth International Conference on Experimental Safety Vehicles, July 1–4, 1985, Oxford*. U.S. Department of Transportation, National Highway Traffic Safety Administration; 1985:85–90.

Nyström S. Slight head injury with severe sequelae—a problem of insurance medicine. *Scandinavian Journal of Rehabilitation Medicine*. 1972;4:73–76.

Obelieniene D, Bovim G, Schrader H, et al. Headache after whiplash: a historical cohort study outside the medico-legal context. *Cephalalgia*. 1998;18(8): 559–564.

Obelieniene D, Schrader H, Bovim G, et al. Pain after whiplash—a prospective controlled inception cohort study. *Journal of Neurology, Neurosurgery, and Psychiatry*. 1999;6:279–284.

Odom GL, Finney W, Woodhall B. Cervical disk lesions. *Journal of the American Medical Association*. 1958;166(1):23–28.

These researchers compared a new radiographic technique, the myelogram, to plain X-rays. They show that "it was not unusual to have narrowing of the disk and spur formation at one level and to have the myelogram negative at this space, with a defect [at a site where the X-ray was normal]. Abnormal changes in the plain roentgenograms of the cervical spine coincided with myelographic defects in only 30% of the cases."

Thus, this study reveals that abnormalities on myelograms cannot, in themselves, explain the symptoms of neck pain or prove nerve involvement by a disc, since there is a poor correlation among the X-rays, the myelogram, and symptoms.

Olin M. Components of complex TM disorders. *Journal of Craniomandibular Disorders: Facial and Oral Pain*. 1990;4(3):193–196.

This author refutes, in part, the theories of S. Weinberg and H. LaPointe and E. Lader that temporomandibular joint injury occurs in rear-end collisions. See also the work of R. Ferrari et al, H. L. Goldberg, A. P. Heise et al, R. P. Howard et al, W. S. Kirk Jr, R. H. Roydhouse, E. W. Small and D. H. West et al.

Olney DB, Marsden AK. The effect of head restraints and seat belts on the incidence of neck injury in car accidents. *Injury*. 1986;17:365–367.

In this study, the authors note there seems to have been little benefit to head restraints in reducing the incidence of whiplash patients. If the mechanism of whiplash is simply neck hyperextension, then head restraints should be effective, but they are not. This means that either the mechanism of whiplash is not hyper-extension or vehicle occupants are using head restraints incorrectly. The idea that car occupants often leave the head restraint in a "down" position (incorrect use) may be irrelevant since C. J. Kahane has revealed that even in the down position head restraints are all designed to be high enough for most women (the ones who most frequently get whiplash) and some men. Further, no one has shown that tall occupants develop whiplash symptoms more frequently than shorter occupants.

Thus, there really is no evidence of any deficiency in head restraints, yet they do not seem to be effective in reducing the incidence of whiplash patients.

See also Chapter 22, R. C. Grunsten et al, W. E. McConnell et al, B. O'Neill et al, C. Thomas et al, and D. H. West et al.

Olsen J. Whiplash in Australia: illness or injury? [letter]. *Medical Journal of Australia*. 1993;158:71.

Olsnes BT. Neurobehavioural findings in whiplash patients with long-lasting symptoms. *Acta Neurologica Scandinavica*. 1989; 80:584–588.

This author reviews the similarities between the cognitive functions of whiplash patients and those of other patients who have chronic pain syndromes unrelated to trauma. There was no difference between the groups in terms of cognitive function, and the author concludes there is no organic (physical) basis for the cognitive symptoms of whiplash patients. See also "Disturbances of Balance and Hearing" in Chapter 7.

Olson VL. Whiplash-associated chronic headache treated with home cervical traction. *Physical Therapy*. 1997;77:417–424.

Although this article deals with the benefits of neck traction, it is not a study but a case report of a single patient. One needs properly controlled studies before considering traction therapy in whiplash patients.

Olsson I, Bunketorp O, Carlsson G, et al. An in-depth study of neck injuries in rear end collisions. In: *Proceedings of the International Research Council on Biokinetics of Impacts (IRCOBI), September 12–13–14, Bron-Lyon, France*. 1990: 269–280.

In this study, the authors consider in detail the possible mechanisms of injury in rear-end collisions, offering explanations of the whiplash injury and why head restraints have not significantly reduced the incidence of whiplash claims. One must note, however, the methodologic issues of concern, as dealt with in Chapter 22.

First, the study is not likely to be representative of the whiplash population because it looked at only 33 occupants, 27 of whom were men (most whiplash patients are women). The results are therefore not readily applicable to other populations of whiplash patients, and a larger number would increase the chance that the conclusions are valid. Second, the authors state that:

> Most modern cars are equipped with head restraints designed to prevent this type of injury. Nevertheless, neck injuries are still common in rear-end collisions, which indicates that the protective equipment is not functioning satisfactorily.

> As a matter of fact, the use of seat belts has been shown to correlate with an increased risk of neck injuries in different types of car accidents.

There are concerns with both of these conclusions. See Chapter 22.

Finally, the authors state that "it is reasonable to believe that the shorter the distance the less the likelihood that the various tissues involved would be strained."

That belief may be partially based on the assumptions about how the acute injury occurs. Neck hyperextension may not be the only mechanism of the acute minor injury. See again Chapter 22.

Ommaya AK. Trauma to the nervous system. *Annals of the Royal College of Surgeons of England*. 1966;39:317–347.

This author looks at monkeys and experimental head injury by firing pistons at their skulls. This caused damage. See below.

Ommaya AK, Faas F, Yarnell P. Whiplash injury and brain damage. *Journal of the American Medical Association*. 1968; 204(4):285–289.

These authors report the results of experimental rear-end collisions with monkeys in little carts. One must note, however, that the experimenters used accelerations greater than 100g (many times that of typical rear-end collisions producing whiplash patients). With these accelerations they could generate concussion in about 10% of the monkeys. Higher accelerations (15 to 50 times typical rear-end collision accidents) could cause brain damage as well. The authors themselves caution against using these results to describe the outcome of human whiplash patients because the accelerations and forces were so great.

Ommaya AK, Hirsch AE, Martinez JL. The role of whiplash in cerebral concussion. In: *Proceedings of the Tenth Stapp Car Crash Conference*. Paper #660804. Warrendale, PA: Society of Automotive Engineers; 1966: 314–324.

These authors show that if a monkey is struck on the head, bending of the neck may play a role in concussion because when one prevents such bending with a collar, concussion incidence is reduced. Thus, they conclude whiplash neck movements may have some relevance to brain injury. One must note, however, that the forces they used on these monkeys were on the order of 910 newtons, whereas in typical collisions producing whiplash patients, the forces are less. The forces in this study are too great to apply the results to whiplash patients. Also, direct skull impact may affect the way the head and neck experience the forces involved, and so again one cannot so readily apply the study results to whiplash patients without head impact.

O'Neill B, Haddon W Jr, Kelley AB, Sorenson WW. Automobile head restraints—frequency of neck injury claims in relation to the presence of head restraints. *American Journal of Public Health*. March 1972:399–406.

In this study, the authors reveal that head restraints are not effective in preventing whiplash, suggesting that the mechanism of whiplash may not be hyperextension (which head restraints could prevent). See also Chapter 22, R. C. Grunsten et al, C. J. Kahane, W. E. McConnell et al, D. B. Olney and A. K. Marsden, C. Thomas et al, and D. H. West et al.

Ono K, Kanno M. Influences of the physical parameters on the risk to neck injuries in low impact speed rear-end collisions. In: *Proceedings of the International IRCOBI Conference on the Biomechanics of Impacts, September 8–10, 1993, Eindhoven, Netherlands*. 1993:201–212.

Ono K, Kanno M. Influences of the physical parameters on the risk to neck injuries in low impact speed rear-end collisions. *Accident Analysis and Prevention*. 1996;28(4):493–499.

Oosterveld WJ, Kortschot HW, Kingma GG, de Jong HAA, Saatci MR. Electronystagmographic findings following cervical whiplash injuries. *Acta Otolaryngologica (Stockholm)*. 1991;111:201–205.

These authors report some abnormal test results in what they label as whiplash patients. The question is whether these abnormal test results derive from an accident injury. There are many reasons to doubt this. First, the patients the authors describe here are a highly select group, with examinations in some cases years after the accident. It may be that their symptoms at the time of the evaluation were due entirely to other disorders. Second, there is no mention of what medications these people were on that might contribute to findings. Third, there is also no control group (some of these findings are present in the general population who have not had an accident). Finally, authors of more recent, better quality studies have not found these abnormalities in their patients.

Oppenheimer A. Pathology, clinical manifestations and treatment of lesions of the intervertebral disks. *New England Journal of Medicine.* 1944;230(4): 95–105.

This author revealed that patients could have severe changes of disc degeneration on X-ray and yet be completely asymptomatic, so that there is a poor correlation between X-ray findings and symptoms.

O'Shaughnessy T. Latent dysfunctions resulting from unresolved trauma-induced head and neck injuries. *Functional Orthodontist.* 1995;12(2):22–24, 26, 28.

See below.

O'Shaughnessy T. Tomographic proof of trauma-induced injury to the TMJoint and other sites in the body. *Functional Orthodontist.* 1995;12(5):20–28.

See below. In this article, there is also the misconception that what is seen on temporomandibular joint imaging is necessarily a source of the patient's pain. The author offers no study data with controls. See R. Ferrari et al, M. M. Tasaki et al, and P. L. Westesson.

O'Shaughnessy T, Levenson R. Basic treatment precepts ensuant to a whiplash episode. *Functional Orthodontist.* 1994;11(5):16–20.

This author deals with the treatment of temporomandibular joint injury in whiplash patients but does so on a theoretical and conjectural basis. He presents no experimental or study data.

Others have refuted many of the concepts in this article. See R. Ferrari et al, H. L. Goldberg, A. P. Heise et al, R. P. Howard et al, W. S. Kirk Jr, M. Olin, R. H. Roydhouse, E. W. Small, and D. H. West et al.

Otremski I, Marsh JL, Wilde BR, McLardy Smith PD, Newman RJ. Soft tissue cervical spinal injuries in motor vehicle accidents. *Injury.* 1989;20:349–351.

Otte A, Ettlin T, Fierz L, Mueller-Brand J. Parieto-occipital hypoperfusion in late whiplash syndrome: first quantitative SPET study using technetium-99m bicisate (ECD). *European Journal of Nuclear Medicine.* 1996;23(1):72–74.

See below.

Otte A, Ettlin TM, Nitzsche EU, et al. PET and SPECT in whiplash syndrome: a new approach to a forgotten brain? *Journal of Neurology, Neurosurgery, and Psychiatry.* 1997;63: 368–372.

See below.

Otte A, Goetze M, Mueller-Brand J. Statistical parametric mapping in whiplash brain: is it only a contusion mechanism? *European Journal of Nuclear Medicine*. 1998;25:306–312.

These authors extend their earlier studies and confirm that the brain imaging abnormalities in whiplash patients are not a result of any brain injury but simply how neck pain affects the posterior part of the brain, because the nerves to the neck muscles and that part of the brain have a common origin.

Otte A, Mueller-Brand J, Fierz L. Brain SPECT findings in late whiplash syndrome. *Lancet*. 1995;345:1513–1514.

These authors use proper controls to demonstrate that it is the presence of neck pain, not brain injury, that produces brain imaging abnormalities. There is no evidence of brain injury in whiplash patients. See also "Disturbances of Balance and Hearing" in Chapter 7.

Otte A, Mueller-Brand J, Nitzsche EU, Wachter K, Ettlin TM. Functional brain imaging in 200 patients after whiplash injury. *Journal of Nuclear Medicine*. 1997;38(6):1102.

This study is of 200 whiplash patients with symptoms of neck pain, headache, visual disturbance, and cognitive dysfunction. It is an extension of the results of the above studies. The authors reiterate that they believe (given the same findings in patients with nontraumatic neck pain) the imaging abnormalities with single photon emission tomography scanning and positron emission tomography scanning are not indicative of brain injury. Rather, they result from the effect that having neck pain has on blood flow in the posterior (occipital) part of the brain. The authors consider a hypothesis of whether imaging abnormalities are almost a "side effect" of having neck pain. The alteration in blood flow to that part of the brain also appears to alter the metabolism of the brain there (see below). The regions of abnormalities, however, could not explain cognitive symptoms being reported.

As yet, there is no definitive evidence that whiplash patients without head impact suffer any form of brain injury. This is not surprising, since volunteers in whiplash experiments and Lithuanian accident victims experience acute whiplash injury but do not appear to report the chronic symptoms that many whiplash claimants do.

See also "Disturbances of Balance and Hearing" in Chapter 7.

Otte D, Südkamp, Appel H. Variations of injury patterns of seat-belt users. In: *Proceedings of the International Congress and Exposition. Restraint Technologies: Front Seat Occupant Protection SP-690, February 23–27, 1987, Detroit, Michigan*. SAE Paper 870226. Warrendale, PA: Society of Automotive Engineers; 1987:61–71.

Paajanen H, Erkintalo M, Kuusela T, Dahlstrom S, Kormano M. Magnetic resonance study of disc degeneration in young low-back pain patients. *Spine*.
1989;14(9):982–985.

In this study of magnetic resonance imaging scans of the lumbar spine in
asymptomatic 20-year-old men, the authors show that 35% have abnormalities.
Thus, one must be cautious in ascribing back pain to these findings because radiologic findings can just as easily be asymptomatic.

Pallis C, Jones AM, Spillane JD. Cervical spondylosis. *Brain*. 1954;77:274–289.

This is one of the early groups showing that many of the findings on neck X-ray
cannot explain symptoms after trauma since one frequently finds them in asymptomatic individuals. In their study of 50 asymptomatic patients over the age of 50
who had no previous injury, the authors found that "75 per cent showed narrowing
of the spinal canal due to various combinations of posterior osteophytosis, subluxation of cervical vertebrae, and [straightening of the normal cervical lordosis]."

Panagiotacopulos ND, Lee JS, Pope MH, et al. Detection of wire EMG activity
in whiplash injuries using wavelets. *Iowa Orthopaedic Journal*. 1997;17:
134–138.

These authors provide evidence to suggest that the cervical muscles, even in
unexpected low-velocity collisions are capable of reacting fast enough to produce
contraction during sudden acceleration. The muscle reaction appears to be initi-
ated by the initial impact.

Pang LQ. The otological aspects of whiplash injuries. *Laryngoscope*. 1971;81:
1381–1387.

In this study, the author reveals abnormalities of hearing in whiplash patients.
The author also admits, however, that since there were no preaccident hearing assessments available, no firm conclusions can be made about the cause of these
abnormalities.

Panjabi MM, Cholewicki J, Nibu K, Babat LB, Dvorak J. Simulation of whiplash
trauma using whole cervical spine specimens. *Spine*. 1998;23:17–24.

In this study, the authors relate a useful cadaveric model to understand how the
spine moves in a rear-end collision. They will apparently be providing data as to
when (in terms of acceleration from impact) ligament tears or other damage
occur in the cadaveric spine. Of course, there are limitations to any study using
cadavers. Clinically, the most useful information is a comparison of when (in
terms of head acceleration or change in velocity) volunteers report symptoms and
what damage occurs in cadavers at that collision severity. See D. Kallieris et al.

Panjabi MM, Cholewicki J, Nibu K, Grauer J, Vahldiek M. Capsular ligament stretches during in vitro whiplash simulations. *Journal of Spinal Disorders.* 1998;11(3):227–232.

These researchers confirm that when cadavers are subjected to the equivalent of a rear-end collision with a head acceleration of 10.5g, they show early evidence of a probable, and minor, ligament sprain. There is no gross tear of the ligament, however. Any damage is microscopic. It is at this same level of head acceleration that human volunteers report acute neck pain in experimental rear-end collisions. See Chapters 5 and 20.

Parker N. Accident litigants with neurotic symptoms. *Medical Journal of Australia.* 1977;2:318–322.

This article deals with some of the factors responsible for symptoms after accidents, namely personal predisposition, litigation, and physician–patient interaction.

Parker RS, Rosenblum A. IQ loss and emotional dysfunctions after mild head injury incurred in a motor vehicle accident. *Journal of Clinical Psychology.* 1996;52(1):32–43.

In this study, the authors document the many emotional and psychological reactions to trauma, which may in turn produce cognitive symptoms. There is no evidence that whiplash patients have a brain injury. See also "Disturbances of Balance and Hearing" in Chapter 7.

Parmar HV, Raymakers R. Neck injuries from rear impact road traffic accidents: prognosis in persons seeking compensation. *Injury.* 1993;24(2):75–78.

These authors examined the prognostic value of radiological findings and concluded that there was "no evidence that radiological spondylosis either appeared prematurely or deteriorated as a result of the findings which contradicts the findings of Watkinson et al. (1991). However, they only reviewed 35 patients."

Parrish RW, Kingsley DPE, Kendall BE, Moseley IF. MRI evaluation of whiplash injuries. *Neuroradiology.* 1991;33(suppl):161–163.

In this study of whiplash patients and controls, the authors found a somewhat higher incidence of magnetic resonance imaging abnormalities of the cervical spine in whiplash patients. The do not state, however, how they selected the whiplash patients (were they referred for MRI because they had abnormal X-rays?), and so it is not clear if they are an appropriate group of patients for study or if they introduced a bias.

Nevertheless, the authors learned that there was absolutely no correlation between duration of symptoms and abnormalities, nor did the presence of signs of physical examination correlate with the MRI findings.

Parsons T. Illness and the role of the physician: a sociological perspective. In: *Personality in Nature, Society, and Culture*, Kluckholm C, Murray HA, eds. New York: Alfred A Knopf; 1967:609–617.

Partheni M, Miliaras G, Constantoyannis C, Voulgaris S, Spiropoulou P, Papadakis P. Whiplash rate of recovery in Greece. *Journal of Rheumatology*. 1999. In press.

Partheni M, Partheni M, Miliaras G, Constantoyannis C, Voulgaris S, Spiropoulou P, Papadakis N. Whiplash injury following car accidents: rate of recovery. Presented at the annual meeting of the North American Spine Society; 1997; New York.

Patrick LM. Studies of hyperextension and hyperflexion injury in volunteers and human cadavers. In: Gurdjian ES, Thomas LM, eds. *Neckache and Backache*. Springfield, IL: Charles C Thomas; 1970:92–119.

This author reviews the experiments showing lack of chronic symptoms or signs of injury in volunteers despite using forces higher than those in most rear-end collisions producing whiplash patients.

Patrick LM, Chou CC. Response of the human neck in flexion, extension and lateral flexion. In: *Vehicle Research Institute Report VRI 7.3*. New York: Society of Automotive Engineers; 1976.

Pearce JMS. Whiplash injury: a reappraisal. *Journal of Neurology, Neurosurgery, and Psychiatry*. 1989;52:1329–1331.

This author reveals that individuals with preexisting disc degeneration of the cervical spine have no greater propensity to whiplash symptoms than those with normal X-rays. As discussed here and in an article in 1992:

> Those with initial radiographic changes, that is, those with preceding spondylosis, have no greater propensity for these symptoms than those without antecedent radiological spondylosis. . . .
>
> . . . Despite much contention there is a dearth of objective evidence that spondylosis is either accelerated or worsened by the injury.

Relative sparing of the younger and over-60 age groups and very poor correlation with radiographic evidence of spondylosis indicate that symptoms are not in the main, dependent on degenerative changes in the cervical spine.

Pearce JMS. Whiplash injury [letter]. *British Medical Journal*. 1990;301:610.

Pearce JMS. Pearce replies [letter]. *Journal of Neurology, Neurosurgery and Psychiatry.* 1991;54(3):284.

Pearce JMS. Whiplash injury: fact or fiction? *Headache Quarterly, Current Treatment and Research.* 1992;3:45–49.

See 1989 article above.

Pearce JMS. Subtle cerebral lesions in "chronic whiplash syndrome"? [letter]. *Journal of Neurology, Neurosurgery and Psychiatry.* 1993;56(12):1328–1329.

This article deals with a paper by T. M. Ettlin et al in which the author suggested that magnetic resonance imaging (MRI) may provide objective evidence for whiplash injury. See "MRI" in Chapter 5.

Pearce JMS. Polemics of chronic whiplash injury. *Neurology.* 1994;44:1993–1997.

Pearce JMS. Reply from the author [letter]. *Neurology.* 1995;45:2117–2118.

Pennie B, Agambar L. Patterns of injury and recovery in whiplash. *Injury.* 1991; 22(1):57–59.

This article addresses why the reporting of chronic symptoms in whiplash may not be due to compensation issues. This article does not deal with, however, many other psychological factors that may affect whiplash patients.

Penning L. Acceleration injury of the cervical spine by hypertranslation of the head. Part I. Effect of normal translation of the head on cervical spine motion: a radiological study. *European Spine Journal.* 1992;1:7–12.

See below.

Penning L. Acceleration injury of the cervical spine by hypertranslation of the head. Part II. Effect of hypertranslation of the head on cervical spine motion: discussion of literature data. *European Spine Journal.* 1992;1:13–19.

This author considers other physical mechanisms responsible for the acute injury in whiplash patients. He proposes that the mechanism of injury that produces serious injuries like spinal cord damage and fractures might also be operating to a lesser extent in whiplash patients. This may be too much of a stretch. But regardless of the mechanism, the vast majority of whiplash patients have a simple muscle or ligament sprain.

Pettersson K, Hildingsson C, Toolanen G, Fagerlund M, Björnebrink J. MRI and neurology in acute whiplash trauma. No correlation in prospective examination of 39 cases. *Acta Orthopedica Scandinavica.* 1994;65(5):525–528.

These authors reveal that the abnormalities on magnetic resonance imaging (MRI) of whiplash patients are the same as in the general population, do not correlate with symptoms, and are therefore not indicative of specific injuries.

They also explain that only rarely are arm symptoms (numbness or pain) due to nerve compression ("pinched nerve").

See "MRI" in Chapter 5.

Pettersson K, Hildingsson C, Toolanen G, Fagerlund M, Björnebrink J. Disc pathology after whiplash injury. A prospective magnetic resonance imaging clinical investigation. *Spine*. 1997; 22:283–288.

In this study, the authors show that without specific, objective neurological signs on examination, magnetic resonance imaging findings (MRI) of disc abnormalities do not have any relevance to symptoms or to outcome in whiplash patients. See "MRI" in Chapter 5.

Pettersson K, Kärrholm J, Toolanen G, Hildingsson C. Decreased width of the spinal canal in patients with chronic symptoms after whiplash injury. *Spine*. 1995;20(15):1664–1667.

In this study, the authors demonstrate an association between outcome of whiplash patients and the width of the spinal canal as judged by X-ray. No attempt was made to correlate the specific symptoms or signs with radiological findings, so one cannot determine a causal relationship between symptoms and radiological findings. The study is also retrospective, rather than prospective, which is in itself a source of some concern. Moreover, there is no information as to whether the patients had signs of nerve root compression, which would separate them from typical whiplash patients (who usually do not have such signs). In other words, it is not known whether one can extend the results of this study to whiplash patients with a normal neurological examination.

Pettersson K, Toolanen G. High-dose methyl-prednisolone prevents extensive sick-leave after whiplash injury. In: Pettersson K., ed. *Whiplash Injury. A Clinical, Radiographic and Psychological Investigation*. Umeå, Sweden; 1996. Umeå University, Thesis.

In this study, the authors examine the benefits of steroid therapy for accident victims with Grade 3 whiplash-associated disorder, that is, where there are objective neurological abnormalities. They included a few Grade 2 patients. The study data indicate that there is benefit if intravenous steroids are given within 8 hours of the injury, but one must recognize that the study results only barely reached statistical significance. (This means that the results approached a level of difference that could almost occur by chance alone.) Nevertheless, the authors are correct in stating that these are promising results for Grade 3 whiplash-associated disorder.

Of course, the vast majority of whiplash patients have only Grade 1 or 2 whiplash-associated disorder. There were too few Grade 2 patients in this study. One cannot extend the results of the study to other whiplash patients, and obviously, the authors did not design the study to look at chronic neck pain.

Pilowsky I. Abnormal illness behaviour. *British Journal of Medical Psychology.* 1969;42:347–351.

Pilowsky I. A general classification of abnormal illness behaviours. *British Journal of Medical Psychology.* 1978;51:131–137.

Pilowksy I. *Abnormal Illness Behaviour.* New York: Wiley; 1997.

Pintar FA, Sances A Jr, Yoganandan N, et al. Biodynamics of the total human cadaveric cervical spine. In: *Proceedings of the Thirty Fourth Stapp Car Crash Conference.* Paper #902309. Warrendale, PA: Society of Automotive Engineers; 1990: 55–72.

Pokorny AD, Moore FJ. Neuroses and compensation. *Archives of Hygiene and Occupational Medicine.* 1953;8:547–563.

Porter KM. Neck sprains after car accidents. *British Medical Journal.* 1989;298: 973–974.

Powell MC, Wilson M, Szypryt P, Symonds EM, Worthington BS. Prevalence of lumbar disc degeneration observed by magnetic resonance in symptomless women. *Lancet.* 1986;2:1366–1367.

In this study of magnetic resonance imaging (MRI) scans of the lumbar spine in asymptomatic women, the authors show that at least one third have abnormalities by the age of 21 to 40. The authors caution that the high incidence of these abnormalities in asymptomatic women should be kept in mind when looking for a cause of a patient's symptoms.

Prasad P, Mital N, King AI, Patrick LM. Dynamic response of the spine during +Gx acceleration. In: *Proceedings of the Nineteenth Stapp Car Crash Conference.* Paper #751172. Warrendale, PA: Society of Automotive Engineers; 1975:869–897.

Preskorn SH. Comparison of the tolerability of bupropion, fluoxetine, imipramine, nefazodone, paroxetine, setaline, and venlafaxine. *Journal of Clinical Psychiatry.* 1995;56(suppl 6):12–21.

Pressman BD, Shellock FG, Schames J, Schames M. MR imaging of temporomandibular joint abnormalities associated with cervical hyperextension/
hyperflexion (whiplash) injuries. *Journal of Magnetic Resonance Imaging.*
1992;2:569–574.

This study has some sources of concern. The authors included 33 patients who
complained of jaw-related symptoms after a rear-end collision. They had abnormalities, but the only control population used was that of the study by Drace and
Enzmann, and this may be a poor control population. It would be useful if the
authors had a more suitable control population or even just imaged whiplash
patients who had no jaw symptoms, to see how many of them had abnormalities.
Moreover, this study is retrospective and represents a referral population. As well,
the abnormalities they cite exist in individuals with no symptoms at all, so these
abnormalities cannot necessarily be held to indicate the cause of the patient's
pain.
See Chapter 6.

Probert TCS, Wiesenfeld D, Reade PC. Temporomandibular pain dysfunction
disorder resulting from road traffic accidents—an Australian study. International *Journal of Oral and Maxillofacial Surgery.* 1994;23:338–341.

These authors reveal that there is a very low incidence of jaw pain or dysfunction in whiplash patients in Australia, pointing out one of a number of examples
of cultural variation in this phenomenon. See Chapter 6.

Provinciali L, Baroni M, Illuminati L, Ceravolo MG. Multimodal treatment to
prevent the late whiplash syndrome. *Scandinavian Journal of Rehabilitation
Medicine.* 1996;28:105–111.

This is one of the few controlled trials of therapy in whiplash. The authors
demonstrate that therapy with postural advice and psychological support is superior to modalities such as ultrasound, electromagnetic therapy, and transcutaneous
electrical nerve stimulation.
See also G. E. Borchgrevink et al, H. Brodin, L. A. McKinney, K. Mealy et al,
and Quebec Task Force review (W. O. Splitzer et al).

Pruce AM. Whiplash injury: what's new? *Southern Medical Journal.* 1964;57:
332–337.

Purves-Stewart J. Discussion on traumatic neurasthenia and the litigation neurosis. *Proceedings of the Royal Society of Medicine.* 1927;21(1):353–364.

Purviance CC. The whiplash injury. *California Medicine.* 1957;86(2):99–103.

In this study with a dummy, the author used experimental rear-end collisions to reveal the neck extension that takes place. There is little applicability of such a test to the human situation, since the human head and neck complex is quite different. As well, the work of R. C. Grunsten et al, W. E. McConnell et al, and D. H. West et al places doubt on the amount of neck extension of humans in rear-end collisions, and the presence of head restraints eliminates (even in the down position) any chance of significant extension. See also Chapter 22.

The Quebec Task Force on Whiplash-Associated Disorders. Scientific monograph on the Quebec Task Force on Whiplash-Associated Disorders. *Spine.* 1995;20(suppl 8):1S–73S.

See W. O. Spitzer et al.

Quinter J. Whiplash in Australia: illness or injury? [letter]. *Medical Journal of Australia.* 1993;158:70.

Radanov BP. Common whiplash—research findings revisited. *Journal of Rheumatology.* 1997;24(4):623–625.

Radanov BP. Dr. Radanov replies [letter]. *Journal of Rheumatology.* 1998;25(7): 1440.

Radanov BP, Begré S, Sturzenegger M, Augustiny KF. Course of psychological variables in whiplash injury—a 2-year follow-up with age, gender, and education pair-matched patients. *Pain.* 1996;64:429–434.

Radanov BP, Di Stefano GD, Schnidrig A, Ballinari P. Role of psychological stress in recovery from common whiplash. *Lancet.* 1991;338:712–715.

See discussion of articles below. The methodology of some aspects of studies by these authors has been criticized by O. Kwan and J. Friel. See also "Pre- and Postaccident Psychosocial Profile" in Chapter 9.

Radanov BP, Di Stefano GD, Schnidrig A, Sturzenegger M. Psychological stress, cognitive performance and disability after common whiplash. *Journal of Psychosomatic Research.* 1993;37(1):1–10.

This study and those below deal with the effects of psychological factors that occur largely after the accident to produce chronic symptoms. These authors also demonstrate that eliminating the litigation process improves the prognosis in whiplash, but chronic symptoms still exist, thus emphasizing that other psychological factors are important as well.

Radanov BP, Di Stefano GD, Schnidrig A, Sturzenegger M. Common whiplash: psychosomatic or somatopsychic? *Journal of Neurology, Neurosurgery, and Psychiatry*. 1994;57:486–490.

Radanov BP, Di Stefano GD, Schnidrig A, Sturzenegger M, Augustiny KF. Cognitive functioning after common whiplash. *Archives of Neurology*. 1993;50: 87–91.

These authors show that cognitive symptoms are not due to physical injury in whiplash patients.

Radanov BP, Dvorak J. Impaired cognitive functioning after whiplash injury of the cervical spine. *Spine*. 1996;21(3):392–397.

These authors review that cognitive impairment is a result of the pain experience, other psychological factors, and medications in whiplash patients rather than a result of any brain injury. The cognitive impairment improves as the patient's pain improves. See also "Disturbances of Balance and Hearing" in Chapter 7.

Radanov BP, Dvorak J, Valach L. Cognitive deficits in patients after soft tissue injury of the cervical spine. *Spine*. 1990; 17(2):127–131.

Radanov BP, Sturzenegger M. Predicting recovery from common whiplash. *European Neurology*. 1996;36:48–51.

Radanov BP, Sturzenegger M, Di Stefano G. Long-term outcome after whiplash injury. *Medicine*. 1995;74(5):281–297.

This study is of the same group of patients as above, with a longer follow-up, and again shows that in a different society, the prognosis of whiplash is better than in North America, partly owing to elimination of the litigation process.

One of the authors' conclusions, however, may be misleading. They conclude that patients with an abnormal X-ray at the time of the accident have a worse outcome compared to patients with a normal X-ray. The number of patients available for studying this aspect was only 27, far too small a sample size to accept the results as valid. Moreover, this conclusion conflicts with those of other, larger studies. Finally, to support their study results on X-ray findings, the authors quote Watkinson et al. (authors of a very flawed study)

Radanov BP, Sturzenegger M, Di Stefano GD, Schnidrig A. Illness behaviour after common whiplash. *Lancet*. 1992;339: 749–750.

Radanov BP, Sturzenegger M, Di Stefano GD, Schnidrig A. Relationship between early somatic, radiological, cognitive and psychological findings and outcome during a one-year follow-up in 117 patients suffering from common whiplash. *British Journal of Rheumatology*. 1994;33:442–448.

Radanov BP, Sturzenegger M, Di Stefano GD, Schnidrig A, Aljinovic M. Factors influencing recovery from headache after common whiplash. *British Medical Journal*. 1993;307: 652–655.

These authors show that posttraumatic headache occurs most often in patients who had headaches prior to the accident. They also show that headache was associated with increased score on the depression scale.

Ramsay J. Nervous disorder after injury. *British Medical Journal*. 1939;2: 385–390.

This early author explains how a neurosis appears to develop suddenly in some patients although that neurosis has been ready for full expression for some time.

Raney AA, Raney RB. Headache: a common symptom of cervical disk lesions. *Archives of Neurology and Psychiatry*. 1948;59:603–621.

Ranjan R, Thomas M, Matas M. Chronic pain and depression: a review. *Comprehensive Psychiatry*. 1984;25(1):96–105.

Ratliff AHC. Whiplash injuries. *Journal of Bone and Joint Surgery [British]*. 1997;79-B:517–519.

Rauschning W, Jonsson HJ. Injuries of the cervical spine in automobile accidents: pathoanatomic and clinical aspects. In: Gunzburg R, Szpalski M, eds. *Whiplash Injuries. Current Concepts in Prevention, Diagnosis, and Treatment of the Cervical Whiplash Syndrome*. Philadelphia: Lippincott-Raven, 1998: 33–52.

These authors offer examples of what might happen to a whiplash victim. The injuries they refer to, however, are seldom seen in whiplash claimants (they occur in only Grade 3 or 4 whiplash-associated disorders). Indeed, some whiplash claimants in low-velocity injuries have experienced a magnitude of force comparable to sneezing (see M. E. Allen et al and "Whiplash Experiments" in Chapter 5). As such, the discussion in this chapter is not applicable to most whiplash claimants.

Rechtman AM, Borden AGB, Gershon-Cohen J. The lordotic curve of the cervical spine. *Clinical Orthopedics*. 1961;20: 208–215.

These are among the first authors to show that the cervical curve seen on X-ray varies considerably in normal individuals. They proved that abnormalities once thought to be a result of whiplash are within the range of findings in the general population.

See also A. G. B. Borden et al.

Redmond AD. Prognostic factors in soft tissue injuries of the cervical spine [letter]. *Injury*. 1992;23(1):71.

This author considers the flaws in the work done by A. F. Watkinson et al, noting, for instance, the small number of patients.

Redmond AD, Prescott MV, Phair IC. Whiplash and surgically treated cervical disc disease [letter]. *Injury*. 1994;25(6):409.

This is a critique of A. J. Hamer et al's study. See also C. L. Colton and S. M. Barnes.

Reilly PA, Travers R, Littlejohn GO. Epidemiology of soft tissue rheumatism: the influence of the law. *Journal of Rheumatology*. 1991;18(10):1448–1449.

These authors raise some important questions regarding the medicolegal and social dilemmas medicine and the law create, not just in whiplash but in other chronic pain syndromes.

Resnick PJ. The detection of malingered mental illness. *Behavioural Sciences and the Law*. 1984;2(1):21–38.

Reynolds GG, Pavot AP, Kenrick MM. Electromyographic evaluation of patients with posttraumatic cervical pain. *Archives of Physical Medicine and Rehabilitation*. 1968;2:170–172.

Although these authors reveal electromyographic abnormalities in whiplash patients, there is no control group of either asymptomatic individuals or individuals with nontraumatic neck pain. It may be that many of the abnormalities noted in this study are also present in normal subjects or in individuals who have neck pain but no trauma. The findings are thus not proof of injury.

Riley LH, Long D, Riley LH Jr. The science of whiplash. *Medicine*. 1995;74(5): 298–299.

Rimel RW, Giordani B, Barth JT, Boll TJ, Jane JA. Disability caused by minor head injury. *Neurosurgery*. 1981;9(3):221–228.

On the basis of poor performance on cognitive testing, these authors conclude that brain damage is the cause of disability in patients with minor head injury. The authors offer only a theoretical explanation for these defects, and the authors ignore that not brain injury but simply the effects of whiplash and depression on cognitive functioning could be causing these cognitive deficits. See also "Disturbances of Balance and Hearing" in Chapter 7.

Roaf R. Lateral flexion injuries of the cervical spine. *Journal of Bone and Joint Surgery*. 1963;45-B(1):36–38.

Robinson DD, Cassar-Pullicino VN. Acute neck sprain after road traffic accident: a long-term clinical and radiological review. *Injury*. 1993;24(2):79–82.

These authors studied whiplash patients several years after their accident to assess if there had been any changes in their neck X-ray not accounted for by aging alone. They found that:

> An acute neck sprain does not lead to cervical spondylosis, accelerated or otherwise, nor does it lead to worsening of pre-existing degenerative changes. In our group there is also no evidence that injury induces further degenerative changes at any particular level nor the development of canal stenosis.

It is important to note, as well, that patients who had degenerative changes at the time of accident did not develop any changes to suggest a deterioration or worsening of degenerative disc disease years later. Yet they had more symptoms in the long term if they had an abnormal X-ray to begin with. How can one explain this? Merely pointing out to patients time and time again that their X-rays are very abnormal may affect their symptoms, and the worse an X-ray looks the more likely the patient may pursue litigation, which in itself can adversely affect the patient.

This study shows that there is no evidence that acute neck sprain causes, worsens, or accelerates disc degeneration. While it was found that those patients who had severe changes on X-ray had more symptoms in the long term, this may be only because they were more likely to be in litigation, or that telling patients they have severely abnormal X-rays may influence anxiety about or fear of long-term disability.

Roca PD. Ocular manifestations of whiplash injuries. In: *Proceedings of the Fifteenth Annual Meeting of the American Association of Automotive Medicine*. 1971:308–319.

In his study of 16 patients, the author deals with the ocular complications of whiplash. There are a number of important sources of concern in this study. Not all patients came from rear-end collisions. There is a low number of patients, and the patients did not have preaccident examinations to confirm that the findings were new. Many of the findings are present in the normal population, and some of the symptoms are subjective, so one cannot verify them.

Roca PD. Ocular manifestations of whiplash injuries. *Annals of Ophthalmology.* January 1972:63–73.

See above.

Romanelli GG, Mock D, Tenebaum HC. Characteristics and response to treatment of posttraumatic temporomandibular disorder: a retrospective study. *Clinical Journal of Pain.* 1992;8:6–17.

These authors show that patients with posttraumatic temporomandibular joint (TMJ) symptoms have more signs of psychological disorder than do patients with nontraumatic TMJ symptoms, suggesting that psychological factors play an important role in whiplash patients with TMJ symptoms.

Romano TJ. Chronic whiplash re-revisited [letter]. *Journal of Rheumatology.* 1998;25(7):1437.

Ronnen HR, de Korte PJ, Brink PRG, et al. Acute whiplash injury: is there a role for MR imaging? A prospective study of 100 patients. *Radiology.* 1996;201: 93–96.

In this study, the authors confirm that magnetic resonance imaging (MRI) of the neck or brain in the first 3 weeks after accident in whiplash patients shows no evidence of significant ligament tears or significant muscle tears (ie, they must be microscopic and minor to not be detected by MRI).

Rosenbaum JF. Comments on "Chronic Pain as a variant of depressive disease. The pain-prone disorder." *Journal of Nervous and Mental Disease.* 1982; 170(7):412–414.

Rosenbluth W, Hicks L. Evaluating low-speed rear-end impact severity and resultant occupant stress parameters. *Journal of Forensics Sciences.* 1994;39(6): 1393–1424.

In this study, the authors reveal that head accelerations less than 5.0g are not expected to produce injury since this head acceleration occurs in many everyday events. See also M. E. Allen et al.

Roth DA. Cervical analgesic discography. *Journal of the American Medical Association.* 1976;235(16):1713–1714.

Rothbart P, Gale GD. Neuropsychological deficits after whiplash [letter]. *Archives of Physical Medicine and Rehabilitation.* 1998;79:469.

Rowe MJ. Normal variability of the brain-stem auditory evoked response in young and old adult subjects. *Electroencephalography and Clinical Neurophysiology*. 1978;44:459–470.

> The brainstem auditory evoked response . . . show[s] a great intra and inter subject variability [in normals].

This author shows that there is considerable variation in these measurements in normal subjects. One should thus be cautious when using this technology to assert, for instance, that there is brain damage in whiplash patients. The changes found in such patients are often also found in normal subjects.

Rowland LP. Thoracic outlet syndrome. In: Rowland LP, ed. *Merrit's Textbook of Neurology*. Philadelphia: Lea & Febiger; 1989:443.

Roydhouse RH. Temporomandibular and mandibular dysfunction—a review. *Canadian Medical Association Journal*. 1971;105:1320–1324.

Roydhouse RH. Whiplash and temporomandibular dysfunction [letter]. *Lancet*. June 1973:1394–1395.

Arguing against whiplash as a cause for temporomandibular joint injury, this author points out that signs such as joint clicking, deviation on opening the jaw, and dental malocclusion may exist in many persons without symptoms or discomfort, so finding them in whiplash patients is not proof of injury. See also R. Ferrari et al, H. L. Goldberg, A. P. Heise et al, R. P. Howard et al, W. S. Kirk Jr, M. Olin, E. W. Small, and D. H. West et al.

Roydhouse RH. Torquing of neck and jaw due to belt restraint in whiplash-type accidents [letter]. *Lancet*. 1985;1:1341.

This author provides a theory as to how the shoulder strap of a seat belt restraint could cause a twisting neck injury. One must note, however, that the author has no experimental data to support this argument. Such a phenomenon has also never been reproduced in the human whiplash experiments. See Chapter 22.

Rubin AM. Author's reply [letter]. *American Journal of Otology*. 1996;17(1):173–174.

Rubin AM, Woolley SM, Dailey VM, Goebel JA. Postural stability following mild head or whiplash injuries. *American Journal of Otology*. 1995;16(2):216–221.

These authors confirm the presence of postural abnormalities in whiplash patients, but they imply that these are due to some brain injury. In actuality,

M. Karlberg et al have demonstrated that the neck pain alone can generate abnormal postural performance of the head and that symptoms result from this.

There are a number of other concerns about the conclusions reached by Rubin et al, and A. Katsarkas discusses these.

Rubin W. Whiplash with vestibular involvement. *Archives of Otolaryngology.* 1973;97:85–87.

This author gives anecdotal evidence as to the basis for vestibular symptoms in whiplash patients. One must note, however, that there is no preaccident examination to prove that these minor abnormalities were not present all along, that there is no control population (normals or individuals with injury not complaining of such symptoms), and that the number of patients is small.

Also, more recent studies have not reported these abnormalities. See also "Disturbances of Balance and Hearing" in Chapter 7.

Rudy DR. Lateral whiplash. *Journal of the American Medical Association.* 1968; 205(9):103.

Ruedmann AD Jr. Automobile safety device—headrest to prevent whiplash injury. *Journal of the American Medical Association.* 1969;164(17):1889.

Ruesch J. Social technique, social status, and social change in illness. In: Kluckholm C, Murray HA, eds. *Personality in Nature, Society, and Culture.* New York: Alfred A Knopf; 1967:123–136.

Ruesch J, Bowman KM. Prolonged post-traumatic syndromes following head injury. *American Journal of Psychiatry.* 1945;102:145–163.

Ruf S, Cecere F, Kupfer J, Pancherz H. Stress-induced changes in the functional electromyographic activity of the masticatory muscles. *Acta Odontologica Scandinavica.* 1997;55:44–48.

In this study, the authors confirm that emotional distress can alter the muscle activity even in otherwise normal subjects and thus lead to many of the symptoms in so-called temporomandibular joint disorders.

Russell LW. Whiplash injuries of the spine. *Journal of the Florida State Medical Association.* 1957;43(11):1099–1104.

Russell R. See Miller H. Discussion on cervical spondylosis. *Proceedings of the Royal Society of Medicine.* 1955;49:197–208.

Ryan GA, Taylor GW, Moore VM, Dolinis J. Neck strain in car occupants. The influence of crash-related factors on initial severity. *Medical Journal of Australia*. 1993;159:651–656.

Ryan GA, Taylor GW, Moore VM, Dolinis J. Neck strain in car occupants: injury status after 6 months and crash-related factors. *Injury*. 1994;25:533–537.

These authors studied a small group of patients (29) to see what factors about the accident itself might predict outcome. They found that the only variable that correlated with outcome at 6 months was awareness of the impending collision: those unaware of the impending collision had a greater tendency to report chronic symptoms than those aware of the impending collision. The significance of this finding is not certain. First, the study included a small group of patients, and it is retrospective. Second, what criteria are used to define who is aware and who is not? Does hearing screeching brakes but not seeing the vehicle about to hit qualify a person as "aware"? Or did the vehicle have to be seen before the collision to classify an accident victim as "aware"? Third, it is not stated who was at fault in each collision. Because a victim of a rear-end collision is perhaps less likely to be aware of the impending collision and to be at fault, this person is more likely to be the one suing the other driver. The increased propensity of litigation in such cases may account for varying outcomes in symptom reporting. Fourth, the medical literature is replete with small, retrospective studies demonstrating associations that others later show (with larger, prospective studies) to be wrong. Lastly, just because one demonstrates an association does not mean one has demonstrated a causal relationship.

Saltzberg B, Burton WD Jr, Burch NR, et al. Evoked potential studies of the effects of impact acceleration on the motor nervous system. *Aviation, Space, and Environmental Medicine*. 1983;54(12):1100–1110.

This study shows that to cause injury to the nervous system, impact accelerations must be at least 70g (and more than this for the head) for several seconds, an experience whiplash patients do not encounter.

Samblanet HL. Whiplash neck injury—management of subjective and objective symptoms. *Osteopathic Profession*. 1956;23:19–23, 42–44.

Sances A Jr, Myklebust J, Cusick JF, et al. Experimental studies of brain and neck injuries. In: *Proceedings of the Twenty Fifth Stapp Car Crash Conference*. Paper #811032. Warrendale, PA: Society of Automotive Engineers; 1981:149–194.

Sances A Jr, Myklebust J, Kostreva D, et al. Pathophysiology of cervical injuries. In: *Proceedings of the Twenty Sixth Stapp Car Crash Conference*. Paper #821153. Warrendale, PA: Society of Automotive Engineers; 1982:41–70.

Sances A Jr, Weber RC, Larson SJ, et al. Bioengineering analysis of head and spine injuries. *Critical Reviews in Biomedical Engineering.* 1981;5:79–118.

This article provides a careful analysis of the accelerations and forces involved in a variety of collisions. The authors noted that 1,621 simulations with 62 humans resulting in head accelerations of greater than 16g (greater than typical rear-end collisions), with no head restraints, resulted in only "some minor neck pain, headache."

Sand T, Bovim G, Helde G. Intracutaneous sterile water injections do not relieve pain in cervicogenic headache. *Acta Neurologica Scandinavica.* 1992;86: 526–528.

In this placebo-controlled, randomized trial, the authors confirm that sterile water injections have no more benefit than placebos in the treatment of whiplash patients.

Sanders RJ, Monsour JW, Gerber WF, Adams WR, Thompson N. Scalenectomy versus first rib resection for treatment of the thoracic outlet syndrome. *Surgery.* 1979;85(1):109–121.

These authors suggest that the thoracic outlet syndrome is a very common entity often due to trauma. They claim that because their surgical procedure was helpful in so many patients, this proves the diagnosis was correct. It does not. They cite no evidence to prove that thoracic outlet syndrome causes the symptoms. Moreover, without a control group (a group of patients who received other treatments or no treatment instead of surgery), there is no way of knowing whether a placebo effect (it can happen with surgery as well as medications), time alone, rest after surgery, or other ongoing coincident therapy is the reason these patients improved.

There is no scientific evidence that thoracic outlet syndrome truly exists in whiplash patients. See J. R. Youmans, A. J. Wilbourn, and M. Cherington et al.

Sano K, Nakamura N, Hirakawa K, Hashizume K. Correlative studies of dynamics and pathology in whip-lash and head injuries. *Scandinavian Journal of Rehabilitation Medicine.* 1972;4:47–54.

Saunders GH, Haggard MP. The clinical assessment of obscure auditory dysfunction—1. Auditory and psychological factors. *Ear and Hearing.* 1989;10(3): 200–208.

Saunders GH, Haggard MP. The influence of personality-related factors upon consultation for two different "marginal" organic pathologies with and without reports of auditory symptomatology. *Ear and Hearing.* 1993;14(4):242–248.

Savastano AA, Larkin DF. Whiplash injuries. *Rhode Island Medical Journal*. 1957;40:220–222.

Sbordone RJ, Long CJ, eds. *The Ecological Validity of Neuropsychological Testing*. Florida: St. Lucie Press; 1995.

Schaefer JH. Whiplash injuries of the neck. *Journal of the American Medical Association*. 1953;153(10):974.

This article is mostly just amusing. The author clarified a few issues regarding the mechanics of whiplash. Speaking of the work done by J. R. Gay and K. H. Abbott, he noted that "in one place the authors mention cars being '. . . driven ahead several hundred feet by the impact . . .' after being hit in the rear by another car. This is incredible if not ridiculous. In the illustration on page 1699 on the 'mechanics of whiplash injury,' the general argument violates basic principles of physics. "

Schaefer went on to explain that hyperextension of the neck was the first event, and the injurious one, and that J. R. Gay and K. H. Abbott (and later N. Gotten) had it backwards. He further commented on their statement that "multiple oscillation of the head and neck occurred in alternate flexion and extension": "In such collisions the human body is rather inert and has about as much capacity for such 'multiple oscillations' as a sack of potatoes. It cannot oscillate like a tuning fork."

Schaefer JH. Importance of whiplash injury. *International Record of Medicine*. 1956;169(1):28–30.

Schaefer JH. Whiplash injury. *Journal of the American Medical Association*. 1956;162(16):1492.

Schmand B, Lindeboom J, Schagen S, et al. Cognitive complaints in patients after whiplash injury: the impact of malingering. *Journal of Neurology, Neurosurgery, and Psychiatry*. 1998;64:339–343.

This is one of the few studies in which the researchers could give a fairly objective measure of the prevalence of malingering when claimants report cognitive dysfunction.

Schneider K, Zernicke RF, Clark G. Modeling of jaw-head-neck dynamics during whiplash. *Journal of Dental Research*. 1989;68(9):1360–1365.

These authors provide some theoretical arguments for how temporomandibular joint injury could occur in whiplash, but one must note how few facts they present. See R. Ferrari et al, H. L. Goldberg, A. P. Heise et al, R. P. Howard et al, W. S. Kirk Jr, M. Olin, R. H. Roydhouse, E. W. Small, and D. H. West et al.

Schofferman J, Wasserman S. Successful treatment of low back pain and neck pain after a motor vehicle accident despite litigation. *Spine.* 1994;19(9): 1007–1010.

These authors indicate quite correctly that the pursuit of monetary compensation is not a major factor in the development of chronic pain in whiplash patients. One must consider other psychological factors to be more influential.

Schrader H, Obelieniene D, Bovim G, et al. Authors' reply [letter]. *Lancet.* 1996;348:125–126.

Schrader H, Obelieniene D, Bovim G, et al. Natural evolution of late whiplash syndrome outside the medicolegal context. *Lancet.* 1996;347:1207–1211.

These authors reveal that if one removes the effects of expecting symptoms (through cultural awareness about whiplash), amplifying symptoms, and engaging in the litigation process or battling with insurance companies, chronic whiplash symptoms do not appear to occur.

Schutt CH, Dohan FC. Neck injury to women in auto accidents. *Journal of the American Medical Association.* 1968;206(12): 2689–2692.

Schwartz DP, Barth JT, Dane JR, et al. Cognitive deficits in chronic pain patients with and without history of head/neck injury: development of a brief screening battery. *Clinical Journal of Pain.* 1987;3:94–101.

In this study, the authors suggest that injury patients with chronic pain have more cognitive deficits than noninjury chronic pain patients. The authors admit that factors such as the psychological distress of the accident victim, stress of litigation, symptom amplification in the accident victim, and exaggeration in the accident victim may also be operating.

The study is thus no proof of any brain injury in whiplash patients. There are other explanations for the cognitive deficits of whiplash or minor head injury patients. See also "Disturbances of Balance and Hearing" in Chapter 7.

Scott HB. Neuroses following railroad injuries. *Kentucky Medical Journal.* 1917;15:322–323.

Scott MW, McConnell WE, Guzman HM, et al. Comparison of human and ATD head kinematics during low-speed rearend impacts. In: *Proceedings of the Thirty Seventh Stapp Car Crash Conference.* Paper #930094. Warrendale, PA: Society of Automotive Engineers; 1993:1–8.

Sehnert KW, Croft AC. Basal metabolic temperature vs. laboratory assessment in "posttraumatic hypothyroidism." *Journal of Manipulative and Physiological Therapeutics*. 1996;19:6–12.

See J. D. Cassidy for criticisms of this study.

Sehnert KW, Croft AC. In reply [letter]. *Journal of Manipulative and Physiological Therapeutics*. 1996;19(6):426–427.

Selecki BR. Whiplash. A specialist's view. *Australian Family Physician*. 1984;13(4):243–247.

This author states that a "very low restraint set close to the neck creates a fulcrum for hyperextension and potentiates or aggravates injury." One must note that no researcher has ever demonstrated this in any of the human whiplash experiments.

Seletz E. Whiplash injuries. *Journal of the American Medical Association*. 1958;168(13):1750–1755.

Seligmann DA, Pullinger AG. A multiple stepwise logistic regression analysis of trauma history and 16 other history and dental cofactors in females with temporomandibular disorders. *Journal of Orofacial Pain*. 1996;10:351–361.

Seligmann H, Podoshin L, Ben-David J, Fradis M, Goldsher M. Drug-induced tinnitus and other hearing disorders. *Drug Safety*. 1996;14(3):198–212.

Serra LL, Gallicchio B, Serra FP, Grillo G, Ferrari M. BAEP and EMG changes from whiplash injuries. *Acta Neurologica*. 1994;16(5–6):262–270.

These authors study 120 whiplash patients and conclude that they can detect nervous system injury by using these neurologic tests. Their conclusion is potentially erroneous because there is no control group (an essential component, as many of the minor abnormalities they describe might be present in the general population). They admit that the changes are minor, and there is no attempt to correlate the test findings with symptoms, so there is no way of even linking the two. This study does not at all confirm the conclusion that nervous system injury explains the symptoms whiplash patients report.

Sethi KD, Swift TR. Arm and neck pain. In: Bradley, WG, ed. *Neurology in Clinical Practice*. Vol I. Boston: Butterworth-Heinemann; 1991:398.

Severy DM, Brink HM, Baird JD. *Backrest and Head Restraint Design for Rear-End Collision Protection*. Paper #680079. Warrendale, PA: Society of Automotive Engineers; 1968:77.

Severy DM, Mathewson JH, Bechtol CO. Controlled automobile rear-end collisions, an investigation of related engineering and medical phenomena. *Canadian Services Medical Journal.* 1955;11:727–759.

This was the first study of head and neck movements in rear-end collision. Unfortunately, the diagrams and photography are from the movements of a dummy's head and neck, which one cannot liken to any reasonable degree to the human head and neck complex. One does not find these extreme movements in human experiments (see R. C. Grunsten et al, W. E. McConnell et al, G. P. Nielsen et al, and D. H. West et al).

Shannon EW. Post traumatic neuroses. *Insurance Counsel Journal.* July 1961:472–475.

Shapiro SK, Torres F. Brain injury complicating whiplash injuries. *Minnesota Medicine.* July 1960:473–476.

These authors show that some patients with whiplash have abnormal electroencephalograms (EEGs). The authors conclude this finding indicates brain injury. One must note, however, that this study has limitations, as F. A. Gibbs, E. S. Gurdjian and L. M. Thomas, and D. E. Jacome describe. Also, later studies have shown that EEGs are within normal range in whiplash patients. There is no evidence of brain injury in whiplash patients. See also "Disturbance of Cognition" in Chapter 7.

Shapiro SL. The otologic symptoms of cervical whiplash injuries. *Eye, Ear, Nose and Throat Monthly.* 1972;51:32–37.

The author of this study offers an anecdotal explanation for the cause of hearing disturbances in whiplash patients, but one must note that the study has too few patients and lacks a control population. Also, there was no preaccident examination of the hearing and balance of these patients.

Shea M, Wittenberg RH, Edwards WT, White AA, Hayes WC. In vitro hyperextension injuries in the human cadaveric cervical spine. *Journal of Orthopaedic Research.* 1992;10(6):911–916.

These authors show that hyperextension can cause neck injury in cadavers, but the forces they use are extreme (as the authors admit). One cannot easily relate this study to what happens in rear-end collisions producing whiplash patients. As well, the cadaver subjects were elderly, and as the authors of this article point out, younger tissues would have greater integrity. Further, they removed the spines from the cadaver bodies, and therefore there is a lack of supporting tissues.

Shkrum MJ, Green RN, Nowak ES. Upper cervical trauma in motor vehicle collisions. *Journal of Forensic Sciences.* 1989;34(2):381–390.

Shorter E. *From the Mind into the Body.* New York: Free Press, 1994.

Shorter E. *From Paralysis to Fatigue.* New York: Maxwell MacMillan; 1992.

This is a historical description of how cultural and medical fashions help develop certain illnesses and how the symptoms are modeled after organic (physical) illness even though they are nonorganic. This book is worth reading in its entirety.

Siegmund GP, Bailey MN, King DJ. Characteristics of specific automobile bumpers in low-velocity impacts. In: *Proceedings of the Thirty Eighth Stapp Car Crash Conference.* Paper #940916. Warrendale, PA: Society of Automotive Engineers; 1994.

Siegmund GP, King DJ, Montgomery DT. Using barrier impact data to determine speed change in aligned, low-speed vehicle-to-vehicle collisions. In: *Proceedings of the Fortieth Stapp Car Crash Conference.* Paper #960887. Warrendale, PA: Society of Automotive Engineers; 1996:147–168.

Siegmund GP, Williamson PB. Speed change (ΔV) of amusement park bumper cars. In: *Proceedings of the Canadian Multidisciplinary Road Safety Conference VIII, June 14–16, 1993, Saskatoon, Saskatchewan.* 1993:299–308.

Simmons JW, Emery SF, McMillin JN, Landa D, Kimmich SJ. Awake discography. A comparison study with magnetic resonance imaging. *Spine.* 1991;16 (6 suppl):S216–S221.

These authors show that "a large number of individual discs identified as abnormal on both MRI (magnetic resonance imaging) and discography caused no symptoms." That the asymptomatic population may have abnormal discography and MRI scans of the lumbar spine is a reminder that abnormalities do not necessarily explain symptoms in patients studied with these techniques. Thus, for example, whiplash patients are said to have injuries when abnormalities are found with various imaging techniques, but this conclusion is erroneous because those same abnormalities frequently occur in individuals with no symptoms.

Simmons RC. Whiplash: big business & serious problem. *For the Defense.* August 1982:14–22.

Simons DJ, Wolff HG. Studies on headache: mechanisms of chronic post–traumatic headache. *Psychosomatic Medicine.* 1946;8:227–242.

These authors explain that the headache of posttraumatic syndrome is no different in its nature and course from other headaches that accompany and follow stressful and untoward life situations.

Simpson RB, Nedzelski JM, Barber HO, Thomas MR. Psychiatric diagnoses in patients with psychogenic dizziness or severe tinnitus. *Journal of Otolaryngology.* 1988;17(6):325–330.

Sims JK, Ebisu RJ, Wong RKM, Wong LMF. Automobile accident occupant injuries. *Journal of the American College of Emergency Physicians.* 1976;5(10): 796–808.

Sjaastad O. Cervicogenic headache. In: Dalessio DJ, Silberstein SD, eds. *Wolff's Headache and Other Head Pain.* 6th ed. New York: Oxford University Press; 1993:203–208.

Slamovits TL, Glaser JS. The pupils and accommodation. In: Duane TE, Jaeger EA, eds. *Clinical Ophthalmology.* Vol 2. London: JB Lippincott Company; 1988:11, 12, 16.

These authors show some of the findings on eye examination that were mistakenly thought of as abnormal by others studying whiplash patients.

Slater E, Roth M. *Clinical Psychiatry.* 3rd ed. London: Bailliere, Tindall, and Cassell; 1969:507–509.

These authors discuss the psychological basis for the symptoms of the postconcussion syndrome (such as headache, giddiness, difficulties in concentration, and anxiety).

Small EW. An investigation into the psychogenic bases of the temporomandibular joint myofascial pain dysfunction syndrome. *Advances in Pain Research and Therapy.* 1976;1: 889–894.

This author demonstrates that psychological factors play a major role in the symptoms of patients complaining of temporomandibular joint pain.

Smed A. Cognitive function and distress after common whiplash injury. *Acta Neurologica Scandinavica.* 1997;95:73–80.

See M. Karlsborg et al.

Smith HW, Solomon HC. Traumatic neuroses in court. *Virginia Law Review.* 1943;30:87–175.

These authors discuss one of the leading questions regarding traumatic neurosis over the first part of the twentieth century.

Smith MD. Relationship of fibromyalgia to site and type of trauma: comment on the articles by Buskila et al and Aaron et al [letter]. *Arthritis and Rheumatism.* 1998;41(2):378.

Smith T, Trojaborg W. Diagnosis of thoracic outlet syndrome. *Archives of Neurology.* 1987;44:1161–1163.

These authors dispute the existence of thoracic outlet syndrome.

Smythe HA, Gladman A, Mader R, Peloso P, Abu-Shakra M. Strategies for assessing pain and pain exaggeration: controlled studies. *Journal of Rheumatology.* 1997;24:1622–1629.

Sneider SE, Winslow OP Jr, Pryor TH. Cervical diskography: is it relevant? *Journal of the American Medical Association.* 1963;185(3):163–165.

These authors examine the diagnostic value of discography for disc degeneration and whiplash injuries, to explain a patient's symptoms. In a study of 56 patients reporting neck or arm pain, they reviewed the relationship between radiographic findings and symptoms. They explain the problem as it had presented itself then.

> While extravasation and fragmentation of the contrast material are evidence of an abnormal annulus and nucleus, the problem of the relevance of these abnormalities to the etiology of neck and extremity symptoms following injury remains without a positive answer. It has not been demonstrated in an explicit manner that an abnormal diskogram shows the pathological cause of these symptoms. In defense of the proposition that it does, it is stated that the injection of dye into an abnormal disk reproduces the patients' symptoms and therefore localises the cause of the disease. Pain following the extravasation of contrast material may merely demonstrate once again that the material is irritating.

> Present knowledge, however, points to the conclusion that cervical diskograms in asymptomatic patients will be virtually the same as the ones found in symptomatic patients. On this basis, the cervical diskogram has virtually no relevance to the nature of cervical and upper extremity pain following trauma.

> There is a progressive degeneration of the nucleus pulposus with age with increasing frequencies of disk narrowing and osteophyte formation as age increase whether or not the patient has symptoms.

Analysis of this series of diskograms in symptomatic patients leads to the conclusion that cervical diskography is usually not relevant. . . . An uncontrolled diagnostic test which gives the same answer for almost all patients with a wide general symptom complex is open to suspicion.

Snow GH. Economic aspects of "whiplash" injury. *California Medicine*. 1964;101(4):260–262.

Snyder RG, Snow CC, Young JW, Price GT, Hanson P. Experimental comparison of trauma in lateral (+Gy), rearward facing (+Gx), and forward facing (−Gx) body orientations when restrained by lap belt only. *Aerospace Medicine*. 1967;38: 889–894.

These authors show that if a baboon undergoes head accelerations greater than 30g, substantial injury may occur. One must note, however, that this grossly exceeds the accelerations most whiplash patients experience.

Further, experiments with baboons are not equivalent to experiments with humans.

Solomon P. The behavioural response to whiplash injury [letter]. *Journal of Bone and Joint Surgery [British]*. 1998;80B(1): 183.

Solomon P, Tunks E. The role of litigation in predicting disability outcomes in chronic pain patients. *Clinical Journal of Pain*. 1991;7(4):300–304.

Sommer HM. Letter to editor. *Spine*. 1997;22(8):928.

Spitzer WO, Skovron ML, Salmi LR, et al. Scientific monograph of the Quebec Task Force on Whiplash-Associated Disorders. *Spine*. 1995;20(suppl 8): 1S–73S.

Squires B, Gargan MF, Bannister GC. Soft-tissue injuries of the cervical spine. *Journal of Bone and Joint Surgery (British)*. 1996;78-B:955–957.

This follow-up of the patients in the Watkinson et al study has the same important biases as that study: the numbers of patients are small and there was a loss of patients from the original group for the study. The authors do not account for the effect of this loss, nor is there a proper study or even control group for determination of X-ray changes over time.

Stalker AM. Traumatic neuroses. Translation of lecture by A Strümpell 1888. In: *Clinical Lectures on Medicine and Surgery*. Third series. 1894:303–325.

This is one of the earliest discussions on traumatic neurosis. It is the translated work of A. Strümpell.

States JD. Soft tissue injuries of the neck. In: *Proceedings of the Twenty Third Stapp Car Crash Conference*. Paper #790135. Warrendale, PA: Society of Automotive Engineers; 1979: 487–493.

States JD, Balcerak JC, Williams JS, et al. Injury frequency and head restraint effectiveness in rear-end impact accidents. In: *Proceedings of the Sixteenth Stapp Car Crash Conference*. Paper #720967. Warrendale, PA: Society of Automotive Engineers; 1972:228–257.

States JD, Korn MW, Masengill JB. The enigma of whiplash injury. *New York State Journal of Medicine*. December 1970: 2971–2978.

Steigerwald DP. Acceleration-deceleration injury as a precipitating cause of temporomandibular joint dysfunction. *American Chiropractic Association*. 1989; 26(11):61–64.

This author reviews the topic of temporomandibular joint problems and whiplash but provides no experimental data to support the arguments.

Steigerwald DP, Croft AC, Edwards JM, et al. *Whiplash and Temporomandibular Disorders. An Interdisciplinary Approach to Case Management*. San Diego: Keiser Publishing; 1992.

These authors proceed on theory to demonstrate that temporomandibular joint (TMJ) injury actually occurs in whiplash patients. None of the theories have been substantiated by scientific studies using volunteers. R. P. Howard et al's research has disproved the theories of injury. What is more, there is no discussion of the fact that with any imaging modality one chooses, the TMJ abnormalities said to be the cause of symptoms in whiplash patients commonly occur in completely asymptomatic subjects. Finally, none of the authors explain why in some countries, TMJ dysfunction is a nonexistent or rare problem in whiplash patients.

Steigerwald DP, Verne SV, Young D. A retrospective evaluation of the impact of temporomandibular joint arthroscopy on the symptoms of headache, neck pain, shoulder pain, dizziness, and tinnitus. *Journal of Craniomandibular Practice*. 1996;14(1): 46–54.

This study uses a very select group of patients, so there is immediate potential for erroneous conclusions. The results cannot thus confirm any possible temporomandibular joint injury in whiplash patients. The study proceeds on the assumption that if a patient complains of jaw symptoms some time after an accident, those symptoms are due to the accident. This may not be true.

Stenger J. Whiplash. *Basal Facts*. 1977;2:128–134.

This author presents theoretical arguments for the symptoms referable to the temporomandibular joint region in whiplash patients. The works of R. Ferrari et al, H. L. Goldberg, A. P. Heise et al, R. P. Howard et al, W. S. Kirk Jr, M. Olin, R. H. Roydhouse, E. W. Small, and D. H. West et al, however, clearly denounce any such theories.

Stewart JR. Statistical evaluation of the effectiveness of federal motor vehicle safety standard 202: head restraints. Contract No.: DOT HS-8-02014. Chapel Hill, NC: Highway Research Center, University of North Carolina; 1980.

Stewart KB, Murray H, Hess RA. Whiplash. *Nursing*. August 1998:33.

Stobbe TJ. Occupational ergonomics and injury prevention. *Occupational Medicine*. 1996;11(3):531–543.

Stock SR, Cole DC, Tugwell P, Streiner D. Review of applicability of existing functional status measures to the study of workers with musculoskeletal disorders of the neck and upper limb. *American Journal of Industrial Medicine*. 1996;29(6):679–688.

Stockard JJ, Stockard JE, Sharbrough FW. Nonpathologic factors influencing brainstem auditory evoked potentials. *American Journal of EEG Technology*. 1978;18:177–209.

These authors review that there are a number of nonpathological or normal causes of variations in auditory evoked potentials. Thus, finding these in whiplash patients does not necessarily point to a physical cause for their symptoms.

Stoke JCJ. The cervical headache. *Central African Journal of Medicine*. 1967; 13(11):261–264.

Stovner LJ. The nosologic status of the whiplash syndrome: a critical review based on a methodological approach. *Spine*. 1996;21(23):2735–2746.

Strauss I, Savitsky N. Head injury—neurologic and psychiatric aspects. *Archives of Neurology and Psychiatry*. 1934;31(5): 893–913.

These authors review the concepts of the psychological basis for railway spine. Strümpell A. See Stalker AM.

Stuck RM. Whiplash injuries. A new approach to the problem. *Medical Times*. 1962;90(5):493–504.

Sturzenegger M, Di Stefano GD, Radanov BP, Schnidrig A. Presenting symptoms and signs after whiplash injury: the influence of accident mechanisms. *Neurology*. 1994;44:688–693.

Svensson MY, Aldman B, Hansson HA, et al. Pressure effects in the spinal canal during whiplash extension motion: a possible cause of injury to the cervical spinal ganglia. In: *Proceedings of the International IRCOBI Conference on the Biomechanics of Impacts. Eindhoven, Netherlands*. SAE Paper 1993-13-0013. 1993:189–200.

Although these study results do indicate that, in pigs at least, one can cause a nervous system injury with the "whiplash motion," these results are hardly applicable to humans. Clearly, human volunteer studies will always be better than animal studies at determining whether there is a specific type of acute injury that produces chronic damage, which is in turn responsible for reporting of chronic symptoms in whiplash patients. The authors of this study state that low-velocity rear-end collisions often cause pain in the neck region and that there is considerable evidence that nervous system injury may be involved in whiplash patients' symptoms. Actually, low-velocity collisions do not cause pain but rather are followed by claims of pain. Moreover, there is no evidence in humans that nervous system injury occurs in whiplash patients reporting pain without specific neurological abnormalities on examination. Since this study was done, many human volunteer experiments have been unable to produce any significant injury when the impact velocity is below 20 km/h. Thus, the data from the large body of low-velocity experimental collisions with human volunteers lead one to dispute the theories in this article.

Svensson MY, Lövsund P, Haland Y, Larsson S. The influence of seat-back and head-restraint properties on the head-neck motion during rear-impact. *Accident Analysis and Prevention*. 1996;28(2):221–227.

Swartzman LC, Teasell RW, Shapiro AP, McDermid AJ. The effect of litigation status on adjustment to whiplash injury. *Spine*. 1997;21(1):53–58.

These authors show that no matter the severity of the initial injury, litigating whiplash patients report their pain as more severe. The authors attempted to determine if the litigants had more psychological distress. They found no difference between litigants and nonlitigants, which is surprising since the litigants are complaining of more severe pain (and should be more distressed). They speculated that patients in litigation will underreport psychological difficulties.

Regarding secondary gain, the authors conclude that secondary gain does not seem to be a significant factor influencing the function of the whiplash patient. They looked at only work status, however. They did not examine social and family responsibilities or duties that the individual may have been freed from. That too is secondary gain and an aspect of functioning in life.

Szabo TJ, Welcher JB. Dynamics of low speed crash tests with energy absorbing bumpers. In: *Proceedings of the Thirty Sixth Stapp Car Crash Conference*. Paper #921573. Warrendale, PA: Society of Automotive Engineers; 1992: 1367–1375.

This study provides accurate data on forces in rear-end collisions and supersedes the work done by Severy (before 1970). This study gives a more realistic account of accelerations at various velocities of collision.

Szabo TJ, Welcher JB, Anderson RD. Human occupant kinematic response to low speed rear-end impacts. In: *Proceedings of the Thirty Eighth Stapp Car Crash Conference*. Paper #940532. Warrendale, PA: Society of Automotive Engineers; 1994:23–35.

Tallents RH, Katzberg RW, Murphy W, Proskin H. Magnetic resonance imaging findings in asymptomatic volunteers and symptomatic patients with temporomandibular disorders. *Journal of Prosthetic Dentistry*. 1996;75:529–533.

Although these authors indicate that temporomandibular joint (TMJ) imaging abnormalities occur more often in individuals who recall a history of trauma, this does not lead immediately to the conclusion that the abnormalities are a result of the trauma. To determine that, one must do a prospective study soon after the traumatic event, with control groups including trauma victims who have no symptoms of so-called TMJ dysfunction (to find out how often they have imaging abnormalities). There should also be a control group of individuals with anxiety, which may alter muscle activity and lead to imaging abnormalities (see B. A. Loughner et al).

Without this type of study design, one cannot readily or reliably conclude that trauma causes the findings in this study's patients.

The study was also not a pure study of accident victims alone; people who had experienced many other types of so-called traumatic events were included.

Tamura T. Cranial symptoms after cervical injury. *Journal of Bone and Joint Surgery*. 1989;71-B:283–287.

This author suggests that the symptoms of headache, vertigo, tinnitus, and ocular problems in whiplash patients are due to a specific nerve injury because surgery corrects the symptoms. The author used myelography to find an abnormality in each patient complaining of symptoms such as headache, vertigo, tinnitus, and ocular problems. He then operated on half of these patients (he does not tell us why just half were operated on) and found that the patients improved. He concluded that because surgery corrected the problem, something physical must have been wrong with the patients. This raises the following question: Can patients have a placebo response to surgery (ie, improve not because of the surgery itself but because of the belief that they were receiving the correct therapy)? To test this properly, one would have to take patients to the operating room and make an incision in their necks, but carry out the operation in only half of them and let the other half believe they had the complete surgery. This is unethical these days, but some have previously done studies with "sham" surgery. The best example is the study of L. A. Cobb in 1959, in which patients received a cardiac procedure for relief of angina (recurrent chest pain due to heart disease). In one group, patients were taken to the operating room, and a large incision was made in their chests. Then the incision was closed with no cardiac surgery, and the patients left thinking that they had the complete procedure. The other patients had the complete procedure. When physicians reevaluated the patients, those who had the sham procedure did as well as those who had the true procedure.

Tarriere C, Sapin C. Biokinetic study of the head to thorax linkage. In: *Proceedings of the Thirteenth Stapp Car Crash Conference*. Warrendale, PA: Society of Automotive Engineers; 1969:365.

In this study with human cadavers, the authors show that one requires forces greater than 2,000 newtons for significant ligament tears. Such forces do not occur in most collisions producing whiplash patients.

Tasaki MM, Westesson PL, Isberg AM, Ren YF, Tallents RH. Classification and prevalence of temporomandibular joint disk displacement in patients and symptom-free volunteers. *American Journal of Orthodontics and Dentofacial Orthopedics*. 1996;109:249–262.

These authors demonstrate that temporomandibular joint disc abnormalities exist in asymptomatic individuals and thereby are not necessarily responsible for pain in whiplash patients. They also demonstrate that a large segment of the population has abnormalities, and these would presumably be present before an accident in many cases.

Taylor AE. An author replies [letter]. *Archives of Physical Medicine and Rehabilitation*. 1998;79:469.

Taylor AE, Cox CA, Mailis A. Persistent neuropsychological deficits following whiplash: evidence for chronic mild traumatic brain injury? *Archives of Physical Medicine and Rehabilitation*. 1996;77:529–535.

These authors confirm that whiplash patients do not have brain injury as a cause for complaints such as poor memory or concentration. The experience of pain, medication, and litigation are all stated to be capable of generating such symptoms.

The authors also point out that the number of whiplash patients complaining of these symptoms does not differ significantly from the number of individuals in the healthy population who have these complaints. The difference is that the whiplash patient attributes the symptoms to the accident.

See also "Disturbance of Cognition" in Chapter 7.

Taylor JR, Finch P. Acute injury of the neck: anatomical and pathological basis of pain. *Annals of the Academy of Medicine of Singapore*. 1993;22(2):187–192.

See below.

Taylor JR, Kakulas BA. Neck injuries [letter]. *Lancet*. 1991;338:1343.

Taylor JR, Twomey LT. Disc injuries in cervical trauma [letter]. *Lancet*. 1990;336:1318.

These authors argue that the acute injury of most whiplash victims is the same as the injury of individuals who die of major trauma.

Taylor JR, Twomey LT. Acute injuries to cervical joints. An autopsy study of neck sprain. *Spine*. 1993;18(9):1115–1122.

These authors found that individuals who die of major trauma in car accidents have evidence of injury of the intervertebral discs in the cervical spine. They suggest that the pathological findings of the cervical spines of individuals who die in car accidents with major trauma are good evidence for the pathology of whiplash patients who survive. They found that patients with major trauma had neck injuries and those who died of natural causes did not. One must note, however, that the authors do not explain how they overcome the obvious difference between what happens in the nonfatal rear-end collision and what happens in accidents that kill people. (Recall that it is absolutely essential for one to apply study results to a similar population.) The population the authors of this article studied (dead people) and whiplash patients are too different for the results to apply to both populations.

Autopsy evidence of those who survive the collision but who die for reasons not due to trauma demonstrate significant ligament and other pathology. However, magnetic resonance imaging (MRI) scans readily detect this type of injury, and such findings are rarely otherwise found in whiplash patients despite their reporting chronic pain. See "MRI" in Chapter 5.

So why are all those patients reporting symptoms if they do not have significant ligament tears?

The authors also state that "neck sprains are common in all Western countries," but they do not explain why reporting of chronic pain after neck sprains is so rare in Lithuania, New Zealand, and Singapore, countries with just as many car accidents. They also refer to the study of S. J. Davis et al with MRIs but do not explain the studies by D. Barton et al, G. E. Borchgrevink et al, C. Hildingsson et al, M. Karlsborg et al, C. Maimaris, R. W. Parrish et al, J. M. S. Pearce, K. Pettersson et al, H. R. Ronnen et al, and F. Voyvodic et al, researchers who looked for such injuries in actual whiplash patients (not people who died of major trauma) and did not find the acute pathology Taylor and Twomey claim occurs.

They also refer to MacNab's studies frequently. And finally, they state that "degenerative changes would . . . contribute to chronic pain and dysfunction of the cervical spine," even though many studies have shown that there is little correlation between degenerative changes of the spine and symptoms.

Teasell RW, Shapiro AP. Whiplash injuries: an update. *Pain Research & Management*. 1998;3(2):81–90.

Teasell RW, Shapiro AP, Mailis A. Medical management of whiplash injuries: an overview. *Spine: State of the Art Reviews*. 1993;7(3):481–499.

These authors point out quite rightly that many of the passive therapies some use to treat whiplash patients either have not been studied or have not been shown in studies to be better than placebo. They also, unfortunately, recommend other therapies that lack proof of benefit.

See Quebec Task Force (W. O. Spitzer et al) for a more recent review of therapy modalities.

Tenicela R, Cook MDR. Treatment of whiplash injuries by nerve block. *Southern Medical Journal*. 1972;65(5):572–574.

On the basis of an attempt to relieve the pain by local anesthesia injections into certain neck joints, these authors conclude that these joints are responsible for the pain of whiplash patients. One must note, however, that there are relevant concerns with the study. The patients were blind to some degree. The physicians were completely unblind. In 1980, Frost et al conducted a more appropriate experiment, a double-blind placebo-controlled study of the benefits of local anesthetic injection in chronic muscular pain. Their study shows that more patients had relief from the placebo than from the local anesthetic. This discrepancy between findings underlines the importance of study design.

Teresi LM, Lufkin RB, Reicher MA, et al. Asymptomatic degenerative disk disease and spondylosis of the cervical spine: MR imaging. *Radiology*. 1987; 164:83–88.

These authors discuss the fact that finding disc degeneration on magnetic resonance imaging scans of the cervical spine cannot, in itself, be an explanation for neck pain because disc degeneration is so often present in asymptomatic individuals.

Thiemeyer JS, Duncan GA, Hollins GG Jr. Whip-lash injuries of the cervical spine. *Virginia Medical Monthly.* 1958;85:171–174.

These authors remind us of the similarities between whiplash and railway spine.

Thomas A. Whiplash—a misnomer. *Trial.* 1965;1:27–30.

Thomas C, Faverjon G, Hartemann F, et al. Protection against rear-end accidents. In: *Proceedings of the International Research Council on the Biomechanics of Impacts (IRCOBI) Conference, Bron, France.* 1982:17–29.

In this study, the authors reveal that mispositioning of the head restraint cannot explain why whiplash occurs, since whiplash occurs in individuals whose vehicles have fixed head restraints. Thus, the claim that the reason head restraints do not prevent whiplash is that they are being misused is incorrect. The authors also show that height of the occupant has no bearing on whiplash incidence.

See also C. J. Kahane, W. E. McConnell et al, D. B. Olney and A. K. Marsden, B. O'Neill et al, D. H. West et al, and Chapter 22.

Thomas DJ, Ewing CL, Majewski PL, et al. Clinical medical effects of head and neck response during biodynamic stress experiments. In: *Advisory Group for Aerospace Research and Development (AGARD) Conference #267, Lisbon, Portugal.* 1979:15.1–15.15.

Thompson GN. Post-traumatic psychoneurosis—a statistical survey. *American Journal of Psychiatry.* 1965;121:1043–1048.

Thomson JEM. The counterfeit phrase of neck lash injuries. *Orthopedics.* 1960; 2:125.

Thomson JEM. The counterfeit phrase of neck lash injuries. *Insurance Counsel Journal.* January 1961:148.

Thomson RW, Romilly DP, Navin FPD, et al. Energy attenuation within the vehicle during low speed collisions. In: *Report to Transport Canada.* August 1989.

These studies suggest a striking speed of at least 15 km/h would produce acute neck injury. This is in keeping with low-velocity collision experiments with human volunteers. See "Whiplash Experiments" in Chapter 5 and Chapter 20.

Thorson J. Neck injuries in road accidents. *Scandinavian Journal of Rehabilitation Medicine*. 1972;4:110–113.

Threadgill FD. Whiplash injury—end-results in 88 cases. *Insurance Counsel Journal*. January 1961:161–163.

Tjell C, Rosenhall U. Smooth pursuit neck torsion test: a specific test for cervical dizziness. *American Journal of Otology*. 1998;19:76–81.

These researchers compared whiplash patients with dizziness to patients with dizziness from neurological diseases who had no neck pain. They found that neck movements affected dizziness and vision in the whiplash patients but not those with neurological disease. This suggests that abnormal neck movements (because of pain) generate these symptoms of dizziness and visual disturbance so commonly reported by whiplash patients.

Toglia JU. Vestibular and medico-legal aspects of closed cranio-cervical trauma. *Scandinavian Journal of Rehabilitation Medicine*. 1972;4:126–132.

This author suggests that electronystagmography can demonstrate physical abnormalities to explain some of the symptoms of whiplash patients. There are some potential concerns here. First, Toglia had no control population. Second, he did not explain whether there was any relationship between the abnormalities on the test procedures and the patient's symptoms. Third, the patients are a highly select group, with examination in some cases years after their accident. It may be that the symptoms at the time of the examination were due entirely to other disorders, and there is no mention of what medications these people were on that might contribute to findings. Finally, very little information is given about the accident severity.

Recent studies of whiplash patients have not reported the abnormalities in this study. See also "Disturbances of Balance and Hearing" in Chapter 7.

Toglia JU, Rosenberg PE, Ronis ML. Vestibular and audiological aspects of whiplash injury and head trauma. *Journal of Forensic Sciences*. 1969;14(2): 219–226.

These authors report apparent abnormalities in patients complaining of whiplash or head trauma. The authors of the article admit, however, that the lack of preaccident examination prevents one from determining when these abnormalities first occurred.

Toglia JU, Rosenberg PE, Ronis ML. Posttraumatic dizziness. *Archives of Oto-laryngology*. 1970;92:485–492.

See above.

Tom-Harald E. Disability 3–5 years after minor head injury. *Journal of the Oslo City Hospitals*. 1987;37:41–48.

Torres F, Shapiro SK. Electroencephalograms in whiplash injury. *Archives of Neurology*. 1961;5:40–47.

These authors argue that on the basis of finding abnormal electroencephalo-grams, they have defined the physical pathology responsible for chronic whiplash symptoms. One must note, however, that the authors did not study normal sub-jects as a control or study a control set of patients who had been in an accident and had no symptoms. They also did not describe whether there was any correla-tion between the findings and symptoms. The works of F. A. Gibbs, E. S. Gurd-jian et al, and D. E. Jacome completely refute the conclusions of this poor study.

Trimble MR. *Post-Traumatic Neurosis. From Railway Spine to Whiplash*. Chich-ester, England: John Wiley & Sons; 1981.

This is a good historic review and discussion about traumatic neurosis, includ-ing railway spine, but not a very thorough discussion of whiplash.

Trout KS. How to read clinical journals: IV. To determine etiology and causation. *Canadian Medical Association Journal*. 1981;124:985–990.

This article, and the series it is a part of, provide a useful methodology for crit-ically reviewing the medical literature. It is worth reading.

Uhlig Y, Weber BR, Grob D, Müntener M. Fiber composition and fiber transfor-mations in neck muscles of patients with dysfunction of the cervical spine. *Journal of Orthopedic Research*. 1995;13(2):240–249.

This study offers the nearest approximation to obtaining biopsies of muscles of whiplash patients. The study patients, however, are representative of only a very small percentage of whiplash patients (a fraction of 1% perhaps); they require surgery, seldom a consideration in whiplash cases and never a consideration in Grade 1 or 2 whiplash-associated disorder.

In patients with spinal cord or nerve injury (which might occur in Grade 3 or 4 whiplash-associated disorder), the results of this study indicate that some changes occur in the muscle fibers of the neck. Of course, how this physiological change affects symptom reporting is not clear. The changes, in fact, may be a re-sult of having neck pain, limiting neck muscle activities, and so on.

Most of the study patients are not accident victims, and the accident victims are not typical of most whiplash patients. There is no data as to when the accident occurred (if it was years ago, the muscle fiber changes could be due to another process than the accident injury). There is no evidence that such muscle fiber changes actually cause symptoms. Thus, the authors' data are interesting, but they do not explain why some whiplash claimants report chronic symptoms.

Clearly, if the acute accident injury caused muscle fiber changes and this then led to pain, one would expect volunteers and Lithuanian accident victims to experience the same phenomenon of chronic pain. They do not.

Unterharnscheidt F. Traumatic alterations in the rhesus monkey undergoing −Gx impact acceleration. Neurotraumatology. 1983;6:151–167.

Van Akkerveeken PF, Vendrig AA. Chronic symptoms after whiplash: a cognitive approach. In: Gunzburg R, Szpalski M, eds. *Whiplash Injuries. Current Concepts in Prevention, Diagnosis, and Treatment of the Cervical Whiplash Syndrome*. Philadelphia: Lippincott-Raven; 1998:183–191.

These authors confirm that the work of B. P. Radanov et al does not exclude the possibility that psychological factors are important in reporting chronic symptoms. There are many psychological factors that Radanov et al did not evaluate.

The authors recommend psychological assessment and therapy for persistent symptoms in whiplash patients.

Van der Donk J, Schouten JSAG, Passichier J, et al. The associations of neck pain with radiological abnormalities of the cervical spine and personality traits in a general population. *Journal of Rheumatology*. 1991;18:1884–1889.

These authors reveal that disc degeneration on X-ray and neck pain do not correlate. Rather, personality traits and a certain psychosocial history were a far better predictor of whether an individual would have neck pain.

Van Goethem JWM, Biltjes IGGM, van den Hauwe L, Parizel PM, De Schepper AMA. Whiplash injuries: is there a role for imaging? *European Journal of Radiology*. 1996;22:30–37.

These authors present a general review of radiology in whiplash patients. They include, however, individuals with fractures and dislocations, whose mechanism of injury or symptoms are not the same as those of most whiplash patients. Also, the authors state that whiplash patients have a higher incidence of preexisting X-ray changes than age-matched controls, but they base this claim on unpublished and unscrutinized data. Since there is no way for the reader to verify the data and their statistical accuracy, one cannot consider the claim valid at this time.

Verhagen AP, Lanser K, de Bie RA, de Vet HC. Whiplash: assessing the validity of diagnostic tests in a cervical sensory disturbance. *Journal of Manipulative and Physiological Therapeutics*. 1996;19(8):508–512.

Versteegen GJ, Kingma J, Meijler WJ, ten Duis HJ. Neck sprain in patients injured in car accidents: a retrospective study covering the period 1970–1994. *European Spine Journal*. 1998;7(3):195–200.

Versteegen GJ, Kingma J, Meijler WJ, ten Duis HJ. Neck sprain not arising from car accidents: a retrospective study covering 25 years. *European Spine Journal*. 1998;7(3):201–205.

Viano DC. Restraint of a belted or unbelted occupant by the seat in rear-end impacts. In: *Proceedings of the Thirty Sixth Stapp Car Crash Conference*. Paper #922522. Warrendale, PA: Society of Automotive Engineers; 1992:165–177.

Viano DC, Gargan MF. Headrest position during normal driving: implication to neck injury risk in rear crashes. *Accident Analysis and Prevention*. 1996; 28(6):665–674.

Although it suggests that properly adjusted head restraints should prevent whiplash injury, this study is done with dummies and therefore fails to explain adequately how head restraints affect living humans in accidents.

Von Werssowetz OF. A new look at whiplash injuries. *Journal of the Tennessee Medical Association*. 1965;58(2):39–44.

Voyvodic F, Dolinis J, Moore VM, et al. MRI of car occupants with whiplash injury. *Neuroradiology*. 1997;39:35–40.

These authors confirm that magnetic resonance imaging has not found evidence of any specific chronic damage following an acute whiplash injury. That is, significant muscle, ligament, or disc injury is not seen in whiplash patients reporting chronic symptoms.

Waddell G, Pilowsky I, Bond MR. Clinical assessment and interpretation of abnormal illness behaviour in low back pain. *Pain*. 1989;39:41–53.

This article addresses features of patients' symptoms and signs that are clues to abnormal illness behavior.

Wagner R. A 30 mph front/rear crash with human test persons. In: *Proceedings of the Twenty Third Stapp Car Crash Conference*. Paper #791030. Warrendale, PA: Society of Automotive Engineers; 1979:827–840.

Walker AE. Chronic post-traumatic headache. *Headache*. 1965;5:67–72.

Wallis BJ, Bogduk N. Faking a profile: can naive subjects simulate whiplash responses? *Pain*. 1996;66:223–227.

Wallis BJ, Lord SM, Barnsley L, Bogduk B. Pain and psychologic symptoms of Australian patients with whiplash. *Spine*. 1996;21(7):804–810.

This study confirms that whiplash patients do indeed experience a great deal of psychological distress. The authors (using the instrument SCL-90-R as a psychological tool) found that whiplash patients had a profile characterized by somatization, obsessive-compulsive behavior, and depression scores not typical of any preexisting personality disorder or neurotic tendency.

The study does not, of course, eliminate psychosocial status as a factor, but the study shows that one need not have a formal personality disorder to develop chronic symptoms.

Wallis BJ, Lord SM, Barnsley L, Bogduk N. The psychological profiles of patients with whiplash-associated disorder. *Cephalalgia*. 1998;18:101–105.

These researchers suggest that the pain of whiplash is not simply the somatic (bodily) component of anxiety. But they then go on to say that this proves the anxiety is due to pain from an organic lesion in the neck, damaged in the accident! This is a very convenient use of their data. Their study is more closely evaluated by Ferrari (1998) and Kwan and Friel (1998) in *Cephalalgia*. The explanations for their results are much more benign than Wallis et al imply.

Wallis BJ, Lord SM, Bogduk N. Resolution of psychological distress of whiplash patients following treatment by radiofrequency neurotomy: a randomized, double-blind, placebo-controlled trial. *Pain*. 1997;73:15–22.

See the studies by Barnsley et al and Lord et al. When one returns to the original papers that describe the patients in these studies, one finds they are not "whiplash patients." They are individuals who had their accident about 6 years ago (some more than 20 years ago), who in some cases were not even in motor vehicle accidents, and who in some cases had no pain with their accident but then reported pain 3 months later. Therefore, what the authors show is simply that people in the general population (these patients are no different from the general population except that they believe their pain was caused by some form of "whiplash injury") can have chronic neck pain. The chronic neck pain in the general population sometimes arises from the facet joint.

This study does not demonstrate that the acute whiplash injury is a facet joint injury. Given the patients selected for this study, this conclusion cannot be drawn.

What the authors also do not point out (but what is shown in the *New England Journal of Medicine* study by S. M. Lord et al 1996) is that the control group had 10 of 12 in litigation and the treatment group had only 4 of 12 in litigation. Clearly, being in litigation can prevent an individual from reporting any improvement of any kind, no matter what treatment occurs. The control group is not a control group when this major confounding variable exists. No amount of statistics removes this obvious and important difference between the two groups.

Walsh TR, Weinstein JN, Spratt KF, et al. Lumbar discography in normal subjects. *Journal of Bone and Joint Surgery*. 1990;72-A(7):1081–1088.

These authors show that 17% of asymptomatic people have abnormal discography of the lumbar spine, a reminder that abnormalities do not necessarily explain symptoms. Those same abnormalities frequently occur in individuals with no symptoms.

Watkinson AF. Prognostic factors in soft tissue injuries of the cervical spine [letter]. *British Medical Journal*. 1990;301:983.

Watkinson AF. Whiplash injury [letter]. *British Medical Journal*. 1990;301:983.

Watkinson A, Gargan MF, Bannister GC. Prognostic factors in soft tissue injuries of the cervical spine. *Injury*. 1991;22(4): 307–309.

This study has a number of important biases.

1. The total number of patients studied by X-ray and followed up 10 years later, after exclusions, is 33. There is always the risk of obtaining an incorrect conclusion when dealing with such small numbers of patients. This always has the potential to introduce bias into a study's results, and such survey studies require much higher numbers of patients. Most studies of neck X-rays in whiplash patients have had at least 100 patients (J. Balla and R. Iansek 1988 had 5,000). The duration of follow-up is irrelevant, since an inadequately sampled population remains inadequate over time.

   The study selected 33 patients from a group of 61 patients in a prior study (S. H. Norris and I. Watt 1983) that were ages 19 to 76 (mean age 37). The authors do not, however, give age ranges and average age of the 33 people in the follow-up group. Were they among the older or younger patients in the prior study?

2. In the reported control group, there were 100 patients, but the authors do not provide the ages of the controls. The authors do not demonstrate that the control population and study population differ only in the fact that the study population had reported an acute whiplash injury 10 years earlier.

3. The authors state that "increased symptomatic degenerative changes after 10 years suggest that the complaints of patients with whiplash injuries are organic." Many studies have shown that there is no correlation between symptoms (without neurologic findings) and degenerative changes on X-ray.

4. The most important concern with this study, however, is much simpler. The 33 patients followed up roughly 10 years after the accident were somewhere in the range of 19 to 76 years old, with a mean age of 37, when examined 10 years prior. That means that in the follow-up X-ray study the youngest patient was at least 29, and the oldest possibly 86. The average age had to be at least 47 by that time, if the study population remained representative of the original 64 patients.

In this group that was now 10 years older, 67 percent had signs of disc degeneration on X-ray. The authors state that this is much higher than expected for an age group less than 40 years old. The authors compare these findings to those of Z. B. Friedenberg and W. T. Miller's study (1963), which showed that about 6 percent of the people younger than 40 years old had signs of disc degeneration. That is true, but the study group members no longer have a mean age of 37. They now have a mean age of 47 (ranging from 29 to 86). Friedenberg showed the expected rate of disc degeneration for this average age of 47 is at least 50%. So when one accounts for this flaw, there is no significant difference between the study group and the general population.

These study flaws and potential deficiencies bring into question the validity of the conclusions made therein.

Watkinson A, Gargan MF, Bannister GC. Author's reply [letter]. *Injury*. 1992; 23(1):71.

Watson DH, Trott PH. Cervical headache: an investigation of natural head posture and upper cervical flexor muscle performance. *Cephalalgia*. 1993; 13:272–284.

Waxman SG, Rizzo MA. The whiplash (hyperextension-flexion) syndrome: a disorder of dorsal root ganglion neurons? *Journal of Neurotrauma*. 1996;13(12): 735–739.

This article deals with the theoretical basis of whiplash symptoms as being an injury to a specific part of the nervous system. The author does not discuss the fact that human whiplash experiments have never produced any chronic symptoms even though acute symptoms are often produced.

Weißner R, Enßlen A. The head-rest—a necessary safety-feature for modern cars. In: *Proceedings of the International IRCOBI/AAAM Conference on the Bio-*

mechanics of Impacts, June 24–26, 1985, Göteborg, Sweden, Bron, France. 269–276.

Weighill VE. Compensation neurosis: a review of the literature. *Journal of Psychosomatic Research.* 1983;27(2):97–104.

Weinberg ED. Whiplash injuries to the neck. *Maryland State Medical Journal.* 1959;8:67–68.

Weinberg S, LaPointe H. Cervical extension-flexion injury (whiplash) and internal derangement of the temporomandibular joint. *Journal of Oral and Maxillofacial Surgery.* 1987;45: 653–656.

These authors offer a theory of how whiplash might cause temporomandibular joint injury. The articles of R. Ferrari et al, H. L. Goldberg, A. P. Heise et al, R. P. Howard et al, W. S. Kirk Jr, M. Olin, R. H. Roydhouse, E. W. Small, and D. H. West et al refute their comments.

Weinberg S, LaPointe H. The authors reply [letter]. *Journal of Oral and Maxillofacial Surgery.* 1988;46(6):519.

Weinberger LM. Trauma or treatment? The role of intermittent traction in the treatment of cervical soft tissue injuries. *Journal of Trauma.* 1976;16(5): 377–382.

Weinberger LM. Cervico-occipital pain and its surgical treatment. *American Journal of Surgery.* 1978;135:243–247.

This author exposes the myth that the pain of whiplash arises, in part, from one of the cervical nerves. This has been a long-held theory and has no basis in fact.

Weiss HD, Stern BJ, Goldberg J. Post-traumatic migraine: chronic migraine precipitated by minor head or neck trauma. *Headache.* 1991;31:451–456.

Weiss MS, Berger MD. Neurophysiological effects of −X impact acceleration. *Aviation, Space, and Environmental Medicine.* 1983;54(11):1023–1027.

These authors show that to cause injury to the nervous system, the impact acceleration must be at least 60g (and more than this for the head) for several seconds—an experience whiplash patients seldom encounter.

Weissman HN. Distortions and deceptions in self-presentation: effects of protracted litigation in personal injury cases. *Behavioral Sciences and the Law.* 1990;8:67–74.

This is a good review of what effects the legal process can have on symptom reporting.

Wenger DS. Crash and live—need cars kill more soldiers than guns? *Journal of the American Medical Association.* 1955;159(14):1347–1350.

Wennmo K, Wennmo C. Drug-related dizziness. *Acta Oto-Laryngologica.* 1988;455(suppl):11–13.

Wessely S, Hotopf M, Sharpe M. *Chronic Fatigue and Its Syndromes.* Oxford, England: Oxford University Press; 1998.

West DH, Gough JP, Harper GTK. Low speed rear-end collision testing using human subjects. *Accident Reconstruction Journal.* 1993;5(3):22–26.

In this study, the authors provide significant evidence arguing against the likelihood that injury occurs in very low velocity rear-end collisions. See also Chapter 20. They also provide objective evidence that temporomandibular joint injury is unlikely to arise from these collisions. See also R. Ferrari et al, H. L. Goldberg, A. P. Heise et al, R. P. Howard et al, W. S. Kirk Jr, M. Olin, R. H. Roydhouse, E. W. Small, and D. H. West et al for criticisms on TMJ injury in whiplash.

Westesson PL. Reliability and validity of imaging diagnosis of temporomandibular joint disorder. *Advances in Dental Research.* 1993;7(2):137–151.

Westesson PL, Eriksson L, Kurita K. Reliability of a negative clinical temporomandibular joint examination: prevalence of disk displacement in asymptomatic temporomandibular joints. *Oral Surgery, Oral Medicine, Oral Pathology.* 1989;68: 551–554.

In this study of asymptomatic subjects with temporomandibular joint (TMJ) arthrograms, the authors reveal that many of the radiological abnormalities on TMJ imaging are common in subjects with no pain. See also Chapter 6.

Westesson PL, Eriksson L, Kurita K. Temporomandibular joint: variation of normal arthrographic anatomy. *Oral Surgery, Oral Medicine, Oral Pathology.* 1990;69:514–519.

See above.

This is a review of various temporomandibular joint imaging modalities. The author demonstrates that regardless of what type of imaging one uses, many abnormalities are found in asymptomatic individuals. These abnormalities are not necessarily responsible for pain in whiplash patients. He also demonstrates that a large segment of the population has abnormalities, and these would presumably be present before an accident in many cases.

Whitworth AB, Fleischhacker WW. Adverse effects of antipsychotic drugs. *International Clinical Psychopharmacology*. 1995;9(suppl 5):21–27.

Wickstrom JK, LaRocca H. Head and neck injuries from acceleration-deceleration forces. In: Ruge D, Wiltse LL, eds. *Spinal Disorders*. Philadelphia: Lea and Febiger; 1977:349–356.

This chapter includes the statement that myelography and discography are useful diagnostic techniques in finding the source of neck pain in whiplash patients. Note, however, that the works of W. E. Hitselberger and R. M. Witten, E. P. Holt Jr, and S. E. Sneider et al show this to be false.

Wickstrom JK, Martinez JL, Johnston D, Tappen NC. In: *Proceedings of the Seventh Stapp Car Crash Conference*. Springfield, IL: Charles C Thomas; 1963: 284–301.

These authors show that if one accelerates bunnies fast enough, they could be killed. It is impossible, of course, to use their data from animals and apply it to humans.

Wickstrom JK, Martinez JL, Rodriguez R Jr, Haines DM. Hyperextension and hyperflexion injuries to the head and neck of primates. In: Gurdjian ES, Thomas LM, eds. *Neckache and Backache*. Springfield, IL: Charles C Thomas; 1970:108–117.

Wickstrom JK, Rodriguez RP, Martinez JL. Experimental production of acceleration injuries of the head and neck. In: *Accident Pathology*. Washington, DC: US Government Printing Office; 1968:185–189.

In this study, the authors attempt to correct the inadequacies of MacNab's studies by using primates in horizontal collisions and actually measuring the head accelerations and forces with various collisions. They subjected these primates to peak head accelerations of 17g to 46g, with collision velocities of 35 to 63 mph. Using the higher velocities, they were able to produce objective damage on dissection.

Wiesel SW, Tsourmas N, Feffer HL, Citrin CM, Patronas N. A study of computer-assisted tomography. I. The incidence of positive CAT scans in an asymptomatic group of patients. *Spine*. 1984;9(6):549–551.

In this study, the authors examine the lumbar spine in asymptomatic individuals and show that 35% have abnormalities. Some of the findings even include herniated discs. Thus, one must be careful in ascribing back pain to these findings alone, because they are so frequent a finding in the asymptomatic population.

Wiesinger H, Guerry D. The ocular aspects of whiplash injury. *Virginia Medical Monthly*. 1962;89:165–168.

This article is an anecdotal report of some cases of minor abnormalities on eye examination in patients complaining of whiplash. Note, however, that the authors neglected to point out that the patients had no prior eye exam to compare to (so the findings, being minor, may have been present before the accident), and they did not describe the incidence of such minor findings in the general population (did not have controls).

Wilbourn AJ. Thoracic outlet syndrome surgery causing severe brachial plexopathy. *Muscle and Nerve*. 1988;11:66–74.

See below.

Wilbourn AJ. The thoracic outlet syndrome is overdiagnosed. *Archives of Neurology*. 1990;47:328–330.

This author cautions readers to be wary of all who claim thoracic outlet syndrome to be the source of symptoms in whiplash patients.

Wiley AM, Evans JG, Lloyd GL, Ha'eri GB. A review of whiplash injuries seen in a medico-legal practice. *Advocates' Quarterly*. 1979–1981;2:239–252.

Wilfling FJ, Wing PC. Disability and the medical/legal process. *The Advocate (Vancouver)*. 1984;42:183–186.

Williams MM, Hawley JA, McKenzie RA, van Wijmen van PM. A comparison of the effects of two sitting postures on back and referred pain. *Spine*. 1991;16(10):1185–1191.

Winston KR. Whiplash and its relationship to migraine. *Headache*. 1987;27: 452–457.

Wismans J, Philippens M, van Oorschot E, Kallieris D, Mattern R. Comparison of human volunteer and cadaver head-neck response in frontal flexion. In: *Proceedings of the Thirty First Stapp Car Crash Conference*. Paper #872194. Warrendale, PA: Society of Automotive Engineers; 1987:1–11.

These and other authors show that cadavers are not as good as living humans at resisting injury, so one must always account for this difference when interpreting results of cadaver experiments. (See also J. R. Cromack and H. H. Ziperman.)

Wolfe F. The fibromyalgia syndrome: a consensus report on fibromyalgia and disability. *Journal of Rheumatology.* 1996;23(3):534–538.

Wood KB, Garvey TA, Gundry C, Heithoff KB. Magnetic resonance imaging of the thoracic spine. *Journal of Bone and Joint Surgery [American].* 1995;77-A (11):1631–1638.

Woods WW. Personal experiences with surgical treatment of 250 cases of cervicobrachial neurovascular compression syndrome. *Journal of the International College of Surgeons.* 1965;44(3):273–283.

Woodward AH. Chronic whiplash syndrome [letter]. *Neurology.* 1995;45:2117.

Woodward MN, Cook JCH, Gargan MF, Bannister GC. Chiropractic treatment of chronic 'whiplash' injuries. *Injury.* 1996;27(9):643–645.

These authors suggest that chiropractic therapy has possible benefits, but this is only a retrospective study with a very select, small number of patients. The authors admit the need for proper, randomized, controlled trials before concluding there is any benefit to chiropractic therapy in whiplash patients. The study by J. D. Cassidy et al failed to reveal any benefit.

Wooley SC, Blackwell B, Winget C. A learning theory model of chronic illness behavior: theory, treatment, and research. *Psychosomatic Medicine.* 1978; 40(5):379–401.

Worsham RA. Acute sprain of the cervical spine. *Southern Medical Journal.* 1963;56:252–256.

Wright JM. Whiplash injuries. Management and complications. *Journal of the American Osteopathic Association.* 1956;55(9): 564–568.

Wright PB, Brady LP. An anatomic evaluation of whiplash injuries. *Clinical Orthopedics.* 1958;11:120–131.

Yagi M. Clinical studies on so-called whiplash injury, especially on the significance of retrograde brachial arteriography. *Nagoya Journal of Medical Science.* 1967;30:177–192.

This author considers abnormalities of the vertebral artery (which supplies the cervical spine) to be the cause of some whiplash symptoms. One must note, however, that the study lacks the proper controls (ie, no asymptomatic individuals from the general population had their vertebral arteries studied to see how many of them had abnormalities in the absence of symptoms). It may be that the abnormalities in the whiplash patients actually occur in the general population and therefore do not signify injury or explain whiplash symptoms. Indeed, W. H. Hardesty et al showed that asymptomatic individuals between the ages of 17 and 73 had widely varying vertebral arteries and numerous apparent abnormalities.

Yamamoto S. A new trend in the study of low back pain in workplaces. *Industrial Health*. 1997;35(2):173–185.

Yarnell PR, Rossie GV. Minor whiplash head injury with major debilitation. *Brain Injury*. 1988;2(3):255–258.

This article shows that auditory evoked potentials and magnetic resonance imaging scans reveal no physical basis for the complaints of whiplash patients.

Yoganandan N, Haffner M, Maiman DJ, et al. Epidemiology and injury biomechanics of motor vehicle related trauma to the human spine. In: *Proceedings of the Thirty Third Stapp Car Crash Conference*. Paper #892438. Warrendale, PA: Society of Automotive Engineers; 1989:223–242.

These authors conclude that whiplash is more common in vehicle occupants wearing seat belts. One must note, however, that there are important concerns with this and similar studies. See Chapter 22.

Youmans JR. *Neurological Surgery*. Vol 4. 3rd ed. Philadelphia: WB Saunders Company; 1990.

This author provides a review of thoracic outlet syndrome and many of the misconceptions regarding this condition. Some try to use thoracic outlet syndrome to explain the symptoms of whiplash, and this author shows what flaws there are in such an attempt.

> The evolution of [thoracic outlet syndrome] is further clouded by concepts that at one time or another reached great popularity, only to fall into disfavor later. Examples include (1) the use of Adson's maneuver to confirm entrapment by the loss of the radial pulse with stretch of the scalenus anticus muscle, which is no longer considered a meaningful test (2) the popularity of the procedure of simple scalenus anticus muscle section, which later proved ineffective in most circumstances and (3) the more recent reliance on the concept that electrical slowing could be demonstrated across the thoracic outlet using standard nerve conduction velocity techniques, a concept that was recently disproved.

Young WH Jr, Masterson JH. Psychology, organicity, and "whiplash." *Southern Medical Journal*. 1962;55:689–693.

Zabrodski R. Few whiplash patients are malingerers. Canadian Family Physician. 1995;41:29–30.

Zaiser-Kaschel H, Kaschel R, Diener CH, Mayer K. Neuropsychological status after whiplash injury. *Journal of Clinical and Experimental Neuropsychology*. 1992;14:393.

Zarlengo AE. Whiplash injuries. *Dicta*. July–August 1959:285–293.

Zatzkin HR, Kveton FW. Evaluation of the cervical spine in whiplash injuries. *Radiology*. 1960;75:577–583.

Literature Review by Topic

Each section in this text is, in itself, a bibliography of important citations for the topic being discussed. Chapter 14 simply lists articles and books for various topics. For specific comments on some of the articles, please see Chapter 13 and the text. Articles for recommended reading are marked with asterisks.

WHIPLASH CULTURES

Awerbuch MS. Whiplash in Australia: illness or injury? *Medical Journal of Australia.* 1992;157:193–196.

Balla JI, Karnaghan J. Whiplash headache. In: Eadie MJ, Lander C, eds. *Proceedings of the Australian Association of Neurologists. Clinical and Experimental Neurology.* 1986:179–182.

Bonk A, Giebel GD, Edelmann M, Huser R. Whiplash outcome in Germany. *Journal of Rheumatology.* 1999;12(1):70–75.

Ferrari R, Russell AS. The whiplash syndrome—common sense revisited. *Journal of Rheumatology.* 1997;24(4):618–623.

Ferrari R, Russell AS. Epidemiology of whiplash—an international dilemma. *Annals of Rheumatic Diseases.* 1999;58:1–5.

Ferrari R, Russell AS. Whiplash—heading for higher ground. A point of view. *Spine.* 1999;1:97–98.

Giebel GD, Edelmann M, Huser R. Neck sprain: physiotherapy versus collar treatment. *Zentralblatt fur Chirurgie.* 1997;122(7):517–521.

Livingston M. Whiplash injury and peer copying. *Journal of the Royal Society of Medicine.* 1993;86:535–536.

Maguire WB. Whiplash in Australia: illness or injury? [letter]. *Medical Journal of Australia.* 1993;158:138.

Mills H, Horne G. Whiplash-man-made disease. *New Zealand Medical Journal.* 1986;99: 373–374.

Obelieniene D, Schrader H, Bovim G, et al. Pain after whiplash—a prospective controlled inception cohort study. *Journal of Neurology, Neurosurgery, and Psychiatry*. 1999;66: 279–284.

Partheni M, Miliaras G, Constantoyannis C, Voulgaris S, Spiropoulou P, Papadakis P. Whiplash injury following car accidents: rate of recovery. Presented at the annual meeting of the North American Spine Society; 1997; New York.

Partheni M, Miliaras G, Constantoyannis C, Voulgaris S, Spiropoulou P, Papadakis P. Whiplash rate of recovery in Greece. *Journal of Rheumatology*. 1999. In press.

Schrader H, Obelieniene D, Bovim G, et al. Natural evolution of late whiplash syndrome outside the medicolegal context. *Lancet*. 1996;347:1207–1211.

RAILWAY SPINE

Carnett JB, Bates W. Railway spine. *Surgical Clinics of North America*. 1932;12: 1369–1386.

Crenshaw AH. Railroad back and other compensable injuries, 1890–1894. *Bulletin*. May 1975:25–27.

Editorial. Railway spine. *Boston Medical and Surgical Journal*. 1883;109(17):400.

*Erichsen JE. *Railway and Other Injuries*. Philadelphia: Henry C Lea; 1867.

Erichsen JE. *Concussion of the Spine*. New York: William Wood and Company; 1886.

Lind JE. Traumatic neurasthenia, especially "railway spine." *Medical Record*. 1937;146: 65–71.

Scott HB. Neuroses following railroad injuries. *Kentucky Medical Journal*. 1917;15:322–323.

*Strauss I, Savitsky N. Head injury—neurologic and psychiatric aspects. *Archives of Neurology and Psychiatry*. 1934;31(5):893–913.

*Trimble MR. *Post-Traumatic Neurosis. From Railway Spine to Whiplash*. Chichester, England: John Wiley & Sons; 1981.

TRAUMATIC NEUROSIS

Arnott DWH. Neurosis and compensation. *Medical Journal of Australia*. 1941;1:24–25.

Behan RC, Hirschfeld AH. The accident process II. Toward more rational treatment of industrial injuries. *Journal of the American Medical Association*. 1963;186(4):300–306.

Behan RC, Hirschfeld AH. Disability without disease or accident. *Archives of Environmental Health*. 1966;12:655–659.

*Buzzard F. Discussion on traumatic neurasthenia and the litigation neurosis. *Proceedings of the Royal Society of Medicine*. 1927;21(1):353–364.

Crenshaw AH. Railroad back and other compensable injuries, 1890–1894. *Bulletin*. May 1975:25–27.

Davidson HA. Neurosis and malingering. *American Journal of Medical Jurisprudence.* 1939;2:94–96.

Denker PG. The prognosis of insured neurotics. *New York State Journal of Medicine.* 1939; 39(1):238–247.

*Foster LJ. Traumatic neurosis. *American Journal of Roentgenology.* 1933;30(1):44–50.

Halliday JL. Psychoneurosis as a cause of incapacity among insured persons. *British Medical Journal.* March 1935(suppl):85–88.

Hirschfeld AH, Behan RC. The accident process I. Etiological considerations of industrial injuries. *Journal of the American Medical Association.* 1963;186(3):193–199.

Huddleston OL. Whiplash injuries. Diagnosis and treatment. *California Medicine.* 1958; 89(5):318–321.

Kamman GR. Traumatic neurosis, compensation neurosis or attitudinal pathosis? *Archives of Neurology and Psychiatry.* 1951;65:593–603.

Keiser L. *The Traumatic Neurosis.* Philadelphia: JB Lippincott Company; 1968.

Kennedy F. Neuroses following accident. *Bulletin of the New York Academy of Medicine.* 1930;6(1):1–17.

Knapp PC. Traumatic neurasthenia and hysteria. *Brain.* 1897;20:385–406.

Lawton F. A judicial view of traumatic neurosis. *Medicolegal Journal.* 1979;47:6–17.

Lind JE. Traumatic neurasthenia, especially "railway spine." *Medical Record.* 1937;146: 65–71.

Miller H. Accident neurosis. *British Medical Journal.* April 1961:919–925.

Miller H. Accident neurosis. Lecture II. *British Medical Journal.* April 1961:992–998.

Moorhead JJ. Traumatic neuroses. *Postgraduate Medicine.* 1947;2:184–187.

Parker N. Accident litigants with neurotic symptoms. *Medical Journal of Australia.* 1977; 2:318–322.

Pokorny AD, Moore FJ. Neuroses and compensation. *Archives of Hygiene and Occupational Medicine.* 1953;8:547–563.

*Purves-Stewart J. Discussion on traumatic neurasthenia and the litigation neurosis. *Proceedings of the Royal Society of Medicine.* 1927;21(1):353–364.

Ramsay J. Nervous disorder after injury. *British Medical Journal.* 1939;2:385–390.

Scott HB. Neuroses following railroad injuries. *Kentucky Medical Journal.* 1917;15: 322–323.

Shannon EW. Post traumatic neuroses. *Insurance Counsel Journal.* July 1961:472–475.

*Smith HW, Solomon HC. Traumatic neuroses in court. *Virginia Law Review.* 1943;30: 87–175.

*Stalker AM. Traumatic neuroses. Translation of lecture by A Strümpell 1888. In: *Clinical Lectures on Medicine and Surgery.* Third series. 1894:303–325.

Strauss I, Savitsky N. Head injury—neurologic and psychiatric aspects. *Archives of Neurology and Psychiatry.* 1934;31(5):893–913.

Thompson GN. Post-traumatic psychoneurosis—a statistical survey. *American Journal of Psychiatry.* 1965;121:1043–1048.

*Trimble MR. *Post-Traumatic Neurosis. From Railway Spine to Whiplash.* Chichester, England: John Wiley & Sons; 1981.

WHIPLASH—GENERAL

Anonymous. Whiplash injury [letter]. *Lancet.* 1991;338:1207–1208.

Babcock JL. Cervical spine injuries. Diagnosis and classification. *Archives of Surgery.* 1976;11:646–651.

Baer N. Fraud worries insurance companies but should concern physicians too, industry says. *Canadian Medical Association Journal.* 1997;156(2):251–256.

*Balla JI, Iansek R. Headaches arising from disorders of the cervical spine. In: Hopkins A, ed. *Headache. Problems in Diagnosis and Management.* London: WB Saunders; 1988: 243–267.

*Barnsley L, Lord SM, Bogduk N. Whiplash injury. *Pain.* 1994;58:283–307.

Barry M. Whiplash injuries. *British Journal of Rheumatology.* 1992;31(9):579–581.

Becker RE. Whiplash injuries. *Academy of Applied Osteopathy—Year Book.* 1958:65–69.

Berry H. Psychological aspects of whiplash injury. In: Wilkins RH, Rengachary SS, eds. *Neurosurgery.* Vol 2. Philadelphia: McGraw-Hill; 1985:1716–1719.

Björnstig U, Hildingsson C, Toolanen G. Soft-tissue injury of the neck in a hospital based material. *Scandinavian Journal of Social Medicine.* 1990;18:263–267.

Borchgrevink GE, Lereim I, Røyneland L, Bjørndal A, Haraldseth O. National health insurance consumption and chronic symptoms following mild neck sprain injuries in car collisions. *Scandinavian Journal of Social Medicine.* 1996;24(4):264–271.

Bosworth DM. Whiplash—an unacceptable medical term. *Journal of Bone and Joint Surgery.* 1959;41-A:16.

Bounds JA. Chronic whiplash syndrome [letter]. *Neurology.* 1995;45:2117.

Braaf MM, Rosner S. Whiplash injury of the neck: symptoms, diagnosis, treatment, and prognosis. *New York State Journal of Medicine.* 1958;58:1501–1507.

Braaf MM, Rosner S. Whiplash injury of neck—fact or fancy? *International Surgery.* 1966;46(2):176–182.

Braaf MM, Rosner S. Trauma of cervical spine as a cause of chronic headache. *Journal of Trauma.* 1975;15(5):441–446.

Braunstein PW, Moore JO. The fallacy of the term "whiplash injury." *American Journal of Surgery.* 1959;97:522–529.

Breck LW, Van Norman RW. Medicolegal aspects of cervical spine sprains. *Clinical Orthopaedics and Related Research.* 1971;74:124–128.

Bring G, Westman G. Chronic posttraumatic syndrome after whiplash injury. *Scandinavian Journal of Primary Health Care.* 1991;9:135–141.

Byrn C, Borenstein P, Linder LE. Treatment of neck and shoulder pain in whip-lash syndrome patients with intracutaneous sterile water injections. *Acta Anaesthesiologica Scandinavica.* 1991;35:52–53.

Byrn C, Olsson I, Falkheden L, et al. Subcutaneous sterile water injections for chronic neck and shoulder pain following whiplash injuries. *Lancet.* 1993;341:449–452.

Cammack KV. Whiplash injuries to the neck. *American Journal of Surgery.* 1957;93: 663–666.

Cassidy JD. Basal metabolic temperature vs. laboratory assessment in "posttraumatic hypothyroidism" [letter]. *Journal of Manipulative and Physiological Therapeutics.* 1996;19(6):425–426.

Christie B. Appeal overturns link between multiple sclerosis and whiplash. *British Medical Journal.* 1998;316:799.

Coppola AR. Neck injury, a reappraisal. *International Surgery.* 1968;50(6):510–515.

Crowe HE. A new diagnostic sign in neck injuries. *Insurance Counsel Journal.* July 1962: 463–466.

Crowe HE. A new diagnostic sign in neck injuries. *California Medicine.* 1964;100(1): 12–13.

Cullum DE. Whiplash in Australia: illness or injury? [letter]. *Medical Journal of Australia.* 1992;157:428–429.

Darragh FN, O'Connor P. Whiplash injury. *Journal of Neurology, Neurosurgery, and Psychiatry.* 1991;54(3):283–284.

*Davis AG. Injuries of the cervical spine. *Journal of the American Medical Association.* 1945;127(3):149–156.

Deans GT, Magalliard JN, Kerr M, Rutherford WH. Neck sprain—a major cause of disability following car accidents. *Injury.* 1987;18:10–12.

Deans GT, Magalliard JN, Rutherford WH. Incidence and duration of neck pain among patients injured in car accidents. *British Medical Journal.* 1986;292:94–95.

DeGravelles WD, Kelley JH. *Injuries Following Rear-End Automobile Collisions.* Springfield, IL: Charles C Thomas; 1969.

DePalma AF, Subin DK. Study of the cervical syndrome. *Clinical Orthopedics.* 1965;38: 135–142.

DeRoy MS. Whiplash injuries. Fact or fallacy? *Medical Times.* 1963;91(10):976–978.

Dolinis J. Risk factors for 'whiplash' in drivers: a cohort study of rear-end traffic crashes. *Injury.* 1997;28(3):173–179.

Dorman TA. Whiplash injury [letter]. *Lancet.* 1991;338:1208.

Dunn EJ, Blazar S. Soft-tissue injuries of the lower cervical spine. In: Griffin PP, ed. *Instructional Course Lectures.* Chicago, IL: American Academy of Orthopaedic Surgeons; 1987:499–512.

Du Toit GT. The post-traumatic painful neck. *Forensic Science.* 1974;3:1–18.

Dvorak J, Valach L, Schmid S. Cervical spine injuries in Switzerland. *Journal of Manual Medicine.* 1989;4:7–16.

Eck DB. Flexion-extension injury of the cervical spine. *Journal of the Medical Society of New Jersey.* 1960;57:300–306.

Editorial. Are the 1956 cars safer? *Consumers' Research Bulletin.* 1956;37:16–19.

Editorial. Crashes cause most neck pain. *AMA News.* December 5, 1956:7.

Editorial. Therapy for whiplash: leave alone. *Medical World News*. 1962;3:69.

Ellerbroek WC. Whiplash injuries and cervical pain. *Headache*. 1966;6(2):73–77.

Ellis SJ. Tremor and other movement disorders after whiplash type injuries. *Journal of Neurology, Neurosurgery, and Psychiatry*. 1997;63:110–112.

Evans RW. Chronic whiplash syndrome [letter]. *Neurology*. 1995;45:2117.

Evans RW. Whiplash around the world. *Headache*. 1995;35:262–263.

Farquhar D. Misconceived ideas [letter]. *Canadian Family Physician*. 1995;41:563.

*Ferrari R, Russell AS. The whiplash syndrome—common sense revisited. *Journal of Rheumatology*. 1997;24(4):618–623.

*Ferrari R, Russell AS. Authors' reply [letter]. *Journal of Rheumatology*. 1998;25(7): 1438–1440.

Flax HJ, Fernández B, Rodríguez-Ramón A. The "whiplash" injury. *Boletin Asociacion medica de Puerto Rico*. 1971;63(6):161–165.

Foley-Nolan D, O'Connor P. Whiplash injury [letter]. *Journal of Neurology, Neurosurgery, and Psychiatry*. 1991;54(3):283–284.

Foreman SM, Croft AC. *Whiplash Injuries. The Cervical Acceleration/Deceleration Syndrome*. Baltimore: Williams & Wilkins; 1988.

Foreman SM, Croft AC. *Whiplash Injuries. The Cervical Acceleration/Deceleration Syndrome*. Baltimore: Williams & Wilkins; 1995.

Forsyth HF. Extension injuries of the cervical spine. *Journal of Bone and Joint Surgery*. 1964;46-A(8):1792–1797.

Frankel CJ. Medical-legal aspect of injuries to the neck. *Journal of the American Medical Association*. 1959;169(3):216–223.

Frankel VH. Whiplash injuries to the neck. In: Hirsch C, Zotterman Y, eds. *Cervical Pain*. Oxford, England: Pergamon Press; 1971:97–112.

Frankel VH. Comments on soft tissue injuries of the neck. In: *Head and Neck Injury Criteria, A Consensus Workshop, National Highway Traffic Safety Administration, 1981, March 26–27, Washington, DC*. 1981:121–122.

Fredin Y, Elert J, Britschgi N, et al. A decreased ability to relax between repetitive muscle contractions in patients with chronic symptoms after whiplash trauma of the neck. *Journal of Musculoskeletal Pain*. 1997;5(2):55–70.

Galasko CSB, Murray PM, Pitcher M, et al. Neck sprains after road traffic accidents: a modern epidemic. *Injury*. 1993;24(3):155–157.

Gargan MF, Bannister GC. Long-term prognosis of soft-tissue injuries of the neck. *Journal of Bone and Joint Surgery*. 1990;72-B:901–903.

Gargan MF, Bannister GC. Soft tissue injuries to the neck [letter]. *British Medical Journal*. 1991;303:786.

Gates EM, Cento D. Studies in cervical trauma. Part 1. *International Surgery*. 1966;46(3): 218–222.

*Gay JR, Abbott KH. Common whiplash injuries of the neck. *Journal of the American Medical Association*. 1953;152(18):1698–1704.

Gebhard JS, Donaldson DH, Brown CW. Soft-tissue injuries of the cervical spine. *Orthopaedic Review*. 1994;(suppl):9–17.

Gelber LJ. Medico-legal aspects of whiplash injuries. *Mississippi Valley Medical Journal.* 1956;78:215–216.

Gelber LJ. Medico-legal aspects of whiplash injuries. *Nassau Medical News.* 1956; 28(8):1–6.

Goff CW, Alden JO. *Traumatic Cervical Syndrome and Whiplash.* Philadelphia: JB Lippincott Company; 1964.

Gordon DA. The rheumatologist and chronic whiplash syndrome. *Journal of Rheumatology.* 1997;24(4):617–618.

Greenfield J, Ilfeld FW. Acute cervical strain. *Clinical Orthopedics and Related Research.* 1977;122:196–200.

Gukelberger M. The uncomplicated post-traumatic cervical syndrome. *Scandinavian Journal of Rehabilitation Medicine.* 1972;4:150–153.

*Gunzburg R, Szpalski M. *Whiplash Injuries. Current Concepts in Prevention, Diagnosis, and Treatment of the Cervical Whiplash Syndrome.* Philadelphia: Lippincott-Raven; 1998.

Guy JE. The whiplash: tiny impact, tremendous injury. *Industrial Medicine and Surgery.* 1968;37:688–691.

Hackett GS. Whiplash injury. *American Practitioner.* 1959;10(8):1333–1336.

Hagström Y, Carlsson J. Prolonged functional impairments after whiplash injury. *Scandinavian Journal of Rehabilitation Medicine.* 1996;28:139–146.

Hamel HA, James OE Jr. Acute traumatic cervical syndrome (whiplash injury). *Southern Medical Journal.* 1962;55:1171–1177.

Hammacher ER, van der Werken C. Acute neck sprain: 'whiplash' reappraised. *Injury.* 1996;27(7):463–466.

Hancock J. Comments on Barnsley et al [letter]. *Pain.* 1995;61:487–495.

Harriton MB. *The Whiplash Handbook.* Springfield, IL: Charles C Thomas; 1989.

Harth M, Teasell RW. Chronic whiplash re-revisited [letter]. *Journal of Rheumatology.* 1998;25(7):1437–1438.

Hartley J. Modern concepts of whiplash injury. *New York State Journal of Medicine.* 1958;58(2):3306–3310.

Hawkes CD. Whiplash injuries of the head and neck. *Archives of Surgery.* 1957;75: 828–833.

Hawkins GW. Flexion and extension injuries of the cervico-capital joints. *Clinical Orthopedics.* 1962;24:22–33.

Heilig D. "Whiplash" mechanics of injury: management of cervical and dorsal involvement. *Journal of the American Osteopathic Association.* 1963;63:113–120.

Hodgson SP, Grundy M. Neck sprains after car accidents [letter]. *British Medical Journal.* 1989;298:1452.

Hohl M. Soft-tissue neck injuries. In: Sherk HH, Dunn EJ, Eismont FJ, et al. *The Cervical Spine.* Philadelphia: JB Lippincott Company; 1989:436–441.

Hone MR. What's in a name? [letter]. *Medical Journal of Australia.* 1997;167:175.

Huddleston OL. Whiplash injuries. Diagnosis and treatment. *California Medicine.* 1958;89(5):318–321.

Hudson AJ. Chronic whiplash [letter]. *Neurology.* 1996;47:615–616.

Immega G. Whiplash injuries increase with seat belt use. *Canadian Family Physician.* 1995;41:203–204.

Jackson R. *The Cervical Syndrome.* 3rd ed. Springfield, IL: Charles C Thomas; 1966.

Jacobs H. Whiplash legitimized by clinical support [letter]. *Canadian Family Physician.* 1995;41:202–203.

James OE Jr, Hamel HA. Whiplash injuries of the neck. *Missouri Medicine.* 1955;52(6): 423–426.

Janecki CJ Jr, Lipke JM. Whiplash syndrome. *American Family Physician.* 1978;17(4): 144–151.

Janes JM, Hooshmand H. Extension-flexion injury of the neck. *Modern Medicine (Review Edition).* 1965;33:894–895.

Janes JM, Hooshmand H. Extension-flexion injury of the neck. *Modern Medicine.* August 1965:128–129.

Johnson G. Hyperextension soft tissue injuries of the cervical spine—a review. *Journal of Accident and Emergency Medicine.* 1996;13:3–8.

Jónsson H Jr, Bring G, Rauschning W, Sahlstedt B. Hidden cervical spine injuries in traffic accident victims with skull fractures. *Journal of Spinal Disorders.* 1991;4(3):251–263.

Juhl M, Kjærgaard-Seerup K. Cervical spine epidemiological investigation. Medical and social consequences. In: *Proceedings of the International IRCOBI Conference on the Biomechanics of Impacts, 1981, Salonde-Provence.* 1981:49–58.

*Kelly M. Whiplash syndrome. *Irish Medical Journal.* 1992;85(3):85–87.

Kenna CJ. The whiplash syndrome. A general practitioner's viewpoint. *Australian Family Physician.* 1984;13(4):256–257.

*Khan H, McCormack D, Burke J, McManus F. Incidental neck symptoms in high energy trauma victims. *Irish Medical Journal.* 1997;90(4):143.

Kinsey FR. Pain in the neck. *Pennsylvania Medical Journal.* 61:1628–1631.

Knight PO, Wheat JD. The whiplash injury—clinical and medico-legal aspects. *Bulletin of the Tulane University Medical Facility.* 1959;18(4):199–214.

Langwieder K, Backaitis SH, Fan W, Partyka S, Ommaya A. Comparative studies of neck injuries of car occupants in frontal collisions in the United States and in the Federal Republic of Germany. In: *Proceedings of the Twenty Fifth Stapp Car Crash Conference.* Paper #811030. Warrendale, PA: Society of Automotive Engineering; 1981:71–127.

La Rocca H. Cervical sprain syndrome. In: Frymoyer JW et al, eds. *The Adult Spine.* Vol 2. New York: Raven Press; 1991:1051–1061.

Lipow EG. Whiplash injuries. *Southern Medical Journal.* 1955;48:1304–1311.

*Livingston M. Neck and back sprains from MVAs: a retrospective study. *British Columbia Medical Journal.* 1991;33(12):654–656.

Livingston M. Wise words of Malleson accordant. *Canadian Family Physician.* 1995;41:204.

Lottes JO, Luh AM, Leydig SM, Fries JW, Burst DO. Whiplash injuries of the neck. *Missouri Medicine.* 1959;56(6):645–650.

Maag U, Laberge-Nadeau C, Xiang-Tong T. Neck sprains in car crashes: incidence, associations, length of compensation and costs to the insurer. In: *Proceedings of the 37th Annual Conference of the Association for the Advancement of Automotive Medicine, 1993, November 4–6, San Antonio, Texas, Des Plaines, Illinois.* 1993:15–26.

*MacNab I. The "whiplash syndrome." *Orthopedic Clinics of North America.* 1971;2(2):389–403.

MacNab I. Acceleration extension injuries of the cervical spine. In: Rothman RH, Simeone FA, eds. *The Spine.* Philadelphia: WB Saunders; 1982:647–660.

Malleson A. Whiplash: folly and fakery. *Humane Medicine.* 1990;6(3):193–196.

Malleson A. Chronic whiplash syndrome. Psychosocial epidemic. *Canadian Family Physician.* 1994;40:1906–1909.

Malleson A. Response [letter]. *Canadian Family Physician.* 1995;41:204–206.

Malleson A. Response [letter]. *Canadian Family Physician.* 1995;41:563, 565.

Marshall HW. Neck injuries. *Boston Medical and Surgical Journal.* 1919;158(4):93–98.

Marshall PD, O'Connor M, Hodgkinson JP. The perceived relationship between neck symptoms and precedent injury. *Injury.* 1995;26:17–19.

Martin GM. Sprains, strains, and whiplash injuries. *Physical Therapy Review.* 1959; 39(12):808–817.

Mayfield FH, Griffith JC. Whiplash injuries. *Journal of the Michigan State Medical Society.* 1957;56:1142–1146, 1161.

McGee FO. Whiplash injury of the cervical spine. *Orthopedics.* 1959;1:105–108, 115–116.

McIntire RT. Whiplash injuries. *Journal of the Medical Association of Alabama.* 1959;29:170.

McKellar CC. "Whiplash"—should we discard the name? *Medical Journal of Australia.* 1979;2:494.

McOsker TC. Neck injury and rear-end collision. *Rhode Island Medical Journal.* 1962;45:252–257.

Merskey H. Chronic whiplash syndrome [letter]. *Neurology.* 1995;45:2116.

Morehouse LE. Body functions and controls in whiplash injuries. *International Record of Medicine.* 1956;169(1):11–13.

Morrow J. Surgical anatomy of whiplash injuries. *International Record of Medicine.* 1956;169(1):14–18.

Nagle DB. Whiplash of the cervical spine. *Radiology.* 1957;69:823–827.

Newman PK. Author's reply [letter]. *British Medical Journal.* 1990;301:610.

Newman PK. Whiplash injury [letter]. *British Medical Journal.* 1990;301:395–396.

Nicholson MW. Whiplash: fact, fantasy or fakery. *Hawaii Medical Journal.* 1974;33(5): 168–170.

Nielsen JM. Whiplash injury with amnesia for life experiences. *Bulletin of Los Angeles Neurological Society.* 1959;24:27–30.

Otremski I, Marsh JL, Wilde BR, McLardy Smith PD, Newman RJ. Soft tissue cervical spinal injuries in motor vehicle accidents. *Injury.* 1989;20:349–351.

Pearce JMS. Whiplash injury [letter]. *British Medical Journal.* 1990;301:610.

Pearce JMS. Pearce replies [letter]. *Journal of Neurology, Neurosurgery, and Psychiatry.* 1991;54(3):284.

*Pearce JMS. Whiplash injury: fact or fiction? *Headache Quarterly, Current Treatment and Research.* 1992;3:45–49.

Pearce JMS. Subtle cerebral lesions in "chronic whiplash syndrome"? [letter]. *Journal of Neurology, Neurosurgery, and Psychiatry.* 1993;56(12):1328–1329.

Pearce JMS. Polemics of chronic whiplash injury. *Neurology.* 1994;44:1993–1997.

Pearce JMS. Reply from the author [letter]. *Neurology.* 1995;45:2117–2118.

Pruce AM. Whiplash injury: what's new? *Southern Medical Journal.* 1964;57:332–337.

*Radanov BP. Common whiplash—research findings revisited. *Journal of Rheumatology.* 1997;24(4):623–625.

Ratliff AHC. Whiplash injuries. *Journal of Bone and Joint Surgery [British].* 1997; 79-B:517–519.

Riley LH, Long D, Riley LH Jr. The science of whiplash. *Medicine.* 1995;74(5):298–299.

Roaf R. Lateral flexion injuries of the cervical spine. *Journal of Bone and Joint Surgery.* 1963;45-B(1):36–38.

Romano TJ. Chronic whiplash re-revisited [letter]. *Journal of Rheumatology.* 1998;25(7): 1437.

Rudy DR. Lateral whiplash. *Journal of the American Medical Association.* 1968;205(9): 103.

Russell LW. Whiplash injuries of the spine. *Journal of the Florida State Medical Association.* 1957;43(11):1099–1104.

Ryan GA, Taylor GW, Moore VM, Dolinis J. Neck strain in car occupants. The influence of crash-related factors on initial severity. *Medical Journal of Australia.* 1993; 159:651–656.

Samblanet HL. Whiplash neck injury—management of subjective and objective symptoms. *Osteopathic Profession.* 1956;23:19–23, 42–44.

Sano K, Nakamura N, Hirakawa K, Hashizume K. Correlative studies of dynamics and pathology in whip-lash and head injuries. *Scandinavian Journal of Rehabilitation Medicine.* 1972;4:47–54.

Savastano AA, Larkin DF. Whiplash injuries. *Rhode Island Medical Journal.* 1957;40:220–222.

Schaefer JH. Whiplash injuries of the neck. *Journal of the American Medical Association.* 1953;153(10):974.

Schaefer JH. Importance of whiplash injury. *International Record of Medicine.* 1956; 169(1):28–30.

Schaefer JH. Whiplash injury. *Journal of the American Medical Association.* 1956; 162(16):1492.

Schutt CH, Dohan FC. Neck injury to women in auto accidents. *Journal of the American Medical Association.* 1968;206(12):2689–2692.

Sehnert KW, Croft AC. Basal metabolic temperature vs. laboratory assessment in "post-traumatic hypothyroidism." *Journal of Manipulative and Physiological Therapeutics.* 1996;19:6–12.

Sehnert KW, Croft AC. In reply [letter]. *Journal of Manipulative and Physiological Therapeutics.* 1996;19(6):426–427.

Selecki BR. Whiplash. A specialist's view. *Australian Family Physician.* 1984;13(4): 243–247.

Seletz E. Whiplash injuries. *Journal of the American Medical Association.* 1958;168(13): 1750–1755.

Shkrum MJ, Green RN, Nowak ES. Upper cervical trauma in motor vehicle collisions. *Journal of Forensic Sciences.* 1989;34(2):381–390.

Simmons RC. Whiplash: big business & serious problem. *For the Defense.* August 1982:14–22.

Snow GH. Economic aspects of "whiplash" injury. *California Medicine.* 1964;101(4): 260–262.

Sommer HM. Letter to editor. *Spine.* 1997;22(8):928.

Squires B, Gargan MF, Bannister GC. Soft-tissue injuries of the cervical spine. *Journal of Bone and Joint Surgery [British].* 1996;78-B:955–957.

States JD, Korn MW, Masengill JB. The enigma of whiplash injury. *New York State Journal of Medicine.* December 1970:2971–2978.

Stovner LJ. The nosologic status of the whiplash syndrome: a critical review based on a methodological approach. *Spine.* 1996;21(23):2735–2746.

Stuck RM. Whiplash injuries. A new approach to the problem. *Medical Times.* 1962;90(5):493–504.

Sturzenegger M, Di Stefano GD, Radanov BP, Schnidrig A. Presenting symptoms and signs after whiplash injury: the influence of accident mechanisms. *Neurology.* 1994;44: 688–693.

Tamura T. Cranial symptoms after cervical injury. *Journal of Bone and Joint Surgery.* 1989;71-B:283–287.

Taylor JR, Kakulas BA. Neck injuries [letter]. *Lancet.* 1991;338:1343.

Taylor JR, Twomey LT. Disc injuries in cervical trauma [letter]. *Lancet.* 1990;336:1318.

Teasell RW, Shapiro AP. Whiplash injuries: an update. *Pain Research & Management.* 1998;3(2):81–90.

Thomas A. Whiplash—a misnomer. *Trial.* 1965;1:27–30.

Thomson JEM. The counterfeit phrase of neck lash injuries. *Orthopedics.* 1960;2:125.

Thomson JEM. The counterfeit phrase of neck lash injuries. *Insurance Counsel Journal.* January 1961:148.

Thorson J. Neck injuries in road accidents. *Scandinavian Journal of Rehabilitation Medicine.* 1972;4:110–113.

Threadgill FD. Whiplash injury—end-results in 88 cases. *Insurance Counsel Journal.* January 1961:161–163.

Von Werssowetz OF. A new look at whiplash injuries. *Journal of the Tennessee Medical Association.* 1965;58(2):39–44.

Watkinson AF. Whiplash injury [letter]. *British Medical Journal.* 1990;301:983.

Weinberg ED. Whiplash injuries to the neck. *Maryland State Medical Journal.* 1959;8:67–68.

Wiley AM, Evans JG, Lloyd GL, Ha'eri GB. A review of whiplash injuries seen in a medico-legal practice. *Advocates'Quarterly.* 1979–1981;2:239–252.

Winston KR. Whiplash and its relationship to migraine. *Headache.* 1987;27:452–457.

Woodward AH. Chronic whiplash syndrome [letter]. *Neurology.* 1995;45:2117.

Worsham RA. Acute sprain of the cervical spine. *Southern Medical Journal.* 1963;56: 252–256.

Wright JM. Whiplash injuries. Management and complications. *Journal of the American Osteopathic Association.* 1956;55(9):564–568.

Wright PB, Brady LP. An anatomic evaluation of whiplash injuries. *Clinical Orthopedics.* 1958;11:120–131.

Yarnell PR, Rossie GV. Minor whiplash head injury with major debilitation. *Brain Injury.* 1988;2(3):255–258.

Zabrodski R. Few whiplash patients are malingerers. *Canadian Family Physician.* 1995; 41:29–30.

Zarlengo AE. Whiplash injuries. *Dicta.* July–August 1959:285–293.

Zatzkin HR, Kveton FW. Evaluation of the cervical spine in whiplash injuries. *Radiology.* 1960;75:577–583.

THEORIES OF INJURY MECHANISM IN WHIPLASH

Berton J. *Whiplash: Test of the Influential Variables.* Paper #680080. Warrendale, PA: Society of Automotive Engineers; 1968:77.

Billig HE Jr. Traumatic neck, head, eye syndrome. *Journal of the International College of Surgeons.* 1953;20(5):558–561.

Billig HE Jr. The mechanism of whiplash injuries. *International Record of Medicine.* 1956;169(1):3–7.

Billig HE Jr. Head, neck, shoulder and arm syndrome following cervical injury. *Journal of the International College of Surgeons.* 1959;32(3):287–297.

Cameron BM, Cree CMN. A critique of the compression theory of whiplash. *Orthopedics.* 1960;2:127–129.

*Davis AG. Injuries of the cervical spine. *Journal of the American Medical Association.* 1945;127(3):149–156.

Dinning TAR. Whiplash in Australia: illness or injury? [letter]. *Medical Journal of Australia.* 1993;158:138, 140.

Fields A. The autonomic nervous system in whiplash injuries. *International Record of Medicine.* 1956;169(1):8–10.

Fleming JFR. The neurosurgeon's responsibility in "whiplash" injuries. *Clinical Neurosurgery*. 1973;20:242–252.

Frankel VH. Pathomechanics of whiplash injuries to the neck. In: Morley TP, ed. *Current Controversies in Neurosurgery*. Philadelphia: WB Saunders; 1976:39–50.

*Gay JR, Abbott KH. Common whiplash injuries of the neck. *Journal of the American Medical Association*. 1953;152(18):1698–1704.

Gissane W. The causes and the prevention of neck injuries to car occupants. *Annals of the Royal College of Surgeons of England*. 1966;39:161–163.

Golding DN. Whiplash injuries. *British Journal of Rheumatology*. 1992;32(2):174.

Kihlberg JK. Flexion-torsion neck injury in rear impacts. In: *Proceedings of the Thirteenth Annual Meeting of the American Association of Automotive Medicine*. 1969:1–16.

Lesoin F, Thomas CE, Lozes G, Villette L, Jomin M. Has the safety-belt replaced the hangman's noose? [letter]. *Lancet*. 1985;1:1341.

Lubin S, Sehmer J. Are automobile head restraints used effectively? *Canadian Family Physician*. 1993;39:1584–1588.

McKeever DC. The mechanics of the so-called whiplash injury. *Orthopedics*. 1960;2:3–6.

Morris F. Do head-restraints protect the neck from whiplash injuries? *Archives of Emergency Medicine*. 1989;6:17–21.

Olsson I, Bunketorp O, Carlsson G, et al. An in-depth study of neck injuries in rear end collisions. In: *Proceedings of the International Research Council on Biokinetics of Impacts (IRCOBI), September 12–13–14, Bron-Lyon, France*. 1990:269–280.

Panagiotacopulos ND, Lee JS, Pope MH, et al. Detection of wire EMG activity in whiplash injuries using wavelets. *Iowa Orthopaedic Journal*. 1997;17:134–138.

Penning L. Acceleration injury of the cervical spine by hypertranslation of the head. Part I. Effect of normal translation of the head on cervical spine motion: a radiological study. *European Spine Journal*. 1992;1:7–12.

Penning L. Acceleration injury of the cervical spine by hypertranslation of the head. Part II. Effect of hypertranslation of the head on cervical spine motion: discussion of literature data. *European Spine Journal*. 1992;1:13–19.

Ruedmann AD Jr. Automobile safety device—headrest to prevent whiplash injury. *Journal of the American Medical Association*. 1969;164(17):1889.

Severy DM, Brink HM, Baird JD. *Backrest and Head Restraint Design for Rear-End Collision Protection*. Paper #680079. Warrendale, PA: Society of Automotive Engineers; 1968:77.

States JD. Soft tissue injuries of the neck. In: *Proceedings of the Twenty Third Stapp Car Crash Conference*. Paper #790135. Warrendale, PA: Society of Automotive Engineers; 1979:487–493.

*States JD, Balcerak JC, Williams JS, et al. Injury frequency and head restraint effectiveness in rear-end impact accidents. In: *Proceedings of the Sixteenth Stapp Car Crash Conference*. Paper #720967. Warrendale, PA: Society of Automotive Engineers; 1972: 228–257.

Svensson MY, Lövsund P, Haland Y, Larsson S. The influence of seat-back and head-restraint properties on the head-neck motion during rear-impact. *Accident Analysis and Prevention*. 1996;28(2):221–227.

Taylor JR, Finch P. Acute injury of the neck: anatomical and pathological basis of pain. *Annals of the Academy of Medicine of Singapore.* 1993;22(2):187–192.

Taylor JR, Twomey LT. Disc injuries in cervical trauma [letter]. *Lancet.* 1990;336:1318.

Taylor JR, Twomey LT. Acute injuries to cervical joints. An autopsy study of neck sprain. *Spine.* 1993;18(9):1115–1122.

Waxman SG, Rizzo MA. The whiplash (hyperextension-flexion) syndrome: a disorder of dorsal root ganglion neurons? *Journal of Neurotrauma.* 1996;13(12):735–739.

WHIPLASH AND POSTURAL PROBLEMS

Harms-Ringdahl K, Ekholm J. Intensity and character of pain and muscular activity levels elicited by maintained extreme flexion position of the lower-cervical-upper thoracic spine. *Scandinavian Journal of Rehabilitation Medicine.* 1986;18:117–126.

Hedman TP, Fernie GR. Mechanical response of the lumbar spine to seated postural loads. *Spine.* 1997;22(7):734–743.

Karlberg M, Johansson R, Magnusson M, Fransson PA. Dizziness of suspected cervical origin distinguished by posturographic assessment of human postural dynamics. *Journal of Vestibular Research.* 1996;6(1):37–47.

*Karlberg M, Magnusson M, Malmström EM, Melander A, Moritz U. Postural and symptomatic improvement after physiotherapy in patients with dizziness of suspected cervical origin. *Archives of Physical Medicine and Rehabilitation.* 1996;77:874–882.

Katsarkas A. Postural stability following mild head or whiplash injuries [letter]. *American Journal of Otology.* 1996;17:172–175.

Magnusson ML, Aleksiev A, Wilder DG, et al. Unexpected load and asymmetric posture as etiologic factors in low back pain. *European Spine Journal.* 1996;5(1):23–35.

*McKenzie RA. *The Cervical and Thoracic Spine.* New Zealand: Spinal Publications Ltd; 1990.

*Middaugh S, Kee W, Nicholson J. Muscle overuse and posture as factors in the development and maintenance of chronic musculoskeletal pain. In: Grzesiak R, Ciccone D, eds. *Psychological Vulnerability to Chronic Pain.* New York: Springer; 1994:55–89.

Rubin AM, Woolley SM, Dailey VM, Goebel JA. Postural stability following mild head or whiplash injuries. *American Journal of Otology.* 1995;16(2):216–221.

Watson DH, Trott PH. Cervical headache: an investigation of natural head posture and upper cervical flexor muscle performance. *Cephalalgia.* 1993;13:272–284.

Williams MM, Hawley JA, McKenzie RA, van Wijmen PM. A comparison of the effects of two sitting postures on back and referred pain. *Spine.* 1991;16(10):1185–1191.

WHIPLASH AND X-RAYS, DISC DEGENERATION

Aprill C, Bogduk N. Cervical zygapophyseal joint pain. *Spine.* 1990;15(6):744–777.

Aprill C, Bogduk N. The prevalence of cervical zygapophyseal joint pain. *Spine.* 1992;17(7):744–777.

Arnold JG Jr. The clinical manifestations of spondylochondrosis (spondylosis) of the cervical spine. *Annals of Surgery.* 1955;141(6):872–889.

*Balla JI. Report to the Motor Accidents Board of Victoria on whiplash injuries, 1984. In: Hopkins A, ed. *Headache. Problems in Diagnosis and Management.* London: WB Saunders: 1988:268–289.

*Balla JI, Iansek R. Headaches arising from disorders of the cervical spine. In: Hopkins A, ed. *Headache. Problems in Diagnosis and Management.* London: WB Saunders; 1988: 243–267.

Barnes SM. Whiplash injury and surgically treated cervical disc disease [letter]. *Injury.* 1994;25(6):409–410.

*Borden AGB, Rechtman AM, Gershon-Cohen J. The normal cervical lordosis. *Radiology.* 1960;74:806–809.

Buonocore E, Hartman JT, Nelson CL. Cineradiograms of cervical spine in diagnosis of soft-tissue injuries. *Journal of the American Medical Association.* 1966;198(1):143–147.

Colton CL. Whiplash injury and surgically treated cervical disc disease [letter]. *Injury.* 1994;25(6):409–410.

*Crowe HE. Whiplash injuries of the cervical spine. In: *Section of Insurance, Negligence, and Compensation Law, Proceedings.* American Bar Association; 1958:176–184.

DeGravelles WD, Kelley JH. *Injuries Following Rear-End Automobile Collisions.* Springfield, IL: Charles C Thomas; 1969.

Elias F. Roentgen findings in the asymptomatic cervical spine. *New York State Journal of Medicine.* 1958;58:3300–3303.

Fineman S, Borrelli FJ, Rubinstein BM, Epstein H, Jacobson HG. The cervical spine: transformation of the normal lordotic pattern into a linear pattern in the neutral posture. *Journal of Bone and Joint Surgery.* 1963;45-A(6):1179–1206.

*Friedenberg ZB, Broder HA, Edeiken JE, Spencer HN. Degenerative disk disease of cervical spine. *Journal of the American Medical Association.* 1960;174(4):375–380.

*Friedenberg ZB, Miller WT. Degenerative disc disease of the cervical spine. A comparative study of asymptomatic and symptomatic patients. *Journal of Bone and Joint Surgery.* 1963;45-A(6):1171–1178.

Gargan MF. What is the evidence for an organic lesion in whiplash injury? *Journal of Psychosomatic Research.* 1995;39(6):777–781.

*Gore DR, Sepic SB, Gardner GM. Roentgenographic findings of the cervical spine in asymptomatic people. *Spine.* 1986;11(6):521–524.

*Gore DR, Sepic SB, Gardner GM, Murray MP. Neck pain: a long-term follow-up of 205 patients. *Spine.* 1987;12(1):1–5.

Griffiths HJ, Olson PN, Everson LI, Winemiller BA. Hyperextension strain or "whiplash" injuries to the cervical spine. *Skeletal Radiology.* 1995;24:263–266.

Hadley LA. Roentgenographic studies of the cervical spine. *American Journal of Roentgenology.* 1944;52(2):173–195.

Hamer AJ. Reply from the authors [letter]. *Injury.* 1994;25(6):410.

Hamer AJ, Gargan MF, Bannister GC, Nelson RJ. Whiplash injury and surgically treated cervical disc disease. *Injury.* 1993;24(8):549–550.

Helliwell PS, Evans PF, Wright V. The straight cervical spine: Does it indicate muscle spasm? *Journal of Bone and Joint Surgery [British]*. 1994;76-B:103–106.

*Hildingsson C, Toolanen G. Outcome after soft-tissue injury of the cervical spine. *Acta Orthopaedica Scandinavica*. 1990;61(4):357–359.

Hohl M. Soft tissue injuries of the neck. *Clinical Orthopedics*. 1975;109:42–49.

Hohl M, Hopp E. Soft tissue injuries of the neck—II: factors influencing prognosis. *Orthopedic Transactions*. 1978;2:29.

Irvine DH, Foster JB, Newell DJ, Klukvin BN. Prevalence of cervical spondylosis in a general practice. *Lancet*. 1965;1:1089–1092.

Jensen OK, Justesen T, Nielsen FF, Brixen K. Functional radiographic examination of the cervical spine in patients with post-traumatic headache. *Cephalalgia*. 1990;10:295–303.

*Juhl JH, Miller SM, Roberts GW. Roentgenographic variations in the normal cervical spine. *Radiology*. 1962;78:591–597.

Keats TE. *An Atlas of Normal Roentgen Variants That May Simulate Disease*. 2nd ed. Chicago: Year Book Medical Publishers Inc; 1980.

Lawrence JS. Disc degeneration. Its frequency and relationship to symptoms. *Annals of Rheumatic Diseases*. 1969;28:121–137.

Lee F, Turner JWA. Natural history and prognosis of cervical spondylosis. *British Medical Journal*. 1963;2:1607–1610.

Marchiori DM, Henderson CNR. A cross-sectional study correlating cervical radiographic degenerative findings to pain and disability. *Spine*. 1997;21(23):2747–2752.

*Miles KA, Maimaris C, Finlay D, Barnes MR. The incidence and prognostic significance of radiological abnormalities in soft tissue injuries to the cervical spine. *Skeletal Radiology*. 1988;17:493–496.

*Miller H, Brain R, Russell WR, O'Connell JEA. Discussion on cervical spondylosis. *Proceedings of the Royal Society of Medicine*. 1955;49:197–208.

Munro D. Relation between spondylosis cervicalis and injury of the cervical spine and its contents. *New England Journal of Medicine*. 1960;262(17):839–846.

Myers A. Degeneration of cervical intervertebral discs following whiplash injury. *Bulletin of the Hospital for Joint Diseases*. 1953;14:74–85.

Norris SH, Watt I. The prognosis of neck injuries resulting from rear-end vehicle collisions. *Journal of Bone and Joint Surgery*. 1983;65-B(5):608–611.

Oppenheimer A. Pathology, clinical manifestations and treatment of lesions of the intervertebral disks. *New England Journal of Medicine*. 1944;230(4):95–105.

Pallis C, Jones AM, Spillane JD. Cervical spondylosis. *Brain*. 1954;77:274–289.

*Pearce JMS. Whiplash injury: a reappraisal. *Journal of Neurology, Neurosurgery, and Psychiatry*. 1989;52:1329–1331.

Pearce JMS. Polemics of chronic whiplash injury. *Neurology*. 1994;44:1993–1997.

Pettersson K, Kärrholm J, Toolanen G, Hildingsson C. Decreased width of the spinal canal in patients with chronic symptoms after whiplash injury. *Spine*. 1995;20(15):1664–1667.

Raney AA, Raney RB. Headache: a common symptom of cervical disk lesions. *Archives of Neurology and Psychiatry*. 1948;59:603–621.

Rechtman AM, Borden AGB, Gershon-Cohen J. The lordotic curve of the cervical spine. *Clinical Orthopedics*. 1961;20:208–215.

Redmond AD. Prognostic factors in soft tissue injuries of the cervical spine [letter]. *Injury*. 1992;23(1):71.

Redmond AD, Prescott MV, Phair IC. Whiplash and surgically treated cervical disc disease [letter]. *Injury*. 1994;25(6):409.

Robinson DD, Cassar-Pullicino VN. Acute neck sprain after road traffic accident: a long-term clinical and radiological review. *Injury*. 1993;24(2):79–82.

Russell R. See Miller H. Discussion on cervical spondylosis. *Proceedings of the Royal Society of Medicine*. 1955;49:197–208.

Van der Donk J, Schouten JSAG, Passichier J, et al. The associations of neck pain with radiological abnormalities of the cervical spine and personality traits in a general population. *Journal of Rheumatology*. 1991;18:1884–1889.

Watkinson AF. Prognostic factors in soft tissue injuries of the cervical spine [letter]. *British Medical Journal*. 1990;301:983.

*Watkinson A, Gargan MF, Bannister GC. Prognostic factors in soft tissue injuries of the cervical spine. *Injury*. 1991;22(4):307–309.

*Watkinson A, Gargan MF, Bannister GC. Authors' reply [letter]. *Injury*. 1992;23(1):71.

WHIPLASH AND DISCOGRAPHY

*Holt EP Jr. Fallacy of cervical discography. *Journal of the American Medical Association*. 1966;188(9):799–801.

*Holt EP Jr. Further reflections on cervical discography. *Journal of the American Medical Association*. 1975;231(6):613–614.

Sneider SE, Winslow OP Jr, Pryor TH. Cervical diskography: is it relevant? *Journal of the American Medical Association*. 1963;185(3):163–165.

Wickstrom J, LaRocca H. Head and neck injuries from acceleration-deceleration forces. In: Ruge D, Wiltse LL, eds. *Spinal Disorders*. Philadelphia: Lea and Febiger; 1977:349–356.

WHIPLASH AND MYELOGRAPHY

*Hitselberger WE, Witten RM. Abnormal myelograms in asymptomatic patients. *Journal of Neurosurgery*. 1968;28:204–206.

Odom GL, Finney W, Woodhall B. Cervical disk lesions. *Journal of the American Medical Association*. 1958;166(1):23–28.

Wickstrom J, LaRocca H. Head and neck injuries from acceleration-deceleration forces. In: Ruge D, Wiltse LL, eds. *Spinal Disorders*. Philadelphia: Lea and Febiger; 1977:349–356.

WHIPLASH AND BONE SCANS

*Barton D, Allen M, Finlay D, Belton I. Evaluation of whiplash injuries by technetium 99^m isotope scanning. *Archives of Emergency Medicine*. 1993;10:197–202.

*Hildingsson C, Hietala SO, Toolanen G. Scintigraphic findings in acute whiplash injury of the cervical spine. *Injury.* 1989;20:265–266.

WHIPLASH AND MAGNETIC RESONANCE IMAGING

Boden SD, McCowin PR, Davis DO, et al. Abnormal magnetic-resonance scans of the lumbar spine in asymptomatic subjects. *Journal of Bone and Joint Surgery.* 1990; 72-A(8):1178–1184.

*Borchgrevink G, Smevik O, Haave I, Lereim I, Haraldseth O. MRI of cerebrum and cervical column within two days after "whiplash" neck sprain injury. In: *Proceedings of the Society of Magnetic Resonance Third Scientific Meeting and Exhibition, 1995, August 19–25, Nice, France.* 1995:243.

Borchgrevink GE, Smevik O, Nordby A, et al. MR imaging and radiography of patients with cervical hyperextension-flexion injuries after car accidents. *Acta Radiologica.* 1995;36:425–428.

Davis SJ, Teresi LM, Bradley GB Jr, Ziemba MA, Bloze AE. Cervical spine hyperextension injuries: MR findings. *Radiology.* 1991;180:245–251.

Fagerlund M, Björnebrink J, Pettersson K, Hildingsson C. MRI in acute phase of whiplash injury. *European Radiology.* 1995;5:297–301.

Gundry CR, Fritts HM. Magnetic resonance imaging of the musculoskeletal system. Part 8. The spine, section 2. *Clinical Orthopaedics and Related Research.* 1997;343: 260–271.

Harris JH, Yeakley JW. Hyperextension-dislocation of the cervical spine. Ligament injuries demonstrated by magnetic resonance imaging. *Journal of Bone and Joint Surgery.* 1992;74(4)-B:567–570.

Jensen MC, Brant-Zawadzki MN, Obuchowski N, et al. Magnetic resonance imaging of the lumbar spine in people without back pain. *New England Journal of Medicine.* 1994;331:69–73.

Jónsson H Jr, Cesarini K, Sahlstedt B, Rauschning W. Findings and outcome in whiplash-type neck distortions. *Spine.* 1994;19(24):2733–2743.

*Karlsborg M, Smed A, Jespersen H, et al. A prospective study of 39 patients with whiplash injury. *Acta Neurologica Scandinavica.* 1997;95:65–72.

*Maimaris C. Neck sprains after car accidents [letter]. *British Medical Journal.* 1989;299:123.

Parrish RW, Kingsley DPE, Kendall BE, Moseley WJ. MRI evaluation of whiplash injuries. *Neuroradiology.* 1991;33(suppl):161–163.

*Pearce JMS. Subtle cerebral lessons in "chronic whiplash syndrome"? *Journal of Neurology, Neurosurgery, and Psychiatry.* 1993;56(12):1328–1329.

*Pettersson K, Hildingsson C, Toolanen G, Fagerlund M, Björnebrink J. MRI and neurology in acute whiplash trauma. No correlation in prospective examination of 39 cases. *Acta Orthopedica Scandinavica.* 1994;65(5):525–528.

*Pettersson K, Hildingsson C, Toolanen G, Fagerlund M, Björnebrink J. Disc pathology after whiplash injury. A prospective magnetic resonance imaging clinical investigation. *Spine.* 1997;22:283–288.

*Ronnen HR, de Korte PJ, Brink PRG, et al. Acute whiplash injury: is there a role for MR imaging? A prospective study of 100 patients. *Radiology*. 1996;201:93–96.

*Teresi LM, Lufkin RB, Reicher MA, et al. Asymptomatic degenerative disk disease and spondylosis of the cervical spine: MR imaging. *Radiology*. 1987;164:83–88.

Van Goethem JWM, Biltjes IGGM, van den Hauwe L, Parizel PM, De Schepper AMA. Whiplash injuries: is there a role for imaging? *European Journal of Radiology*. 1996;22:30–37.

Voyvodic F, Dolinis J, Moore VM, et al. MRI of car occupants with whiplash injury. *Neuroradiology*. 1997;39:35–40.

Wood KB, Garvey TA, Gundry C, Heithoff KB. Magnetic resonance imaging of the thoracic spine. *Journal of Bone and Joint Surgery [American]*. 1995;77-A(11):1631–1638.

WHIPLASH AND COMPUTED TOMOGRAPHY

Antinnes JA, Dvorak J, Hayek J, Panjabi MM, Grob D. The value of functional computed tomography in the evaluation of soft-tissue injury in the upper cervical spine. *European Spine Journal*. 1994;3:98–101.

WHIPLASH AND THERMOGRAPHY

*Awerbuch MS. Thermography—its current diagnostic status in musculoskeletal medicine. *Medical Journal of Australia*. 1991;154:441–444.

*Awerbuch MS. Thermography—wither the niche? *Medical Journal of Australia*. 1991;154:444–447.

WHIPLASH EXPERIMENTS—ANIMAL

Boismare F, Boquet J, Moore N, Chretien P, Saligaut C, Daoust M. Hemodynamic, behavioural and biochemical disturbances induced by an experimental cranio-cervical injury (whiplash) in rats. *Journal of the Autonomic Nervous System*. 1985;13:137–147.

Domer FR, King Liu Y, Chandran KB, Krieger KW. Effect of hyperextension-hyperflexion (whiplash) on the function of the blood-brain barrier of rhesus monkeys. *Experimental Neurology*. 1979;63:304–310.

Dunsker SB. Hyperextension and hyperflexion injuries of the cervical spine. In: SB Dunsker, ed. *Seminars in Neurological Surgery: Cervical Spondylosis*. New York: Raven Press; 1981:135–143.

Ewing CL. Injury criteria and human tolerance for the neck. In: Saczalski K, ed. *Aircraft Crashworthiness*. Charlottesville, VA: University Press of Virginia; 1975:141–151.

Gennarelli TA, Segawa H, Wald U, et al. Physiological response to angular acceleration of the head. In: Grossman RG, Gildenberg PL, eds. *Head Injury: Basic and Clinical Aspects*. New York: Raven Press; 1982:128–140.

Gosch HH, Gooding E, Schneider RC. An experimental study of cervical spine and cord injuries. *Journal of Trauma.* 1972;12(2):570–576.

Liu YK, Chandran KB, Heath RG, Unterharnscheidts F. Subcortical EEG changes in rhesus monkeys following experimental hyperextension-hyperflexion (whiplash). *Spine.* 1984;9(4):329–338.

Liu YK, Wickstrom JK, Saltzberg B, et al. Subcortical EEG changes in rhesus monkeys following experimental whiplash. *26th Annual Conference on Engineering in Medicine and Biology.* 1973;15:404.

*MacNab I. Acceleration injuries of the cervical spine. *Journal of Bone and Joint Surgery.* 1964;46-A(8):1797–1799.

MacNab I. Whiplash. *Modern Medicine of Canada.* 1966;21:43–55.

MacNab I. Whiplash injuries of the neck. *Manitoba Medical Review.* 1966;46:172–174.

*MacNab I. Acceleration extension injuries of the cervical spine. *Advocates' Quarterly.* 1979–1981;2:77–93.

Ommaya AK. Trauma to the nervous system. *Annals of the Royal College of Surgeons of England.* 1966;39:317–347.

Ommaya AK, Faas F, Yarnell P. Whiplash injury and brain damage. *Journal of the American Medical Association.* 1968;204(4):285–289.

Saltzberg B, Burton WD Jr, Burch NR, et al. Evoked potential studies of the effects of impact acceleration on the motor nervous system. *Aviation, Space, and Environmental Medicine.* 1983;54(12):1100–1110.

Sances A Jr, Myklebust J, Cusick JF, et al. Experimental studies of brain and neck injuries. In: *Proceedings of the Twenty Fifth Stapp Car Crash Conference.* Paper #811032. Warrendale, PA: Society of Automotive Engineers; 1981:149–194.

Sances A Jr, Myklebust J, Kostreva D, et al. Pathophysiology of cervical injuries. In: *Proceedings of the Twenty Sixth Stapp Car Crash Conference.* Paper #821153. Warrendale, PA: Society of Automotive Engineers; 1982:41–70.

Svensson MY, Aldman B, Hansson HA, et al. Pressure effects in the spinal canal during whiplash extension motion: a possible cause of injury to the cervical spinal ganglia. In: *Proceedings of the International IRCOBI Conference on the Biomechanics of Impacts, Eindhoven, Netherlands.* SAE Paper 1993-13-0013. 1993:189–200.

Unterharnscheidt F. Traumatic alterations in the rhesus monkey undergoing -Gx impact acceleration. *Neurotraumatology.* 1983;6:151–167.

Weiss MS, Berger MD. Neurophysiological effects of -X impact acceleration. *Aviation, Space, and Environmental Medicine.* 1983;54(11):1023–1027.

Wickstrom J, LaRocca H. Head and neck injuries from acceleration-deceleration forces. In: Ruge D, Wiltse LL, eds. *Spinal Disorders.* Philadelphia: Lea and Febiger; 1977:349–356.

Wickstrom J, Martinez JL, Johnston D, Tappen NC. In: *Proceedings of the Seventh Stapp Car Crash Conference.* Warrendale, PA: Society of Automotive Engineers; 1963:284–301.

Wickstrom JK, Martinez JL, Rodriguez R Jr, Haines DM. Hyperextension and hyperflexion injuries to the head and neck of primates. In: Gurdjian ES, Thomas LM, eds. *Neckache and Backache.* Springfield, IL: Charles C Thomas; 1970:108–117.

Wickstrom J, Rodriguez RP, Martinez JL. Experimental production of acceleration injuries of the head and neck. In: *Accident Pathology*. Washington, DC: US Government Printing Office; 1968:185–189.

WHIPLASH EXPERIMENTS—DUMMY

Hu AS, Bean SP, Zimmerman RM. Response of belted dummy and cadaver to rear impact. In: *Proceedings of the Twenty First Stapp Car Crash Conference*. Paper #770929. Warrendale, PA: Society of Automotive Engineers; 1977:589–625.

Kallieris D, Schmidt G. Neck response and injury assessment using cadavers and the USSID for far-side lateral impacts of rear seat occupants with inboard-anchored shoulder belts. In: *Proceedings of the Thirty Fourth Stapp Car Crash Conference*. Paper #902313. Warrendale, PA: Society of Automotive Engineers; 1990:93–99.

Muzzy WH, Lustick L. Comparison of kinematic parameters between hybrid II head and neck system with human volunteers for -Gx acceleration profiles. In: *Proceedings of the Twentieth Stapp Car Crash Conference*. Paper #760801. Warrendale, PA: Society of Automotive Engineers; 1976:45–74.

Navin FDP, Macnabb MJ, Romilly DP, Thomson RW. An investigation into vehicle and occupant response subjected to low-speed rear impacts. In: *Proceedings of the Multidisciplinary Road Safety Conference VI*. 1989:159–169.

Purviance CC. The whiplash injury. *California Medicine*. 1957;86(2):99–103.

Severy DM, Mathewson JH, Bechtol CO. Controlled automobile rear-end collisions, an investigation of related engineering and medical phenomena. *Canadian Services Medical Journal*. 1955;11:727–759.

Thomson RW, Romilly DP, Navin FPD, et al. Energy attenuation within the vehicle during low speed collisions. In: *Report to Transport Canada*. August 1989.

WHIPLASH EXPERIMENTS—HUMAN CADAVER

Abel MS, Wagner RF. Moderately severe whiplash injuries of the cervical vertebrae and their radiologic diagnosis. *American Medical Association Scientific Exhibits*. 1957: 287–295.

Bendjellal F, Tarriere C, Gillet D, et al. Head and neck responses under high G-level lateral deceleration. In: *Proceedings of the Thirty First Stapp Car Crash Conference*. Paper #872196. Warrendale, PA: Society of Automotive Engineers; 1987: 29–47.

Cholewicki J, Panjabi MM, Nibu K, et al. Head kinematics during in vitro whiplash simulation. *Accident Analysis and Prevention*. 1998;30(4):469–479.

Clemens HJ, Burow K. Experimental investigation on injury mechanisms of cervical spine at frontal and rear-front vehicle impacts. In: *Proceedings of the Sixteenth Stapp Car Crash Conference*. Paper #720960. Warrendale, PA: Society of Automotive Engineers; 1972:76–102.

*Cromack JR, Ziperman HH. Three-point belt induced injuries: a comparison between laboratory surrogates and real world accident victims. In: *Proceedings of the Nineteenth*

Stapp Car Crash Conference. Paper #751141. Warrendale, PA: Society of Automotive Engineers; 1975:1–24.

*Gadd CW, Culver CC. A study of responses and tolerances of the neck. In: *Proceedings of the Fifteenth Stapp Car Crash Conference.* Warrendale, PA: Society of Automotive Engineers; 1971:256.

Hu AS, Bean SP, Zimmerman RM. Response of belted dummy and cadaver to rear impact. In: *Proceedings of the Twenty First Stapp Car Crash Conference.* Paper #770929. Warrendale, PA: Society of Automotive Engineers; 1977:589–625.

Kallieris D, Mattern R, Miltner E, Schmidt G, Stein K. Considerations for a neck injury criterion. In: *Proceedings of the Thirty Fifth Stapp Car Crash Conference.* Paper #912916. Warrendale, PA: Society of Automotive Engineers; 1991:401–417.

Kallieris D, Schmidt G. Neck response and injury assessment using cadavers and the US-SID for far-side lateral impacts of rear seat occupants with inboard-anchored shoulder belts. In: *Proceedings of the Thirty Fourth Stapp Car Crash Conference.* Paper #902313. Warrendale, PA: Society of Automotive Engineers; 1990:93–99.

Lange W. Mechanical and physiological response of the human cervical vertebral column to severe impacts applied to the torso. In: *Symposium on Biodynamic Models and Their Applications, Wright-Patterson Air Force Base, Ohio.* 1970:141.

McElhaney JH, Myers BS. Biomechanical aspects of cervical trauma. In: Nahum AM, Melvin JW, eds. *Accidental Injury. Biomechanics and Prevention.* New York: Springer-Verlag; 1993:323–325.

McElhaney JH, Paver JG, McCrackin JH, Maxwell GM. Cervical spine compression responses. In: *Proceedings of the Twenty Seventh Stapp Car Crash Conference.* Warrendale, PA: Society of Automotive Engineers; 1983:163–178.

Panjabi MM, Cholewicki J, Nibu K, Babat LB, Dvorak J. Simulation of whiplash trauma using whole cervical spine specimens. *Spine.* 1998;23:17–24.

Panjabi MM, Cholewicki J, Nibu K, Grauer J, Vahldiek M. Capsular ligament stretches during in vitro whiplash simulations. *Journal of Spinal Disorders.* 1998;11(3):227–232.

*Patrick LM. Studies of hyperextension and hyperflexion injury in volunteers and human cadavers. In: Gurdjian ES, Thomas LM, eds. *Neckache and Backache.* Springfield, IL: Charles C Thomas; 1970:92–119.

Sances A Jr, Myklebust J, Kostreva D, et al. Pathophysiology of cervical injuries. In: *Proceedings of the Twenty Sixth Stapp Car Crash Conference.* Paper #821153. Warrendale, PA: Society of Automotive Engineers; 1982:41–70.

Shea M, Wittenberg RH, Edwards WT, White AA, Hayes WC. In vitro hyperextension injuries in the human cadaveric cervical spine. *Journal of Orthopaedic Research.* 1992; 10(6):911–916.

Tarriere C, Sapin C. Biokinetic study of the head to thorax linkage. In: *Proceedings of the Thirteenth Stapp Car Crash Conference.* Warrendale, PA: Society of Automotive Engineers; 1969:365.

Wismans J, Philippens M, van Oorschot E, Kallieris D, Mattern R. Comparison of human volunteer and cadaver head-neck response in frontal flexion. In: *Proceedings of the Thirty First Stapp Car Crash Conference.* Paper #872194. Warrendale, PA: Society of Automotive Engineers; 1987:1–11.

WHIPLASH EXPERIMENTS—VOLUNTEER

*Allen ME, Weir-Jones I, Motiuk DR, et al. Acceleration perturbations of daily living. A comparison to 'whiplash.' *Spine.* 1994;19(11):1285–1290.

*Bailey MN. Assessment of impact severity in minor motor vehicle collisions. *Journal of Musculoskeletal Pain.* 1996;4(4):21–38.

Bailey MN, Wong BC, Lawrence JM. Data and methods for estimating the severity of minor impacts. In: *Proceedings of the Thirty Ninth Stapp Car Crash Conference.* Paper #950352. Warrendale, PA: Society of Automotive Engineers; 1995:139–173.

Brault JR, Wheeler JB, Siegmund GP, Brault EJ. Clinical response of human subjects to rear-end automobile collisions. *Archives of Physical Medicine and Rehabilitation.* 1998;79:72–80.

*Castro WHM, Schilgen M, Meyer S, et al. Do "whiplash injuries" occur in low-speed rear impacts? *European Spine Journal.* 1997;6:366–375.

Clarke TD, Gragg CD, Sprouffske JF, et al. Human head linear and angular accelerations during impact. In: *Proceedings of the Fifteenth Stapp Car Crash Conference.* Paper #710857. Warrendale, PA: Society of Automotive Engineers; 1971:269–286.

*DuBois RA, McNally BF, DiGregorio JS, Phillips GJ. Low velocity car-to-bus test impacts. *Accident Reconstruction Journal.* 1996;8(5):44–51.

Ewing CL. Injury criteria and human tolerance for the neck. In: Saczalski K, ed. *Aircraft Crashworthiness.* Charlottesville, VA: University Press of Virginia; 1975:141–151.

Ewing CL, Thomas DJ. Torque versus angular displacement response of human head to -Gx impact acceleration. In: *Proceedings of the Seventeenth Stapp Car Crash Conference.* Paper #730976. Warrendale, PA: Society of Automotive Engineers; 1973:309–342.

Ewing CL, Thomas DJ, Beeler GW Jr, et al. Dynamic response of the head and neck of the living human to -Gx impact acceleration. In: *Proceedings of the Twelfth Stapp Car Crash Conference.* Paper #680792. Warrendale, PA: Society of Automotive Engineers; 1968:424–439.

Ewing CL, Thomas DJ, Beeler GW Jr, et al. Living human dynamic response to -Gx impact acceleration. In: *Proceedings of the Thirteenth Stapp Car Crash Conference.* Paper #690817. Warrendale, PA: Society of Automotive Engineers; 1969:400–415.

Ewing CL, Thomas DJ, Lustick L, et al. The effect of the initial position of the head and neck on the dynamic response of the human head and neck to -Gx impact acceleration. In: *Proceedings of the Nineteenth Stapp Car Crash Conference.* Paper #751157. Warrendale, PA: Society of Automotive Engineers; 1975:487–512.

Ewing CL, Thomas DJ, Lustick L, et al. The effect of duration, rate of onset, and peak sled acceleration on the dynamic response of the human head and neck. In: *Proceedings of the Twentieth Stapp Car Crash Conference.* Paper #760800. Warrendale, PA: Society of Automotive Engineers; 1976:3–41.

Ewing CL, Thomas DJ, Majewski PL, et al. Measurement of head, T1, and pelvic response to -Gx impact acceleration. In: *Proceedings of the Twenty First Stapp Car Crash Conference.* Paper #770927. Warrendale, PA: Society of Automotive Engineers; 1977:509–545.

*Gough JP. Human occupant dynamics in low-speed rear end collisions: an engineering perspective. *Journal of Musculoskeletal Pain.* 1996;4(4):11–19.

*Grunsten RC, Gilbert NS, Mawn SV. The mechanical effects of impact acceleration on the unconstrained human head and neck complex. *Contemporary Orthopaedics.* 1989;18(2):199–202.

Gurdjian ES, Thomas LM, eds. *Neckache and Backache.* Springfield, IL: Charles C Thomas; 1970.

Hodgson VR. Tolerance of the neck to impact acceleration. In: *Technical Report 9.* Contract no. N00014-75-C-1015. Washington, DC: Department of Navy; 1979.

Howard RP, Bowles AP, Guzman HM, Krenrich SW. Head, neck, and mandible dynamics generated by "whiplash." *Accident Prevention and Analysis.* 1998;30(4):525–534.

*Kahane CJ. *Evaluation of Head Restraints: Federal Motor Vehicle Safety Standard 202.* Washington, DC: National Highway Traffic Safety Administration, Office of Program Evaluation; 1982.

Kassirer MR, Manon N. Head banger's whiplash. *Clinical Journal of Pain.* 1993;9: 138–141.

Kwan O. Rear-end auto collisions. Another view [letter]. *Archives of Physical Medicine and Rehabilitation.* 1998;79:721–722.

Matsushita T, Sato TB, Hirabayashi K, et al. X-ray study of the human neck motion due to head inertia loading. In: *Proceedings of the Thirty Eighth Stapp Car Crash Conference.* Paper #942208. Warrendale, PA: Society of Automotive Engineers; 1994:55–64.

*McConnell WE, Howard RP, Guzman HM, et al. Analysis of human test subject kinematic responses to low velocity rear end impacts. In: *Proceedings of the Thirty Seventh Stapp Car Crash Conference.* Paper #930889. Warrendale, PA: Society of Automotive Engineers; 1993:21–30.

*McConnell WE, Howard RP, Van Poppel J, et al. Human head and neck kinematics after low velocity rear-end impacts—understanding "whiplash." In: *Proceedings of the Thirty Ninth Stapp Car Crash Conference.* Paper #952724. Warrendale, PA: Society of Automotive Engineers; 1995:215–238.

Melville PH. "Research" in car crashes [letter]. *Canadian Medical Association Journal.* 1963;89:275.

*Mertz HJ, Patrick LM. Investigation of the kinematics of whiplash. In: *Proceedings of the Eleventh Stapp Car Crash Conference.* Paper #670919. Warrendale, PA: Society of Automotive Engineers; 1967:175–206.

*Mertz HJ, Patrick LM. Strength and response of the human neck. In: *Proceedings of the Fifteenth Stapp Car Crash Conference.* Paper #710855. Warrendale, PA: Society of Automotive Engineers; 1971:2903–2928.

Meyer S, Weber M, Castro W, Schilgen M, Peuker C. The minimal collision velocity for whiplash. In: Gunzburg R, Szpalski M, eds. *Whiplash Injuries. Current Concepts in Prevention, Diagnosis, and Treatment of the Cervical Whiplash Syndrome.* Philadelphia: Lippincott-Raven; 1998:95–115.

Muzzy WH, Lustick L. Comparison of kinematic parameters between hybrid II head and neck system with human volunteers for -Gx acceleration profiles. In: *Proceedings of the

Twentieth Stapp Car Crash Conference. Paper #760801. Warrendale, PA: Society of Automotive Engineers; 1976:45–74.

Nielsen GP, Gough JP, Little DM, West DH, Baker VT. Human subject responses to repeated low speed impacts using utility vehicles. In: *Proceedings of the Forty First Stapp Car Crash Conference.* Paper #970394. Warrendale, PA: Society of Automotive Engineers; 1997:189–212.

Nygren A, Gustafsson H, Tingvall C. Effects of different types of headrests in rear-end collisions. In: *Proceedings of the Tenth International Conference on Experimental Safety Vehicles, July 1–4, 1985, Oxford.* U.S. Department of Transportation, National Highway Traffic Safety Administration; 1985:85–90.

Ono K, Kanno M. Influences of the physical parameters on the risk to neck injuries in low impact speed rear-end collisions. In: *Proceedings of the International IRCOBI Conference on the Biomechanics of Impacts, September 8–10, 1993, Eindhoven, Netherlands.* 1993:201–212.

Ono K, Kanno M. Influences of the physical parameters on the risk to neck injuries in low impact speed rear-end collisions. *Accident Analysis and Prevention.* 1996;28(4): 493–499.

*Patrick LM. Studies of hyperextension and hyperflexion injury in volunteers and human cadavers. In: Gurdjian ES, Thomas LM, eds. *Neckache and Backache.* Springfield, IL: Charles C Thomas; 1970:92–119.

*Patrick LM, Chou CC. Response of the human neck in flexion, extension and lateral flexion. In: *Vehicle Research Institute Report VRI 7.3.* New York: Society of Automotive Engineers; 1976.

Rosenbluth W, Hicks L. Evaluating low-speed rear-end impact severity and resultant occupant stress parameters. *Journal of Forensics Sciences.* 1994;39(6):1393–1424.

Sances A Jr, Weber RC, Larson SJ, et al. Bioengineering analysis of head and spine injuries. *Critical Reviews in Biomedical Engineering.* 1981;5:79–118.

Scott MW, McConnell WE, Guzman HM, et al. Comparison of human and ATD head kinematics during low-speed rearend impacts. In: *Proceedings of the Thirty Seventh Stapp Car Crash Conference.* Paper #930094. Warrendale, PA: Society of Automotive Engineers; 1993:1–8.

Severy DM, Mathewson JH, Bechtol CO. Controlled automobile rear-end collisions, an investigation of related engineering and medical phenomena. *Canadian Services Medical Journal.* 1955;11:727–759.

Siegmund GP, Bailey MN, King DJ. Characteristics of specific automobile bumpers in low-velocity impacts. In: *Proceedings of the Thirty Eighth Stapp Car Crash Conference.* Paper #940916. Warrendale, PA: Society of Automotive Engineers; 1994.

Siegmund GP, King DJ, Montgomery DT. Using barrier impact data to determine speed change in aligned, low-speed vehicle-to-vehicle collisions. In: *Proceedings of the Fortieth Stapp Car Crash Conference.* Paper #960887. Warrendale, PA: Society of Automotive Engineers; 1996:147–168.

Siegmund GP, Williamson PB. Speed change (ΔV) of amusement park bumper cars. In: *Proceedings of the Canadian Multidisciplinary Road Safety Conference VIII, June 14–16, 1993, Saskatoon, Saskatchewan.* 1993:299–308.

Snyder RG, Snow CC, Young JW, Price GT, Hanson P. Experimental comparison of trauma in lateral (+Gy), rearward facing (+Gx), and forward facing (-Gx) body orientations when restrained by lap belt only. *Aerospace Medicine.* 1967;38:889–894.

Szabo TJ, Welcher J. Dynamics of low speed crash tests with energy absorbing bumpers. In: *Proceedings of the Thirty Sixth Stapp Car Crash Conference.* Paper #921573. Warrendale, PA: Society of Automotive Engineers; 1992:1367–1375.

Szabo TJ, Welcher JB, Anderson RD. Human occupant kinematic response to low speed rear-end impacts. In: *Proceedings of the Thirty Eighth Stapp Car Crash Conference.* Paper #940532. Warrendale, PA: Society of Automotive Engineers; 1994:23–35.

Thomas DJ, Ewing CL, Majewski PL, et al. Clinical medical effects of head and neck response during biodynamic stress experiments. In: *Advisory Group for Aerospace Research and Development (AGARD) Conference #267, Lisbon, Portugal.* 1979:15. 1–15.15.

Wagner R. A 30 mph front/rear crash with human test persons. In: *Proceedings of the Twenty Third Stapp Car Crash Conference.* Paper #791030. Warrendale, PA: Society of Automotive Engineers; 1979:827–840.

Weißner R, Enßlen A. The head-rest—a necessary safety-feature for modern cars. In: *Proceedings of the International IRCOBI/AAAM Conference on the Biomechanics of Impacts, June 24–26, 1985, Göteborg, Sweden, Bron, France.* 269–276.

*West DH, Gough JP, Harper GTK. Low speed rear-end collision testing using human subjects. *Accident Reconstruction Journal.* 1993;5(3):22–26.

Wismans J, Philippens M, van Oorschot E, Kallieris D, Mattern R. Comparison of human volunteer and cadaver head-neck response in frontal flexion. In: *Proceedings of the Thirty First Stapp Car Crash Conference.* Paper #872194. Warrendale, PA: Society of Automotive Engineers; 1987:1–11.

WHIPLASH EXPERIMENTS—LOW-VELOCITY COLLISIONS

*Bailey M. Assessment of impact severity in minor motor vehicle collisions. *Journal of Musculoskeletal Pain.* 1996;4(4):21–38.

Bailey MN, Wong BC, Lawrence JM. Data and methods for estimating the severity of minor impacts. In: *Proceedings of the Thirty Ninth Stapp Car Crash Conference.* Paper #950352. Warrendale, PA: Society of Automotive Engineers; 1995:139–173.

Brault JR, Wheeler JB, Siegmund GP, Brault EJ. Authors' reply [letter]. *Archives of Physical Medicine and Rehabilitation.* 1998;79:722–723.

Brault JR, Wheeler JB, Siegmund GP, Brault EJ. Authors' reply [letter]. *Archives of Physical Medicine and Rehabilitation.* 1998;79:1024.

Brault JR, Wheeler JB, Siegmund GP, Brault EJ. Clinical response of human subjects to rear-end automobile collisions. *Archives of Physical Medicine and Rehabilitation.* 1998;79:72–80.

*Castro WHM, Schilgen M, Meyer S, et al. Do "whiplash injuries" occur in low-speed rear impacts? *European Spine Journal.* 1997;6:366–375.

*DuBois RA, McNally BF, DiGregorio JS, Phillips GJ. Low velocity car-to-bus test impacts. *Accident Reconstruction Journal.* 1996;8(5):44–51.

Ferrari R. Rear-end auto collisions [letter]. *Archives of Physical Medicine and Rehabilitation.* 1998;79:721.

Garmoe W. Rear-end collisions [letter]. *Archives of Physical Medicine and Rehabilitation.* 1998;79:1024.

Geigl BC, Steffan H, Leinzinger P, Roll, Mühlbauer M, Bauer G. The movement of head and cervical spine during rear-end impact. In: *Proceedings of the International IRCOBI Conference on the Biomechanics of Impact, 1994, Lyon, France.* 127–137.

*Gough JP. Human occupant dynamics in low-speed rear end collisions: an engineering perspective. *Journal of Musculoskeletal Pain.* 1996;4(4):11–19.

Howard RP, Bowles AP, Guzman HM, Krenrich SW. Head, neck, and mandible dynamics generated by "whiplash." *Accident Prevention and Analysis.* 1998;30(4):525–534.

Matsushita T, Sato TB, Hirabayashi K, et al. X-ray study of the human neck motion due to head inertia loading. In: *Proceedings of the Thirty Eighth Stapp Car Crash Conference.* Paper #942208. Warrendale, PA: Society of Automotive Engineers; 1994:55–64.

*McConnell WE, Howard RP, Guzman HM, et al. Analysis of human test subject kinematic responses to low velocity rear end impacts. In: *Proceedings of the Thirty Seventh Stapp Car Crash Conference.* Paper #930889. Warrendale, PA: Society of Automotive Engineers; 1993:21–30.

*McConnell WE, Howard RP, Van Poppel J, et al. Human head and neck kinematics after low velocity rear-end impacts—understanding "whiplash." In: *Proceedings of the Thirty Ninth Stapp Car Crash Conference.* Paper #952724. Warrendale, PA: Society of Automotive Engineers; 1995:215–238.

Meyer S, Weber M, Castro W, Schilgen M, Peuker C. The minimal collision velocity for whiplash. In: Gunzburg R, Szpalski M, eds. *Whiplash Injuries. Current Concepts in Prevention, Diagnosis, and Treatment of the Cervical Whiplash Syndrome.* Philadelphia: Lippincott-Raven; 1998:95–115.

*Nielsen GP, Gough JP, Little DM, West DH, Baker VT. Human subject responses to repeated low speed impacts using utility vehicles. In: *Proceedings of the Forty First Stapp Car Crash Conference.* Paper #970394. Warrendale, PA: Society of Automotive Engineers; 1997:189–212.

Ono K, Kanno M. Influences of the physical parameters on the risk to neck injuries in low impact speed rear-end collisions. In: *Proceedings of the International IRCOBI Conference on the Biomechanics of Impacts, September 8–10, 1993, Eindhoven, Netherlands.* 1993:201–212.

Ono K, Kanno M. Influences of the physical parameters on the risk to neck injuries in low impact speed rear-end collisions. *Accident Analysis and Prevention.* 1996;28(4):493–499.

Rosenbluth W, Hicks L. Evaluating low-speed rear-end impact severity and resultant occupant stress parameters. *Journal of Forensics Sciences.* 1994;39(6):1393–1424.

Scott MW, McConnell WE, Guzman HM, et al. Comparison of human and ATD head kinematics during low-speed rearend impacts. In: *Proceedings of the Thirty Seventh Stapp Car Crash Conference.* Paper #930094. Warrendale, PA: Society of Automotive Engineers; 1993:1–8.

Siegmund GP, Bailey MN, King DJ. Characteristics of specific automobile bumpers in low-velocity impacts. In: *Proceedings of the Thirty Eighth Stapp Car Crash Conference.* Paper #940916. Warrendale, PA: Society of Automotive Engineers; 1994.

Siegmund GP, King DJ, Montgomery DT. Using barrier impact data to determine speed change in aligned, low-speed vehicle-to-vehicle collisions. In: *Proceedings of the Fortieth Stapp Car Crash Conference.* Paper #960887. Warrendale, PA: Society of Automotive Engineers; 1996:147–168.

Siegmund GP, Williamson PB. Speed change (ΔV) of amusement park bumper cars. In: *Proceedings of the Canadian Multidisciplinary Road Safety Conference VIII, June 14–16, 1993, Saskatoon, Saskatchewan.* 1993;299–308.

Szabo TJ, Welcher J. Dynamics of low speed crash tests with energy absorbing bumpers. In: *Proceedings on the Thirty Sixth Stapp Car Crash Conference.* Paper #921573. Warrendale, PA: Society of Automotive Engineers; 1992:1367–1375.

Szabo TJ, Welcher JB, Anderson RD. Human occupant kinematic response to low speed rear-end impacts. In: *Proceedings of the Thirty Eighth Stapp Car Crash Conference.* Paper #940532. Warrendale, PA: Society of Automotive Engineers; 1994:23–35.

*West DH, Gough JP, Harper GTK. Low speed rear-end collision testing using human subjects. *Accident Reconstruction Journal.* 1993;5(3):22–26.

WHIPLASH AND THE TEMPOROMANDIBULAR JOINT

Brady C, Taylor D, O'Brien M. Whiplash and temporomandibular joint dysfunction. *Journal of the Irish Dental Association.* 1993;39(3):69–72.

Braun BL, DiGiovanna A, Schiffman E, Bonnema J, Friction J. A cross-sectional study of temporomandibular joint dysfunction in post-cervical trauma patients. *Journal of Craniomandibular Disorders: Facial and Oral Pain.* 1992;6:24–31.

Brooke RI, Lapointe HJ. Temporomandibular joint disorders following whiplash. *Spine: State of the Art Reviews.* 1993;7(3):443–454.

Brooke RI, Stenn PG. Postinjury myofascial pain dysfunction syndrome. Its etiology and prognosis. *Oral Surgery, Oral Medicine, and Oral Pathology.* 1978;45(6):846–850.

Brooks SL, Westesson P, Eriksson L, Hansson LG, Barsotti JB. Prevalence of osseous changes in the temporomandibular joint of asymptomatic persons without internal derangement. *Oral Surgery, Oral Medicine, and Oral Pathology.* 1992;73:122–126.

Burgess J. Symptom characteristics in TMD patients reporting blunt trauma and/or whiplash injury. *Journal of Craniomandibular Disorders: Facial and Oral Pain.* 1991;5(4):251–257.

Burgess J, Dworkin SF. Litigation and post-traumatic TMD: how patients report treatment outcome. *Journal of the American Dental Association.* 1993;124:105–110.

Burgess JA, Kolbinson DA, Lee PT, Epstein JB. Motor vehicle accidents and TMDs: assessing the relationship. *Journal of the American Dental Association.* 1996;127:1767–1772.

Bush FM, Dolwick MF. *The Temporomandibular Joint and Related Orofacial Disorders.* Philadelphia: JB Lippincott; 1995:72–73.

Cannistraci AJ, Fritz G. Dental applications of biofeedback. In: Basmajian JV, ed. *Biofeedback Principles and Practice for Clinicians.* 3rd ed. Baltimore: Williams & Wilkins; 1989:297–310.

Christensen LV, McKay DC. Reflex jaw motions and jaw stiffness pertaining to whiplash injury of the neck. *Journal of Craniomandibular Practice.* 1997;15(3):242–260.

De Boever JA, Keersmaekers K. Trauma in patients with temporomandibular disorders: frequency and treatment outcome. *Journal of Oral Rehabilitation.* 1996;23:91–96.

De Wijer A, Steenks MH, Bosman F, Helders PJM, Faber J. Symptoms of the stomatognathic system in temporomandibular and cervical spine disorders. *Journal of Oral Rehabilitation.* 1996;23:733–741.

De Wijer A, Steenks MH, De Leeuw JRJ, Bosman F, Helders PJM. Symptoms of the cervical spine in temporomandibular and cervical spine disorders. *Journal of Oral Rehabilitation.* 1996;23:742–750.

Drace JE, Enzmann DR. Defining the normal temporomandibular joint: closed-, partially open-, and open-mouth MR imaging of asymptomatic subjects. *Radiology.* 1990;177:67–71.

Epstein JB. Temporomandibular disorders, facial pain and headache following motor vehicle accidents. *Canadian Dental Association Journal.* 1992;58(6):488–495.

Ernest EA III. The orthopedic influence of the TMJ apparatus in whiplash: report of a case. *General Dentistry.* 1979;27(2):62–64.

Ferrari R, Leonard M. Whiplash and temporomandibular disorders. *Journal of the American Dental Association.* 1998;129:1739–1745.

Ferrari R, Schrader H, Obelieniene D. Prevalence of temporomandibular disorders associated with whiplash injury in Lithuania. *Oral Surgery, Oral Medicine, Oral Pathology.* 1999. In press.

*Frankel VH. Temporomandibular joint pain syndrome following deceleration injury to the cervical spine. *Bulletin of the Hospital for Joint Diseases.* 1965;26:47–51.

Garcia R Jr, Arrington JA. The relationship between cervical whiplash and temporomandibular joint injuries: an MRI study. *Journal of Craniomandibular Practice.* 1996;14(3):233–239.

Gillies GT. Temporomandibular joint injury potential imposed by the low-velocity extension-flexion maneuver [letter]. *Journal of Oral and Maxillofacial Surgery.* 1995;53:263.

Goldberg HL. Trauma and the improbable anterior displacement. *Journal of Craniomandibular Disorders: Facial and Oral Pain.* 1990;4(2):131–134.

Goldberg MB, Mock D, Ichise M, et al. Neuropsychologic deficits and clinical features of posttraumatic temporomandibular disorders. *Journal of Orofacial Pain.* 1996;10:126–140.

Greco CM, Rudy TE, Turk DC, Herlich A, Zaki HH. Traumatic onset of temporomandibular disorders: positive effects of a standardized conservative treatment program. *Clinical Journal of Pain.* 1997;13:337–347.

Gross A, Gale EN. A prevalence study of the clinical signs associated with mandibular dysfunction. *Journal of the American Dental Association.* 1983;107:932–936.

Grzesiak RC. Psychologic considerations in temporomandibular dysfunction. *Dental Clinics of North America.* 1991;35(1):209–226.

*Heise AP, Laskin DM, Gervin AS. Incidence of temporomandibular joint symptoms following whiplash injury. *Journal of Oral and Maxillofacial Surgery.* 1992;50:825–828.

*Howard RP, Benedict JV, Raddin JH, Smith HL. Assessing neck extension-flexion as a basis for temporomandibular joint dysfunction. *Journal of Oral and Maxillofacial Surgery.* 1991;49:1210–1213.

*Howard RP, Bowles AP, Guzman HM, Krenrich SW. Head, neck, and mandible dynamics generated by "whiplash." *Accident Prevention and Analysis.* 1998;30(4):525–534.

*Howard RP, Hatsell CP, Guzman HM. Temporomandibular joint injury potential imposed by the low-velocity extension-flexion maneuver. *Journal of Oral and Maxillofacial Surgery.* 1995;53:256–262.

Katzberg RW, Westesson PL, Tallents R, Drake CM. Orthodontics and temporomandibular joint derangement. *American Journal of Orthodontics and Dentofacial Orthopedics.* 1996;109:515–520.

Kircos LT, Ortendahl DA, Mark AS, Arakawa M. Magnetic resonance imaging of the TMJ disc in asymptomatic volunteers. *Journal of Oral and Maxillofacial Surgery.* 1987;45:852–854.

Kirk WS Jr. Whiplash as a basis for TMJ dysfunction. *Journal of Oral and Maxillofacial Surgery.* 1992;50:427–428.

*Kolbinson DA, Epstein JB, Burgess JA. Temporomandibular disorders, headaches, and neck pain following motor vehicle accidents and the effects of litigation: review of the literature. *Journal of Orofacial Pain.* 1996;10:101–125.

Kolbinson DA, Epstein JB, Burgess JA, Senthilselvan A. Temporomandibular disorders, headaches, and neck pain following motor vehicle accidents: a pilot investigation of persistence and litigation effects. *Journal of Prosthetic Dentistry.* 1997;77(1):46–53.

Kolbinson DA, Epstein JB, Senthilselvan A, Burgess JA. A comparison of TMD patients with or without prior motor vehicle accident involvement: initial signs, symptoms, and diagnostic characteristics. *Journal of Orofacial Pain.* 1997;11:206–214.

Kolbinson DA, Epstein JB, Senthilselvan A, Burgess JA. A comparison of TMD patients with or without prior motor vehicle accident involvement: treatment and outcomes. *Journal of Orofacial Pain.* 1997;11:337–345.

Kolbinson DA, Epstein JB, Senthilselvan A, Burgess JA. Effect of impact and injury characteristics on post-motor vehicle accident temporomandibular disorders. *Oral Surgery, Oral Medicine, Oral Pathology, Oral Radiology, and Endodontics.* 1998;85(6):665–673.

Krogstad BS, Jokstad A, Dahl BL, Soboleva U. Somatic complaints, psychologic distress, and treatment outcome in two groups of TMD patients, one previously subjected to whiplash injury. *Journal of Orofacial Pain.* 1998;12:136–144.

Kronn E. The incidence of TMJ dysfunction in patients who have suffered a cervical whiplash injury following a traffic accident. *Journal of Orofacial Pain.* 1993;7: 209–213.

Kupperman A. Whiplash and disc derangement [letter]. *Journal of Oral and Maxillofacial Surgery.* 1988;46(6):519.

*Lader E. Cervical trauma as a factor in the development of TMJ dysfunction and facial pain. *Journal of Craniomandibular Disorders.* 1983;1(2):85–90.

Levandoski RR. Mandibular whiplash. Part 1, An extension-flexion injury of the temporomandibular joints. *Functional Orthodontist.* January/February 1993:26–29, 32–33.

Levandoski RR. Mandibular whiplash. Part 2, An extension-flexion injury of the temporomandibular joints. *Functional Orthodontist.* January/February 1993:45–51.

Loughner BA, Gremillion HA, Larkin LH, Mahan PE, Watson RE. Muscle attachment to the lateral aspect of the articular disk of human temporomandibular joint. *Oral Surgery, Oral Medicine, Oral Pathology.* 1996;82:139–144.

*Lupton DE. Psychological aspects of temporomandibular joint dysfunction. *Journal of the American Dental Association.* 1969;79:131–136.

Mannheimer J, Attanasio R, Cinotti WR, Pertes R. Cervical strain and mandibular whiplash: Effects upon the craniomandibular apparatus. *Clinical Preventative Dentistry.* 1989;11(1):29–32.

McKay DC, Christensen LV. Whiplash injuries of the temporomandibular joint in motor vehicle accidents: speculations and facts. *Journal of Oral Rehabilitation.* 1998;25(10): 731–746.

*Moody PM, Kemper JT, Okesen JP, et al. Recent life changes and myofascial pain syndrome. *Journal of Prosthetic Dentistry.* 1982;48(3):328–330.

*Muir CB, Goss AN. The radiologic morphology of asymptomatic temporomandibular joints. *Oral Surgery, Oral Medicine, Oral Pathology.* 1990;70:349–354.

Muir CB, Goss AN. The radiologic morphology of painful temporomandibular joints. *Oral Surgery, Oral Medicine, Oral Pathology.* 1990;70:355–359.

Olin M. Components of complex TM disorders. *Journal of Craniomandibular Disorders: Facial and Oral Pain.* 1990;4(3):193–196.

O'Shaughnessy T. Latent dysfunctions resulting from unresolved trauma-induced head and neck injuries. *Functional Orthodontist.* 1995;12(2):22–24, 26, 28.

O'Shaughnessy T. Tomographic proof of trauma-induced injury to the TMJoint and other sites in the body. *Functional Orthodontist.* 1995;12(5):20–28.

O'Shaughnessy T, Levenson R. Basic treatment precepts ensuant to a whiplash episode. *Functional Orthodontist.* 1994;11(5):16–20.

Pressman BD, Shellock FG, Schames J, Schames M. MR imaging of temporomandibular joint abnormalities associated with cervical hyperextension/hyperflexion (whiplash) injuries. *Journal of Magnetic Resonance Imaging.* 1992;2:569–574.

Probert TCS, Wiesenfeld D, Reade PC. Temporomandibular pain dysfunction disorder resulting from road traffic accidents—an Australian study. *International Journal of Oral and Maxillofacial Surgery.* 1994;23:338–341.

Romanelli GG, Mock D, Tenebaum HC. Characteristics and response to treatment of post-traumatic temporomandibular disorder: a retrospective study. *Clinical Journal of Pain.* 1992;8:6–17.

*Roydhouse RH. Temporomandibular and mandibular dysfunction—a review. *Canadian Medical Association Journal*. 1971;105:1320–1324.

*Roydhouse RH. Whiplash and temporomandibular dysfunction [letter]. *Lancet*. June 1973:1394–1395.

Ruf S, Cecere F, Kupfer J, Pancherz H. Stress-induced changes in the functional electromyographic activity of the masticatory muscles. *Acta Odontologica Scandinavica*. 1997;55:44–48.

Schneider K, Zernicke RF, Clark G. Modeling of jaw-head-neck dynamics during whiplash. *Journal of Dental Research*. 1989;68(9):1360–1365.

Seligman DA, Pullinger AG. A multiple stepwise logistic regression analysis of trauma history and 16 other history and dental cofactors in females with temporomandibular disorders. *Journal of Orofacial Pain*. 1996;10:351–361.

*Small EW. An investigation into the psychogenic bases of the temporomandibular joint myofascial pain dysfunction syndrome. *Advances in Pain Research and Therapy*. 1976;1:889–894.

Steigerwald DP. Acceleration-deceleration injury as a precipitating cause of temporomandibular joint dysfunction. *American Chiropractic Association*. 1989;26(11):61–64.

Steigerwald DP, Croft AC, Edwards JM, et al. *Whiplash and Temporomandibular Disorders. An Interdisciplinary Approach to Case Management*. San Diego: Keiser Publishing; 1992.

Steigerwald DP, Verne SV, Young D. A retrospective evaluation of the impact of temporomandibular joint arthroscopy on the symptoms of headache, neck pain, shoulder pain, dizziness, and tinnitus. *Journal of Craniomandibular Practice*. 1996;14(1):46–54.

Stenger J. Whiplash. *Basal Facts*. 1977;2:128–134.

Tallents RH, Katzberg RW, Murphy W, Proskin H. Magnetic resonance imaging findings in asymptomatic volunteers and symptomatic patients with temporomandibular disorders. *Journal of Prosthetic Dentistry*. 1996;75:529–533.

*Tasaki MM, Westesson PL, Isberg AM, Ren YF, Tallents RH. Classification and prevalence of temporomandibular joint disk displacement in patients and symptom-free volunteers. *American Journal of Orthodontics and Dentofacial Orthopedics*. 1996;109: 249–262.

*Weinberg S, LaPointe H. Cervical extension-flexion injury (whiplash) and internal derangement of the temporomandibular joint. *Journal of Oral and Maxillofacial Surgery*. 1987;45:653–656.

Weinberg S, LaPointe H. The authors reply [letter]. *Journal of Oral and Maxillofacial Surgery*. 1988;46(6):519.

*Westesson PL. Reliability and validity of imaging diagnosis of temporomandibular joint disorder. *Advances in Dental Research*. 1993;7(2):137–151.

*Westesson P, Eriksson L, Kurita K. Reliability of a negative clinical temporomandibular joint examination: prevalence of disk displacement in asymptomatic temporomandibular joints. *Oral Surgery, Oral Medicine, Oral Pathology*. 1989;68:551–554.

*Westesson P, Eriksson L, Kurita K. Temporomandibular joint: variation of normal arthrographic anatomy. *Oral Surgery, Oral Medicine, Oral Pathology*. 1990;69:514–519.

WHIPLASH AND BALANCE/DIZZINESS/VERTIGO

Alund M, Ledin T, Ödkvist L, Larson SE. Dynamic posturography among patients with common neck disorders. *Journal of Vestibular Research*. 1993;3:383–389.

Alvord LS. Psychological status of patients undergoing electronystagmography. *Journal of the American Academy of Audiology*. 1991;2(4):261–265.

Chester JB Jr. Whiplash, postural control, and the inner ear. *Spine*. 1991;16(7):716–720.

Claussen CF, Claussen E. Neurootological contributions to the diagnostic follow-up after whiplash injuries. *Acta Otolaryngolica*. 1995;520(suppl):53–56.

Conte A, Caruso G, Mora R. Static and dynamic posturography in prevalent laterally directed whiplash injuries. *European Archives of Otorhinolaryngology*. 1997;254: 186–192.

Ferrari R, Russell AS. Development of persistent neurological symptoms in patients with simple neck sprain. *Arthritis Care & Research*. 1999;12(1):70 –76.

Fischer AJEM, Huygen PLM, Folgering HT, Verhagen WIM, Theunissen EJJM. Hyperactive VOR and hyperventilation after whiplash injury. *Acta Otolaryngolica (Stockholm)*. 1995;520(suppl):49–52.

*Fischer AJEM, Verhagen WIM, Huygen PLM. Whiplash injury. A clinical review with emphasis on neuro-otological aspects. *Clinical Otolaryngology*. 1997;22:192–201.

Fitzgerald DC. Head trauma: hearing loss and dizziness. *Journal of Trauma*. 1996;40(3): 488–496.

Fitz-Ritzon D. Assessment of cervicogenic vertigo. *Journal of Manipulative and Physiological Therapeutics*. 1991;14(3):193–198.

Furman JM, Jacob RG. Psychiatric dizziness. *Neurology*. 1997;48:1161–1166.

Gimse R, Bjørgen IA, Straume A. Driving skills after whiplash. *Scandinavian Journal of Psychology*. 1997;38:165–170.

Gimse R, Bjørgen IA, Tjell C, Tyssedal JS, Bø K. Reduced cognitive functions in a group of whiplash patients with demonstrated disturbances in the posture control system. *Journal of Clinical and Experimental Neuropsychology*. 1997;19(6):838–849.

*Gimse R, Tjell C, BjØrgen IA, Saunte C. Disturbed eye movements after whiplash due to injuries to the posture control system. *Journal of Clinical and Experimental Neuropsychology*. 1996;18(2):178–186.

Hayes PE, Kristoff CA. Adverse reactions to five new antidepressants. *Clinical Pharmacy*. 1986;5(6):471–480.

Heikkilä H, Aström PG. Cervicocephalic kinesthetic sensibility in patients with whiplash injury. *Scandinavian Journal of Rehabilitation Medicine*. 1996;28:133–138.

Heikkilä H, Wenngren BI. Cervicocephalic kinesthetic sensibility, active range of cervical motion, and oculomotor function in patients with whiplash injury. *Archives of Physical Medicine and Rehabilitation*. 1998;79:1089–1094.

Hinoki M. Vertigo due to whiplash injury: a neurotological approach. *Acta Otolaryngologica (Stockholm)*. 1985;419(suppl):9–29.

Karlberg M, Johansson R, Magnusson M, Fransson PA. Dizziness of suspected cervical origin distinguished by posturographic assessment of human postural dynamics. *Journal of Vestibular Research*. 1996;6(1):37–47.

*Karlberg M, Magnusson M, Malmström EM, Melander A, Moritz U. Postural and symptomatic improvement after physiotherapy in patients with dizziness of suspected cervical origin. *Archives of Physical Medicine and Rehabilitation*. 1996;77:874–882.

Katsarkas A. Postural stability following mild head or whiplash injuries [letter]. *American Journal of Otology*. 1996;17:172–175.

Lader MH. Tolerability and safety: essentials in antidepressant pharmacotherapy. *Journal of Clinical Psychiatry*. 1996;57(suppl 2):39–44.

Landy PJB. Neurological sequelae of minor head and neck injuries. *Injury*. 1998;29(3): 199–206.

Loudon JK, Ruhl M, Field E. Ability to reproduce head position after whiplash injury. *Spine*. 1997;22(8):865–868.

Oosterveld WJ, Kortschot HW, Kingma GG, de Jong HAA, Saatci MR. Electronystagmographic findings following cervical whiplash injuries. *Acta Otolaryngologica (Stockholm)*. 1991;111:201–205.

Preskorn SH. Comparison of the tolerability of bupropion, fluoxetine, imipramine, nefazodone, paroxetine, setaline, and venlafaxine. *Journal of Clinical Psychiatry*. 1995;56(suppl 6):12–21.

Rubin AM. Author's reply [letter]. *American Journal of Otology*. 1996;17(1):173–174.

Rubin AM, Woolley SM, Dailey VM, Goebel JA. Postural stability following mild head or whiplash injuries. *American Journal of Otology*. 1995;16(2):216–221.

Rubin W. Whiplash with vestibular involvement. *Archives of Otolaryngology*. 1973; 97:85–87.

Serra LL, Gallicchio B, Serra FP, Grillo G, Ferrari M. BAEP and EMG changes from whiplash injuries. *Acta Neurologica*. 1994;16(5–6):262–270.

Simpson RB, Nedzelski JM, Barber HO, Thomas MR. Psychiatric diagnoses in patients with psychogenic dizziness or severe tinnitus. *Journal of Otolaryngology*. 1988;17(6): 325–330.

Toglia JU, Rosenberg PE, Ronis ML. Posttraumatic dizziness. *Archives of Otolaryngology*. 1970;92:485–492.

Verhagen AP, Lanser K, de Bie RA, de Vet HC. Whiplash: assessing the validity of diagnostic tests in a cervical sensory disturbance. *Journal of Manipulative and Physiological Therapeutics*. 1996;19(8):508–512.

Wennmo K, Wennmo C. Drug-related dizziness. *Acta Oto-Laryngologica*. 1988; 455(suppl):11–13.

Whitworth AB, Fleischhacker WW. Adverse effects of antipsychotic drugs. *International Clinical Psychopharmacology*. 1995;9(suppl 5):21–27.

Yagi M. Clinical studies on so-called whiplash injury, especially on the significance of retrograde brachial arteriography. *Nagoya Journal of Medical Science*. 1967;30:177–192.

WHIPLASH AND THE EAR

Aplin DY, Kane JM. Personality and experimentally simulated hearing loss. *British Journal of Audiology*. 1985;19:251–255.

Braaf MM, Rosner S. Meniere-like syndrome following whiplash injury of the neck. *Journal of Trauma*. 1962;2:494–501.

Brien JA. Ototoxicity associated with salicylates. A brief review. *Drug Safety*. 1993;9(2): 143–148.

Chrisman OD, Gervais RF. Otologic manifestations of the cervical syndrome. *Clinical Orthopedics*. 1962;24:34–39.

Erlandsson IS, Rubinstein B, Axelsson A, Carlsson SG. Psychological dimensions in patients with disabling tinnitus and craniomandibular disorders. *British Journal of Audiology*. 1991;25:15–24.

Ferrari R, Russell AS. Development of persistent neurological symptoms in patients with simple neck sprain. *Arthritis Care & Research*. 1999;12(1):70–76.

Jung TT, Rhee CK, Lee CS, Park YS, Choi DC. Ototoxicity of salicylate, nonsteroidal antiinflammatory drugs, and quinine. *Otolaryngologic Clinics of North America*. 1993; 26(5):791–810.

Pang LQ. The otological aspects of whiplash injuries. *Laryngoscope*. 1971;81:1381–1387.

*Saunders GH, Haggard MP. The clinical assessment of obscure auditory dysfunction—1. Auditory and psychological factors. *Ear and Hearing*. 1989;10(3):200–208.

*Saunders GH, Haggard MP. The influence of personality-related factors upon consultation for two different "marginal" organic pathologies with and without reports of auditory symptomatology. *Ear and Hearing*. 1993;14(4):242–248.

Seligman H, Podoshin L, Ben-David J, Fradis M, Goldsher M. Drug-induced tinnitus and other hearing disorders. *Drug Safety*. 1996;14(3):198–212.

Shapiro SL. The otologic symptoms of cervical whiplash injuries. *Eye, Ear, Nose and Throat Monthly*. 1972;51:32–37.

Simpson RB, Nedzelski JM, Barber HO, Thomas MR. Psychiatric diagnoses in patients with psychogenic dizziness or severe tinnitus. *Journal of Otolaryngology*. 1988;17(6): 325–330.

Tjell C, Rosenhall U. Smooth pursuit neck torsion test: a specific test for cervical dizziness. *American Journal of Otology*. 1998;19:76–81.

Toglia JU, Rosenberg PE, Ronis ML. Vestibular and audiological aspects of whiplash injury and head trauma. *Journal of Forensic Sciences*. 1969;14(2):219–226.

WHIPLASH AND THE EYE

Burke JP, Orton HP, West J, et al. Whiplash and its effects on the visual system. *Graefe's Archive for Clinical and Experimental Ophthalmology*. 1992;230:335–339.

Ferrari R, Russell AS. Development of persistent neurological symptoms in patients with simple neck sprain. *Arthritis Care & Research*. 1999;12(1):70–76.

Fite JD. Neuro-ophthalmologic syndromes in automobile accidents. *Southern Medical Journal*. 1970;63:567–570.

Freed S, Fishman Hellerstein L. Visual electrodiagnostic findings in mild traumatic brain injury. *Brain Injury*. 1997;11(1):25–36.

Gibson WJ. The eye and whiplash injuries. *Journal of the Florida State Medical Association.* 1968;55(10):917–918.

*Gimse R, Tjell C, BjØrgen IA, Saunte C. Disturbed eye movements after whiplash due to injuries to the posture control system. *Journal of Clinical and Experimental Neuropsychology.* 1996;18(2):178–186.

Girling WNM. Whiplash injuries. Their effect on accommodation convergence, peripheral and central field together with treatment used. *Concilium Ophthalmologicum (Belgium).* 1958;18(2):1550–1557.

Haslett RS, Duvall-Young J, McGalliard JN. Traumatic retinal angiopathy and seat belts: pathogenesis of whiplash injury. *Eye.* 1994;8:615–617.

Heikkliä H, Wenngren BI. Cervicocephalic kinesthetic sensibility, active range of cervical motion, and oculomotor function in patients with whiplash injury. *Archives of Physical Medicine and Rehabilitation.* 1998;79:1089–1094.

Hildingsson C, Wenngren BI, Bring G, Toolanen G. Oculomotor problems after cervical spine injury. *Acta Orthopaedica Scandinavica.* 1989;60(5):513–516.

*Hildingsson C, Wenngren BI, Toolanen G. Eye motility dysfunction after soft-tissue injury of the cervical spine. *Acta Orthopedica Scandinavica.* 1993;64(2):129–132.

Horwich H. The ocular effects of whiplash injury. *Transactions of the Section of Ophthalmology of the American Medical Association.* 1956:86–90.

Horwich H, Kasner D. The effect of whiplash injuries on ocular functions. *Southern Medical Journal.* 1962;55:69–71.

Jaanus SD. Ocular side effects of selected systemic drugs. *Optometry Clinics.* 1992;2(4): 73–96.

Kelley JS, Hoover RE, George T. Whiplash maculopathy. *Archives of Ophthalmology.* 1978;96:834–835.

Lader MH. Tolerability and safety: essentials in antidepressant pharmacotherapy. *Journal of Clinical Psychiatry.* 1996;57(suppl 2):39–44.

Middleton JM. Ophthalmic aspects of whiplash injuries. *International Record of Medicine.* 1956;169(1):19–20.

Preskorn SH. Comparison of the tolerability of bupropion, fluoxetine, imipramine, nefazodone, paroxetine, setaline, and venlafaxine. *Journal of Clinical Psychiatry.* 1995; 56(suppl 6):12–21.

Roca PD. Ocular manifestations of whiplash injuries. In: *Proceedings of the Fifteenth Annual Meeting of the American Association of Automotive Medicine.* 1971:308–319.

Roca PD. Ocular manifestations of whiplash injuries. *Annals of Ophthalmology.* January 1972:63–73.

Slamovits TL, Glaser JS. The pupils and accommodation. In: Duane TE, Jaeger EA, eds. *Clinical Ophthalmology.* Vol 2. London: JB Lippincott Company; 1988:11, 12, 16.

Tjell C, Rosenhall U. Smooth pursuit neck torsion test: a specific test for cervical dizziness. *American Journal of Otology.* 1998;19:76–81.

Wiesinger H, Guerry D. The ocular aspects of whiplash injury. *Virginia Medical Monthly.* 1962;89:165–168.

WHIPLASH AND BRAIN INJURY

Alexander MP. In the pursuit of proof of brain damage after whiplash injury. *Neurology.* 1998;51:336–340.

Bicik I, Radanov BP, Schäfer N, et al. PET with [18]fluorodeoxyglucose and hexamethyl-propylene amine oxime SPECT in late whiplash syndrome. *Neurology.* 1998;51: 345–350.

Bohnen N, Jolles J, Verhey FRJ. Persistent neuropsychological deficits in cervical whiplash patients without direct headstrike. *Acta Neurologica Belgium.* 1993;93:23–31.

Borchgrevink G, Smevik O, Haave I, Lereim I, Haraldseth O. MRI of cerebrum and cervical column within two days after "whiplash" neck sprain injury. In: *Proceedings of the Society of Magnetic Resonance Third Scientific Meeting and Exhibition, 1995, August 19–25, Nice, France.* 1995:243.

Di Stefano GD, Radanov BP. Course of attention and memory after common whiplash: a two-year prospective study with age, education and gender pair-matched patients. *Acta Neurologica Scandinavica.* 1995;91:346–352.

Ferrari R, Russell AS. Development of persistent neurological symptoms in patients with simple neck sprain. *Arthritis Care & Research.* 1999;12(1):70 –76.

Karlsborg M, Smed A, Jespersen H, et al. A prospective study of 39 patients with whiplash injury. *Acta Neurologica Scandinavica.* 1997;95:65–72.

Landy PJB. Neurological sequelae of minor head and neck injuries. *Injury.* 1998; 29(3):199–206.

*Lees-Haley PR, Brown RS. Neuropsychological complaint base rates of 170 personal injury claimants. *Archives of Clinical Neuropsychology.* 1993;8:203–209.

Olsnes BT. Neurobehavioural findings in whiplash patients with long-lasting symptoms. *Acta Neurologica Scandinavica.* 1989;80:584–588.

Otte A, Ettlin TM, Nitzsche EU, et al. PET and SPECT in whiplash syndrome: a new approach to a forgotten brain? *Journal of Neurology, Neurosurgery, and Psychiatry.* 1997;63:368–372.

*Otte A, Mueller-Brand J, Fierz L. Brain SPECT findings in late whiplash syndrome. *Lancet.* 1995;345:1513–1514.

*Otte A, Mueller-Brand J, Nitzsche EU, Wachter K, Ettlin TM. Functional brain imaging in 200 patients after whiplash injury. *Journal of Nuclear Medicine.* 1997;38(6):1102.

*Radanov BP, Dvorak J. Impaired cognitive functioning after whiplash injury of the cervical spine. *Spine.* 1996;21(3):392–397.

*Ronnen HR, de Korte PJ, Brink PRG, et al. Acute whiplash injury: is there a role for MR imaging? A prospective study of 100 patients. *Radiology.* 1996;201:93–96.

Rothbart P, Gale GD. Neuropsychological deficits after whiplash [letter]. *Archives of Physical Medicine and Rehabilitation.* 1998;79:469.

Schwartz DP, Barth JT, Dane JR, et al. Cognitive deficits in chronic pain patients with and without history of head/neck injury: development of a brief screening battery. *Clinical Journal of Pain.* 1987;3:94–101.

*Taylor AE. An author replies [letter]. *Archives of Physical Medicine and Rehabilitation.* 1998;79:469.

*Taylor AE, Cox CA, Mailis A. Persistent neuropsychological deficits following whiplash: evidence for chronic mild traumatic brain injury? *Archives of Physical Medicine and Rehabilitation*. 1996;77:529–535.

WHIPLASH AND HEADACHE

Balla JI, Iansek R. Headaches arising from disorders of the cervical spine. In: Hopkins A, ed. *Headache. Problems in Diagnosis and Management*. London: WB Saunders; 1988:243–267.

Ferrari R. Whiplash-associated headache [letter]. *Cephalalgia*. 1998;18(8):585–586.

Friedman AP, Ransohoff J. Post-traumatic headache. *Trauma*. 1964;5:33–61.

Haas DC. Chronic posttraumatic headache. In: Olesen J, Tfelt-Hansen P, Welch KMA, eds. *The Headaches*. New York: Raven Press; 1993:629–637.

Haas DC. Chronic post-traumatic headaches classified and compared with natural headaches. *Cephalalgia*. 1996;16:486–493.

Iansek R, Heywood J, Karnaghan J, Balla JI. Cervical spondylosis and headaches. *Clinical and Experimental Neurology*. 1986;23:175–178.

Kwan O, Friel J. The dilemma of whiplash [letter]. *Cephalalgia*. 1998;18(8):586–587.

Landy PJB. Neurological sequelae of minor head and neck injuries. *Injury*. 1998; 29(3):199–206.

Obelieniene D, Bovim G, Schrader H, et al. Headache after whiplash: a historical cohort study outside the medico-legal context. *Cephalalgia*. 1998;18(8):559–564.

Radanov BP, Sturzenegger M, Di Stefano GD, Schnidrig A, Aljinovic M. Factors influencing recovery from headache after common whiplash. *British Medical Journal*. 1993; 307:652–655.

Wallis BJ, Lord SM, Barnsley L, Bogduk N. The psychological profiles of patients with whiplash-associated disorder. *Cephalalgia*. 1998;18:101–105.

WHIPLASH AND THORACIC OUTLET SYNDROME

*Adams RD, Victor M. *Principles of Neurology*. 4th ed. New York: McGraw-Hill; 1989: 174.

*Caldwell JW, Crane CR, Krusen EM. Nerve conduction studies: an aid in the diagnosis of the thoracic outlet syndrome. *Southern Medical Journal*. 1971;64(2):210–212.

Capistrant TD. Thoracic outlet syndrome in whiplash injury. *Annals of Surgery*. 1977;185:175–178.

Capistrant TD. Thoracic outlet syndrome in cervical strain injury. *Minnesota Medicine*. 1986;69:13–17.

Cherington M. A conservative point of view of the thoracic outlet syndrome. *American Journal of Surgery*. 1989;158:394–395.

Cherington M, Cherington C. Thoracic outlet syndrome: reimbursement patterns and patient profiles. *Neurology*. 1992;42:943–945.

Cherington M, Happer I, Machanic B, Parry L. Surgery for thoracic outlet syndrome may be hazardous to your health. *Muscle and Nerve.* 1986;9:632–634.

*Cuetter AC, Bartoszek DM. The thoracic outlet syndrome: controversies, overdiagnosis, overtreatment, and recommendations for management. *Muscle and Nerve.* 1989;12: 410–419.

Ferrari R, Russell AS. Development of persistent neurological symptoms in patients with simple neck sprain. *Arthritis Care & Research.* 1999;12(1)70–76.

Hachinski V. The thoracic outlet syndrome. *Archives of Neurology.* 1990;47:330.

*Nelson DA. Thoracic outlet syndrome and dysfunction of the temporomandibular joint: proved pathology or pseudosyndromes? *Perspectives in Biology and Medicine.* 1990;33(4):567–576.

*Rowland LP. Thoracic outlet syndrome. In: Rowland LP, ed. *Merrit's Textbook of Neurology.* Philadelphia: Lea & Febiger; 1989:443.

Sanders RJ, Monsour JW, Gerber WF, Adams WR, Thompson N. Scalenectomy versus first rib resection for treatment of the thoracic outlet syndrome. *Surgery.* 1979;85(1):109–121.

Sethi KD, Swift TR. Arm and neck pain. In: *Neurology in Clinical Practice.* Vol I. Boston: Butterworth-Heinemann; 1991:398.

Smith T, Trojaborg W. Diagnosis of thoracic outlet syndrome. *Archives of Neurology.* 1987;44:1161–1163.

Wilbourn AJ. Thoracic outlet syndrome surgery causing severe brachial plexopathy. *Muscle and Nerve.* 1988;11:66–74.

Wilbourn AJ. The thoracic outlet syndrome is overdiagnosed. *Archives of Neurology.* 1990;47:328–330.

Woods WW. Personal experiences with surgical treatment of 250 cases of cervicobrachial neurovascular compression syndrome. *Journal of the International College of Surgeons.* 1965;44(3):273–283.

*Youmans JR. *Neurological Surgery.* Vol 4. 3rd ed. Philadelphia: WB Saunders; 1990.

WHIPLASH AND ELECTRONYSTAGMOGRAPHY OR ELECTROMYOGRAPHY

Compere WE Jr. Electronystagmographic findings in patients with "whiplash" injuries. *Laryngoscope.* 1968;78:1226–1233.

Dell'Osso LF, Daroff RB, Troost BT. Nystagmus and saccadic intrusions and oscillations. In: Duane TE, Jaeger EA, eds. *Clinical Ophthalmology.* Vol 2. London: JB Lippincott Company; 1988:13, 17.

Oosterveld WJ, Kortschot HW, Kingma GG, de Jong HAA, Saatci MR. Electronystagmographic findings following cervical whiplash injuries. *Acta Otolaryngologica (Stockholm).* 1991;111:201–205.

Reynolds GG, Pavot AP, Kenrick MM. Electromyographic evaluation of patients with posttraumatic cervical pain. *Archives of Physical Medicine and Rehabilitation.* 1968; 2:170–172.

Serra LL, Gallicchio B, Serra FP, Grillo G, Ferrari M. BAEP and EMG changes from whiplash injuries. *Acta Neurologica.* 1994;16(5–6):262–270.

WHIPLASH AND SPECT OR PET SCANS (BRAIN IMAGING)

Kischka U, Ettlin T, Plohmann A, Stahl H. SPECT findings in patients with whiplash injury of the neck. *Neurology.* 1994;44(suppl 2):763P.

Otte A, Ettlin T, Fierz L, Mueller-Brand J. Parieto-occipital hypoperfusion in late whiplash syndrome: first quantitative SPET study using technetium-99m bicisate (ECD). *European Journal of Nuclear Medicine.* 1996;23(1):72–74.

Otte A, Ettlin TM, Nitzsche EU, et al. PET and SPECT in whiplash syndrome: a new approach to a forgotten brain? *Journal of Neurology, Neurosurgery, and Psychiatry.* 1997;63:368–372.

*Otte A, Goetze M, Mueller-Brand J. Statistical parametric mapping in whiplash brain: is it only a contusion mechanism? *European Journal of Nuclear Medicine.* 1998;25: 306–312.

*Otte A, Mueller-Brand J, Fierz L. Brain SPECT findings in late whiplash syndrome. *Lancet.* 1995;345:1513–1514.

*Otte A, Mueller-Brand J, Nitzsche EU, Wachter K, Ettlin TM. Functional brain imaging in 200 patients after whiplash injury. *Journal of Nuclear Medicine.* 1997;38(6):1102.

WHIPLASH AND BRAINSTEM AUDITORY EVOKED POTENTIALS

Chappa KH, Gladstone KJ, Young RR. Brain stem auditory evoked responses. *Archives of Neurology.* 1979;36:81–87.

Noseworthy JH, Miller J, Murray TJ, Regan D. Auditory brainstem response in postconcussion syndrome. *Archives of Neurology.* 1981;38:275–278.

*Rowe MJ. Normal variability of the brain-stem auditory evoked response in young and old adult subjects. *Electroencephalography and Clinical Neurophysiology.* 1978;44: 459–470.

Serra LL, Gallicchio B, Serra FP, Grillo G, Ferrari M. BAEP and EMG changes from whiplash injuries. *Acta Neurologica.* 1994;16(5–6):262–270.

*Stockard JJ, Stockard JE, Sharbrough FW. Nonpathologic factors influencing brainstem auditory evoked potentials. *American Journal of EEG Technology.* 1978;18:177–209.

WHIPLASH AND ELECTROENCEPHALOGRAPHY (EEG)

Ewing CL, Thomas DJ, Beeler GW Jr, et al. Dynamic response of the head and neck of the living human to -Gx impact acceleration. In: *Proceedings of the Twelfth Stapp Car Crash Conference.* Paper #680792. Warrendale, PA: Society of Automotive Engineers; 1968:424–439.

Gibbs FA. Objective evidence of brain disorder in cases of whiplash injury. *Clinical Electroencephalography.* 1971;2(2):107–110.

*Jacome DE. EEG in whiplash: a reappraisal. *Clinical Electroencephalography.* 1987; 18(1):41–45.

*Jacome DE, Risko M. EEG features in post-traumatic syndrome. *Clinical Electroencephalography.* 1984;15(4):214–221.

Serra LL, Gallicchio B, Serra FP, Grillo G, Ferrari M. BAEP and EMG changes from whiplash injuries. *Acta Neurologica*. 1994;16(5–6):262–270.

*Shapiro SK, Torres F. Brain injury complicating whiplash injuries. *Minnesota Medicine*. July 1960:473–476.

*Torres F, Shapiro SK. Electroencephalograms in whiplash injury. *Archives of Neurology*. 1961;5:40–47.

WHIPLASH AND HEAD RESTRAINTS

Carlsson G, Nilsson S, Nilsson-Ehle A, et al. Neck injuries in rear end car collisions. Biomechanical considerations to improve head restraints. In: *Proceedings of the International IRCOBI/AAAM Conference on the Biomechanics of Injury, 1985, June 24–26, Göteborg, Sweden, Bron, France*. 1985:277–289.

*Grunsten RC, Gilbert NS, Mawn SV. The mechanical effects of impact acceleration on the unconstrained human head and neck complex. *Contemporary Orthopaedics*. 1989;18(2):199–202.

*Kahane CJ. *Evaluation of Head Restraints: Federal Motor Vehicle Safety Standard 202*. Washington, DC: National Highway Traffic Safety Administration, Office of Program Evaluation; 1982.

*Lövsund P, Nygren A, Salen B, Tingvall C. Neck injuries in rear end collisions among front and rear seat occupants. In: *Proceedings of the International IRCOBI Conference on the Biomechanics of Impacts, 1988, September 14–16, Bergisch, Gladbach, Germany, Bron, France*. 1988:319–325.

*McConnell WE, Howard RP, Guzman HM, et al. Analysis of human test subject kinematic responses to low velocity rear end impacts. In: *Proceedings of the Thirty Seventh Stapp Car Crash Conference*. Paper #930889. Warrendale, PA: Society of Automotive Engineers; 1993:21–30.

*Olney DB, Marsden AK. The effect of head restraints and seat belts on the incidence of neck injury in car accidents. *Injury*. 1986;17:365–367.

*O'Neill B, Haddon W Jr, Kelley AB, Sorenson WW. Automobile head restraints—frequency of neck injury claims in relation to the presence of head restraints. *American Journal of Public Health*. March 1972:399–406.

Schrader H, Obelieniene D, Bovim G, et al. Natural evolution of late whiplash syndrome outside the medicolegal context. *Lancet*. 1996;347:1207–1211.

Stewart JR. Statistical evaluation of the effectiveness of federal motor vehicle safety standard 202: head restraints. Contract No.: DOT HS-8-02014. Chapel Hill, NC: Highway Research Center, University of North Carolina; 1980.

*Thomas C, Faverjon G, Hartemann F, et al. Protection against rear-end accidents. In: *Proceedings of the International Research Council on the Biomechanics of Impacts (IRCOBI) Conference, Bron, France*. 1982:17–29.

Viano DC, Gargan MF. Headrest position during normal driving: implication to neck injury risk in rear crashes. *Accident Analysis and Prevention*. 1996;28(6):665–674.

*West DH, Gough JP, Harper GTK. Low speed rear-end collision testing using human subjects. *Accident Reconstruction Journal*. 1993;5(3):22–26.

WHIPLASH AND SEAT BELTS

Bourbeau R, Desjardins D, Maag U, Laberge-Nadeau C. *Neck Injuries amongst Front Seat Belted and Unbelted Car Occupants (Seat Belts and Neck Injuries)*. Publication #818. Centre de recherche sur les transports; 1992.

Bourbeau R, Desjardins D, Maag U, Laberge-Nadeau C. Neck injuries among belted and unbelted occupants of the front seat of cars. *Journal of Trauma*. 1993;35(5):794–799.

Caldwell IW. Seat belts and head rests. *British Medical Journal*. 1972;2:163.

Christian MS. Non-fatal injuries sustained by seatbelt wearers: a comparative study. *British Medical Journal*. 1976;2:1310–1311.

Deans GT, Magalliard JN, Kerr M, Rutherford WH. Neck sprain—a major cause of disability following car accidents. *Injury*. 1987;18:10–12.

De Fonseka CP. Neck injuries in seatbelt wearers [letter]. *British Medical Journal*. 1977;1:168.

Faverjon G, Henry C, Thomas C, Tarriere C. Head and neck injuries for belted front occupants in real frontal crashes: patterns and risks. In: *Proceedings of the International IRCOBI Conference on the Biomechanics of Impacts, September 14–16, 1988, Bergisch, Gladbach, Germany, Bron, France*. 301–317.

Gissane W. Seat belts and head rests [letter]. *British Medical Journal*. 1972;2:288.

Gissane W, Bull JP. A seat belt syndrome? [letter]. *British Medical Journal*. 1974;1:394.

Maag U, Desjardins D, Bourbeau R, Laberge-Nadeau C. Seat belts and neck injuries. In: *Proceedings of the International Research Council on the Biomechanics of Impacts (IRCOBI) Conference, 1990, Bron, France*. 1990:1–13.

Nygren A. Injuries to car occupants—some aspects of the interior safety of cars. *Acta Otolaryngologica*. 1984;395(suppl):1–164.

Otte D, Südkamp N, Appel H. Variations of injury patterns of seat-belt users. In: *Proceedings of the International Congress and Exposition. Restraint Technologies: Front Seat Occupant Protection SP-690, February 23–27, 1987, Detroit, Michigan*. SAE Paper 870226. Warrendale, PA: Society of Automotive Engineers; 1987:61–71.

Roydhouse RH. Torquing of neck and jaw due to belt restraint in whiplash-type accidents [letter]. *Lancet*. 1985;1:1341.

Schrader H, Obelieniene D, Bovim G, et al. Natural evolution of late whiplash syndrome outside the medicolegal context. *Lancet*. 1996;347:1207–1211.

Yoganandan N, Haffner M, Maiman DJ, et al. Epidemiology and injury biomechanics of motor vehicle related trauma to the human spine. In: *Proceedings of the Thirty Third Stapp Car Crash Conference*. Paper #892438. Warrendale: PA: Society of Automotive Engineers; 1989:223–242.

PSYCHOLOGY OF WHIPLASH—GENERAL

*Balla JI, Karnaghan J. Whiplash headache. In: Eadie MJ, Lander C, eds. *Proceedings of the Australian Association of Neurologists. Clinical and Experimental Neurology*. 1986:179–182.

Bankes MJK, Noble LM. The behavioural response to whiplash injury [letter]. *Journal of Bone and Joint Surgery [British]*. 1998;80-B:555–558.

Bannister GC, Main C. Authors' reply [letter]. *Journal of Bone and Joint Surgery [British]*. 1998;80-B:555.

Berry H. Psychological aspects of chronic neck pain following hyperextension-flexion strains of the neck. In: Morley TP, ed. *Current Controversies in Neurosurgery*. Philadelphia: WB Saunders; 1976:51–60.

Berry H. Psychological aspects of whiplash injury. In: Wilkins RH, Rengachary SS, eds. *Neurosurgery*. Vol 2. Philadelphia: McGraw-Hill; 1985:1716–1719.

BjØrgen IA. Late whiplash syndrome [letter]. *Lancet*. 1996;348:124.

Braaf MM, Rosner S. Symptomatology and treatment of injuries of the neck. *New York State Journal of Medicine*. 1955;55(1):237–242.

*Carette S. Whiplash injury and chronic neck pain. *New England Journal of Medicine*. 1994;330(15):1083–1084.

Champion GD. Whiplash in Australia: illness or injury? *Medical Journal of Australia*. 1992;157:574.

Cole ES. Psychiatric aspects of compensable injury. *Medical Journal of Australia*. 1970;1:93–100.

Culpan R, Taylor C. Psychiatric disorders following road traffic and industrial injuries. *Australian and New Zealand Journal of Psychiatry*. 1973;7:32–39.

de Mol BA, Heijer T. Late whiplash syndrome [letter]. *Lancet*. 1996;348:124–125.

Di Stefano GD, Radanov BP. Course of attention and memory after common whiplash: a two-year prospective study with age, education and gender pair-matched patients. *Acta Neurologica Scandinavica*. 1995;91:346–352.

Editorial. Neck injury and the mind. *Lancet*. 1991;338:728–729.

Ellertsson AB, Sigurjonsson K, Thorsteinsson T. Clinical and radiographic study of 100 cases of whiplash injury. *Proceedings of the 22nd Scandinavian Congress of Neurology*. *Acta Neurologica Scandinavica Supplementum*. 1978;67:269.

Ettlin TM, Kischka U, Reichmann S, et al. Cerebral symptoms after whiplash injury of the neck: a prospective clinical and neuropsychological study of whiplash injury. *Journal of Neurology, Neurosurgery, and Psychiatry*. 1992;55:943–948.

*Evans RW. Some observations on whiplash injuries. *Neurologic Clinics*. 1992;10(4): 975–997.

Ferrari R. Whiplash-associated headache [letter]. *Cephalalgia*. 1998;18(8):585–586.

Ferrari R, Russell AS. The whiplash syndrome—common sense revisited. *Journal of Rheumatology*. 1997;24(4):618–623.

Ferrari R, Russell AS. Authors' reply [letter]. *Journal of Rheumatology*. 1998;25(7): 1438–1440.

Field H. Post-traumatic syndrome [letter]. *Journal of the Royal Society of Medicine*. 1981;74:630.

Freeman MD, Croft AC. Late whiplash syndrome [letter]. *Lancet*. 1996;348:125.

Freeman MD, Croft AC, Rossignol AM. "Whiplash associated disorders: redefining whiplash and its management" by the Quebec Task Force. A critical evaluation. *Spine.* 1998;23:1043–1049.

Gargan MF, Bannister GC, Main C, Hollis S. The behavioural response to whiplash injury. *Journal of Bone and Joint Surgery [British].* 1997;79-B:523–526.

Gorman WF. The alleged whiplash "injury." *Arizona Medicine.* 1974;31(6):411–413.

Gorman WF. Whiplash—a neuropsychiatric injury. *Arizona Medicine.* 1974;31(6):414–416.

Gorman WF. "Whiplash": fictive or factual? *Bulletin of the American Academy of Psychiatry and Law.* 1979;7:245–248.

*Gregory GF, Crockett DJ. Chronic benign pain syndrome: A legal and psychological overview. *Advocate.* 1988;46(3):369–378.

*Gurdjian ES, Thomas LM, eds. *Neckache and Backache.* Springfield, IL: Charles C Thomas; 1970.

Harder S, Veilleux M, Suissa S. The effect of socio-demographic and crash-related factors on the prognosis of whiplash. *Journal of Clinical Epidemiology.* 1998;51(5):377–384.

Hodge JR. The whiplash injury. A discussion of this phenomenon as a psychosomatic illness. *Ohio State Medical Journal.* 1964;60:762–766.

Hodge JR. The whiplash neurosis. *Psychosomatics.* 1971;12:245–249.

Hoffman BF. The demographic and psychiatric characteristics of 110 personal injury litigants. *Bulletin of the American Academy of Psychiatry and Law.* 1991;19(3): 227–236.

*Karlsborg M, Smed A, Jespersen H, et al. A prospective study of 39 patients with whiplash injury. *Acta Neurologica Scandinavica.* 1997;95:65–72.

*Kelly R. The post-traumatic syndrome. *Pahlavi Medical Journal.* 1972;3:530–547.

*Kelly R. The post-traumatic syndrome: an iatrogenic disease. *Forensic Science.* 1975; 6:17–24.

Kessels RPC, Keyser A, Verhagen WIM, van Luitelaar ELJM. The whiplash syndrome: a psychophysiological and neuropsychological study towards attention. *Acta Neurologica Scandinavica.* 1998;97:188–193.

Kischka U, Ettlin T, Heim S, Schmid G. Cerebral symptoms following whiplash injury. *European Neurology.* 1991;31:136–140.

Krusen EM Jr, Krusen UL. Cervical syndrome especially the tension-neck problem: clinical study of 800 cases. *Archives of Physical Medicine and Rehabilitation.* 1955;36: 518–523.

*Kwan O, Friel J. The dilemma of whiplash [letter]. *Cephalalgia.* 1998;18(8):586–587.

*Kwan O, Friel J. Comment on Radanov et al [letter]. *Journal of Rheumatology.* 1999. In press.

Lee J, Giles K, Drummond PD. Psychological disturbances and an exaggerated response to pain in patients with whiplash injury. *Journal of Psychosomatic Research.* 1993; 37(2):105–110.

Leopold RL, Dillon H. Psychiatric considerations in whiplash injuries of the neck. *Pennsylvania Medical Journal.* 1960;63(3):385–389.

Livingston M. Whiplash injury [letter]. *Lancet.* 1991;338:1208.

Livingston M. Whiplash injury and peer copying. *Journal of the Royal Society of Medicine*. 1993;86:535–536.

*Livingston M. Whiplash injury: some continuing problems. *Humane Medicine*. 1993; 9(4):274–281.

Magnússon T. Extracervical symptoms after whiplash trauma. *Cephalalgia*. 1994; 14:223–227.

*Malt UF, Olafsen OM. Psychological appraisal and emotional response to physical injury: a clinical, phenomenological study of 109 adults. *Psychiatric Medicine*. 1992; 10(3):117–134.

Mayou R. Medico-legal aspects of road traffic accidents. *Journal of Psychosomatic Research*. 1995;39(6):789–798.

Mayou R, Bryant B. Outcome of 'whiplash' neck injury. *Injury*. 1996;27(9):617–623.

McIntire RT. Whiplash injuries. *Journal of the Medical Association of Alabama*. 1959; 29:170.

McNeal HJ. "Whiplash"—an unrealistic psychological word. *Insurance Counsel Journal*. April 1963:275–278.

Merskey H. Psychiatry and the cervical sprain syndrome. *Canadian Medical Association Journal*. 1984;130:1119–1121.

Merskey H. Psychological consequences of whiplash. *Spine: State of the Art Reviews*. 1993;7(3):471–480.

Modlin HC. The postaccident anxiety syndrome: psychosocial aspects. *American Journal of Psychiatry*. 1967;123(8):1008–1012.

Norris JW. Whiplash injury [letter]. *Lancet*. 1991;338:1207–1208.

Olsnes BT. Neurobehavioural findings in whiplash patients with long-lasting symptoms. *Acta Neurologica Scandinavica*. 1989;80:584–588.

Parker RS, Rosenblum A. IQ loss and emotional dysfunctions after mild head injury incurred in a motor vehicle accident. *Journal of Clinical Psychology*. 1996;52(1): 32–43.

Radanov BP. Dr. Radanov replies [letter]. *Journal of Rheumatology*. 1998;25(7):1440.

*Radanov BP, Begré S, Sturzenegger M, Augustiny KF. Course of psychological variables in whiplash injury—a 2-year follow-up with age, gender, and education pair-matched patients. *Pain*. 1996;64:429–434.

Radanov BP, Di Stefano GD, Schnidrig A, Ballinari P. Role of psychological stress in recovery from common whiplash. *Lancet*. 1991;338:712–715.

Radanov BP, Di Stefano GD, Schnidrig A, Sturzenegger M. Psychological stress, cognitive performance and disability after common whiplash. *Journal of Psychosomatic Research*. 1993;37(1):1–10.

Radanov BP, Di Stefano GD, Schnidrig A, Sturzenegger M. Common whiplash: psychosomatic or somatopsychic? *Journal of Neurology, Neurosurgery, and Psychiatry*. 1994;57:486–490.

Radanov BP, Di Stefano GD, Schnidrig A, Sturzenegger M, Augustiny KF. Cognitive functioning after common whiplash. *Archives of Neurology*. 1993;50:87–91.

*Radanov BP, Dvorak J. Impaired cognitive functioning after whiplash injury of the cervical spine. *Spine*. 1996;21(3):392–397.

Radanov BP, Dvorak J, Valach L. Cognitive deficits in patients after soft tissue injury of the cervical spine. *Spine*. 1990;17(2):127–131.

Radanov BP, Sturzenegger M, Di Stefano GD. Long-term outcome after whiplash injury. *Medicine*. 1995;74(5):281–297.

Radanov BP, Sturzenegger M, Di Stefano GD, Schnidrig A. Illness behaviour after common whiplash. *Lancet*. 1992;339:749–750.

*Radanov BP, Sturzenegger M, Di Stefano GD, Schnidrig A. Relationship between early somatic, radiological, cognitive and psychological findings and outcome during a one-year follow-up in 117 patients suffering from common whiplash. *British Journal of Rheumatology*. 1994;33:442–448.

Radanov BP, Sturzenegger M, Di Stefano GD, Schnidrig A, Aljinovic M. Factors influencing recovery from headache after common whiplash. *British Medical Journal*. 1993; 307:652–655.

*Schmand B, Lindeboom J, Schagen S, et al. Cognitive complaints in patients after whiplash injury: the impact of malingering. *Journal of Neurology, Neurosurgery, and Psychiatry*. 1998;64:339–343.

Schrader H, Obelieniene D, Bovim G, et al. Authors' reply [letter]. *Lancet*. 1996; 348: 125–126.

*Schrader H, Obelieniene D, Bovim G, et al. Natural evolution of late whiplash syndrome outside the medicolegal context. *Lancet*. 1996;347:1207–1211.

*Smed A. Cognitive function and distress after common whiplash injury. *Acta Neurologica Scandinavica*. 1997;95:73–80.

Solomon P. The behavioural response to whiplash injury [letter]. *Journal of Bone and Joint Surgery [British]*. 1998;80B(1):183.

*Taylor AE, Cox CA, Mailis A. Persistent neuropsychological deficits following whiplash: evidence for chronic mild traumatic brain injury? *Archives of Physical Medicine and Rehabilitation*. 1996;77:529–535.

*Van Akkerveeken PF, Vendrig AA. Chronic symptoms after whiplash: a cognitive approach. In: Gunzburg R, Szpalski M, eds. *Whiplash Injuries. Current Concepts in Prevention, Diagnosis, and Treatment of the Cervical Whiplash Syndrome*. Philadelphia: Lippincott-Raven; 1998:183–191.

Wallis BJ, Bogduk N. Faking a profile: can naive subjects simulate whiplash responses? *Pain*. 1996;66:223–227.

Wallis BJ, Lord SM, Barnsley L, Bogduk B. Pain and psychologic symptoms of Australian patients with whiplash. *Spine*. 1996;21(7):804–810.

Wallis BJ, Lord SM, Barnsley L, Bogduk N. The psychological profiles of patients with whiplash-associated disorder. *Cephalalgia*. 1998;18:101–105.

Young WH Jr, Masterson JH. Psychology, organicity, and "whiplash." *Southern Medical Journal*. 1962;55:689–693.

Zaiser-Kaschel H, Kaschel R, Diener CH, Mayer K. Neuropsychological status after whiplash injury. *Journal of Clinical and Experimental Neuropsychology*. 1992;14:393.

SYMPTOM EXPECTATION

*Aubrey JB, Dobbs AR, Rule BG. Laypersons' knowledge about the sequelae of minor head injury and whiplash. *Journal of Neurology, Neurosurgery, and Psychiatry.* 1989;52:842–846.

Barsky AJ. Amplification, somatization, and the somatoform disorders. *Psychosomatics.* 1992;33(1):28–34.

Barsky AJ, Goodson JD, Lane RS, Cleary PD. The amplification of somatic symptoms. *Psychosomatic Medicine.* 1988;50:510–519.

*Mittenberg W, DiGiulio DV, Perrin S, Bass AE. Symptoms following mild head injury: expectation as aetiology. *Journal of Neurology, Neurosurgery, and Psychiatry.* 1992;55:200–204.

*Schrader H, Obelieniene D, Bovim G, et al. Natural evolution of late whiplash syndrome outside the medicolegal context. *Lancet.* 1996;347:1207–1211.

SYMPTOM AMPLIFICATION

Arntz A, De Jong P. Anxiety, attention and pain. *Journal of Psychosomatic Research.* 1993;37(4):423–432.

Barsky AJ. Amplification, somatization, and the somatoform disorders. *Psychosomatics.* 1992;33(1):28–34.

Barsky AJ, Goodson JD, Lane RS, Cleary PD. The amplification of somatic symptoms. *Psychosomatic Medicine.* 1988;50:510–519.

Ferrari R. Rear-end auto collisions [letter]. *Archives of Physical Medicine and Rehabilitation.* 1998;79:721.

Ferrari R, Russell AS. Neck injury and chronic pain syndromes: comment on article by Buskila et al [letter]. *Arthritis and Rheumatism.* 1998;41(4):758–759.

Mayou R. Somatization. *Psychotherapy and Psychosomatics.* 1993;59:69–83.

SYMPTOM ATTRIBUTION

This is a brief list of some recent review articles that cite the rather frequent occurrence of neck and back pain in a variety of occupations. Presumably, many whiplash patients are in these occupations and have had or will have neck and back pain from them. They will have likely not remembered any significant neck or back pain episodes from their occupation before the accident—because they had no reason to. After the accident, when hypervigilance for symptoms begins, these same episodes will continue, be amplified, and then be misattributed to the accident.

Hagberg M. ABC of work related disorders. Neck and arm disorders. *British Medical Journal.* 1996;313(7054):419–422.

Hartigan C, Miller L, Liewehr SC. Rehabilitation of acute and subacute low back and neck pain in the work-injured patient. *Orthopedic Clinics of North America*. 1996;27(4): 841–860.

Jayson MI. ABC of work related disorders. Back pain. *British Medical Journal*. 1996;313(7053):355–358.

Stobbe TJ. Occupational ergonomics and injury prevention. *Occupational Medicine*. 1996;11(3):531–543.

Stock SR, Cole DC, Tugwell P, Streiner D. Review of applicability of existing functional status measures to the study of workers with musculoskeletal disorders of the neck and upper limb. *American Journal of Industrial Medicine*. 1996;29(6):679–688.

Yamamoto S. A new trend in the study of low back pain in workplaces. *Industrial Health*. 1997;35(2):173–185.

PSYCHOLOGY OF WHIPLASH—EFFECTS OF PRE- AND POSTTRAUMATIC PSYCHOSOCIAL PROFILE

*Balla JI. The late whiplash syndrome. *Australian and New Zealand Journal of Surgery*. 1980;50(6):610–614.

*Balla JI. Report to the Motor Accidents Board of Victoria on whiplash injuries, 1984. In: Hopkins A, ed. *Headache. Problems in Diagnosis and Management*. London: WB Saunders; 1988:268–289.

Borchgrevink GE, Stiles TC, Borchgrevink PC, Lereim I. Personality profile among symptomatic and recovered patients with neck sprain injury, measured by MCMI-I acutely and 6 months after car accidents. *Journal of Psychosomatic Research*. 1997;42(4): 357–367.

Braaf MM, Rosner S. Symptomatology and treatment of injuries of the neck. *New York State Journal of Medicine*. 1955;55(1):237–242.

*Drottning M, Staff PH, Levin L, Malt UF. Acute emotional response to common whiplash predicts subsequent pain complaints. A prospective study of 107 subjects sustaining whiplash injury. *Nordic Journal of Psychiatry*. 1995;49:293–299.

Farbman AA. Neck sprain. Associated factors. *Journal of the American Medical Association*. 1973;223(9):1010–1015.

Friedman AP, Ransohoff J. Post-traumatic headache. *Trauma*. 1964;5:33–61.

Grzesiak RC, Ciccone DS. *Psychological Vulnerability to Chronic Pain*. New York: Springer Publishing; 1994.

Hirschfeld AH, Behan RC. The accident process I. Etiological considerations of industrial injuries. *Journal of the American Medical Association*. 1963;186(3):193–199.

Hodge JR. The whiplash injury. A discussion of this phenomenon as a psychosomatic illness. *Ohio State Medical Journal*. 1964;60:762–766.

*Imboden JB, Canter A, Cluff LE. Convalescence from influenza. *Archives of Internal Medicine*. 1961;108:115–121.

Kay DWK, Kerr TA, Lassman LP. Brain trauma and the postconcussional syndrome. *Lancet.* 1971;2:1052–1055.

*Kwan O, Friel J. Comment on Radanov et al [letter]. *Journal of Rheumatology.* 1999. In press.

Mayou R, Bryant B, Duthie R. Psychiatric consequences of road traffic accidents. *British Medical Journal.* 1993;307:647–651.

*Radanov BP, Sturzenegger M, Di Stefano GD, Schnidrig A. Relationship between early somatic, radiological, cognitive and psychological findings and outcome during a one-year follow-up in 117 patients suffering from common whiplash. *British Journal of Rheumatology.* 1994;33:442–448.

*Ruesch J, Bowman KM. Prolonged post-traumatic syndromes following head injury. *American Journal of Psychiatry.* 1945;102:145–163.

Slater E, Roth M. *Clinical Psychiatry.* 3rd ed. London: Bailliere, Tindall, and Cassell; 1969:507–509.

*Small EW. An investigation into the psychogenic bases of the temporomandibular joint myofascial pain dysfunction syndrome. *Advances in Pain Research and Therapy.* 1976;1:889–894.

PSYCHOLOGY OF WHIPLASH—EFFECTS OF INSURANCE BATTLES, LITIGATION, AND COMPENSATION

Abbott KH. Whiplash injuries [letter]. *Journal of the American Medical Association.* 1956;162(9):917.

Abbott KH. Neck sprain syndrome. *Medical Arts and Sciences.* 1959;13:139–153.

Awerbuch MS. In reply [letter]. *Medical Journal of Australia.* 1992;157:574.

*Awerbuch MS. Whiplash in Australia: illness or injury? *Medical Journal of Australia.* 1992;157:193–196.

Awerbuch MS. Whiplash in Australia: illness or injury? [letter]. *Medical Journal of Australia.* 1992;157:502.

*Balla JI. The late whiplash syndrome: a study of an illness in Australia and Singapore. *Culture, Medicine and Psychiatry.* 1982;6:191–210.

*Balla JI. Report to the Motor Accidents Board of Victoria on whiplash injuries, 1984. In: Hopkins A, ed. *Headache. Problems in Diagnosis and Management.* London: WB Saunders; 1988:256–289.

*Balla JI, Moraitis S. Knights in armour. A follow-up study of injuries after legal settlement. *Medical Journal of Australia.* 1970;2:355–361.

Beals RK. Compensation and recovery from injury. *Western Journal of Medicine.* 1984;140(2):233–237.

*Buzzard F. Discussion on traumatic neurasthenia and the litigation neurosis. *Proceedings of the Royal Society of Medicine.* 1927;21(1):353–364.

Cook JB. The post-concussional syndrome and factors influencing recovery after minor head injury admitted to hospital. *Scandinavian Medical Journal.* 1972;4:27–30.

Cornes P. Return to work of road accident victims claiming compensation for personal injury. *Injury.* 1992;23(4):256–260.

DePalma AF, Rothman RH, Levitt RL, Hammond NL. The natural history of severe cervical disc degeneration. *Acta Orthopaedica Scandinavica.* 1972;43:392–396.

Goldney RD. "Not cured by verdict": a re-evaluation of the literature. *Australian Journal of Forensic Science.* 1989;20:295–300.

*Gotten N. Survey of one hundred cases of whiplash injury after settlement of litigation. *Journal of the American Medical Association.* 1956;162(9):865–867.

Graham GJ, Butler DS. Whiplash in Australia: illness or injury? [letter]. *Medical Journal of Australia.* 1992;157:429.

Hayes JG. Whiplash in Australia: illness or injury? [letter]. *Medical Journal of Australia.* 1992;157:429.

Huddleston OL. Whiplash injuries. Diagnosis and treatment. *California Medicine.* 1958;89(5):318–321.

Kelly R. The post-traumatic syndrome [letter]. *Journal of the Royal Society of Medicine.* 1981;74:242–245.

*Kelly R, Smith BN. Post-traumatic syndrome: another myth discredited. *Journal of the Royal Society of Medicine.* 1981;74:275–277.

Kinloch BM. Whiplash in Australia: illness or injury? [letter]. *Medical Journal of Australia.* 1993;158:70–71.

Lewy E. Contribution to the problem of compensation neurosis. *Bulletin of the Menninger Clinic.* 1940;4:88–92.

Livingston M. Whiplash injury: misconceptions and remedies. *Australian Family Physician.* 1992;21(11):1642–1644.

MacNab I. The whiplash syndrome. *Clinical Neurosurgery.* 1973;20:232–241.

Maguire WB. Whiplash in Australia: illness or injury? [letter]. *Medical Journal of Australia.* 1993;158:138.

Mayou R, Radanov BP. Whiplash neck injury. *Journal of Psychosomatic Research.* 1996;40(5):461–474.

McDermott FT. Reduction in cervical "whiplash" after new motor vehicle accident legislation in Victoria. *Medical Journal of Australia.* 1993;158:720–721.

*Mendelson G. Not "cured by a verdict." Effect of legal settlement on compensation claimants. *Medical Journal of Australia.* 1982;2:132–134.

Mendelson G. Follow-up studies of personal injury litigants. *International Journal of Law and Psychiatry.* 1984;7:179–188.

Miller H. Accident neurosis. *British Medical Journal.* April 1961:919–925.

Miller H. Accident neurosis. Lecture II. *British Medical Journal.* April 1961:992–998.

Mills H, Horne G. Whiplash—manmade disease. *New Zealand Medical Journal.* 1986; 99:373–374.

Moldofsky H, Wong MTH, Lue FA. Litigation, sleep symptoms and disabilities in postaccident pain (fibromyalgia). *Journal of Rheumatology.* 1993;20:1935–1940.

Olsen J. Whiplash in Australia: illness or injury? [letter]. *Medical Journal of Australia*. 1993;158:71.

Parmar HV, Raymakers R. Neck injuries from rear impact road traffic accidents: prognosis in persons seeking compensation. *Injury*. 1993;24(2):75–78.

Pennie B, Agambar L. Patterns of injury and recovery in whiplash. *Injury*. 1991; 22(1):57–59.

Quinter J. Whiplash in Australia: illness or injury? [letter]. *Medical Journal of Australia*. 1993;158:70.

*Radanov BP, Sturzenegger M, Di Stefano GD, Schnidrig A. Relationship between early somatic, radiological, cognitive and psychological findings and outcome during a one-year follow-up in 117 patients suffering from common whiplash. *British Journal of Rheumatology*. 1994;33:442–448.

Reilly PA, Travers R, Littlejohn GO. Epidemiology of soft tissue rheumatism: the influence of the law. *Journal of Rheumatology*. 1991;18(10):1448–1449.

Schmand B, Lindeboom J, Schagen S, et al. Cognitive complaints in patients after whiplash injury: the impact of malingering. *Journal of Neurology, Neurosurgery, and Psychiatry*. 1998;64:339–343.

Schofferman J, Wasserman S. Successful treatment of low back pain and neck pain after a motor vehicle accident despite litigation. *Spine*. 1994;19(9):1007–1010.

Solomon P, Tunks E. The role of litigation in predicting disability outcomes in chronic pain patients. *Clinical Journal of Pain*. 1991;7(4):300–304.

Swartzman LC, Teasell RW, Shapiro AP, McDermid AJ. The effect of litigation status on adjustment to whiplash injury. *Spine*. 1997;21(1):53–58.

Thiemeyer JS, Duncan GA, Hollins GG Jr. Whip-lash injuries of the cervical spine. *Virginia Medical Monthly*. 1958;85:171–174.

Versteegen GJ, Kingma J, Meijler WJ, ten Duis HJ. Neck sprain in patients injured in car accidents: a retrospective study covering the period 1970–1994. *European Spine Journal*. 1998;7(3):195–200.

Versteegen GJ, Kingma J, Meijler WJ, ten Duis HJ. Neck sprain not arising from car accidents: a retrospective study covering 25 years. *European Spine Journal*. 1998;7(3): 201–205.

Weighill VE. Compensation neurosis: a review of the literature. *Journal of Psychosomatic Research*. 1983;27(2):97–104.

Weissman HN. Distortions and deceptions in self-presentation: effects of protracted litigation in personal injury cases. *Behavioral Sciences and the Law*. 1990;8:67–74.

PSYCHOLOGY OF WHIPLASH—EFFECTS OF THE PATIENT–PHYSICIAN RELATIONSHIP

Abbott KH. Neck sprain syndrome. *Medical Arts and Sciences*. 1959;13:139–153.

Bremner DN, Gillingham FJ. Patterns of convalescence after minor head injury. *Royal College of Surgeons of Edinburgh Journal*. 1974;19:94–97.

Livingston M. Whiplash injury and peer copying. *Journal of the Royal Society of Medicine.* 1993;86:535–536.

Mayou R. Somatization. *Psychotherapy and Psychosomatics.* 1993;59:69–83.

Parker N. Accident litigants with neurotic symptoms. *Medical Journal of Australia.* 1977;2:318–322.

ILLNESS BEHAVIOR AND ADOPTION OF THE SICK ROLE

Barsky AJ, Klerman GL. Overview: hypochondriasis, bodily complaints, and somatic styles. *American Journal of Psychiatry.* 1983;140(3):273–283.

*Blumer D, Heilbronn M. Chronic pain as a variant of depressive disease. The pain-prone disorder. *Journal of Nervous and Mental Disease.* 1981;170(7):381–406.

Ciccone DS, Grzesiak RC. Psychological dysfunction in chronic cervical pain. In: Tollison CD, Satterthwaite JR, eds. *Painful Cervical Trauma.* Baltimore: Williams & Wilkins; 1992:89.

*Cluff LE, Trever RW, Imboden JB, Canter A. Brucellosis. *Archives of Internal Medicine.* 1959;103:398–414.

*Ferrari R, Kwan O, Friel J. Illness behaviour and adoption of the sick role in whiplash claimants. *Forensics* [serial online]. 1999. In press. Available from http://www. acfe.com.

Fishbain DA. Secondary gain concept. Definition problems and its abuse in medical practice. *American Pain Society Journal.* 1994;3(4):264–273.

*Ford CV. *The Somatizing Disorders. Illness as a Way of Life.* New York: Elsevier Biomedical; 1983.

*Grzesiak RC, Ciccone DS. *Psychological Vulnerability to Chronic Pain.* New York: Springer Publishing; 1994.

Halliday JL. *Psychosocial Medicine. A Study of the Sick Society.* New York: WW Norton and Company; 1948.

Hirschfeld AH, Behan RC. The accident process III. Disability: acceptable and unacceptable. *Journal of the American Medical Association.* 1966;197(2):85–89.

*Imboden JB, Canter A, Cluff LE. Convalescence from influenza. *Archives of Internal Medicine.* 1961;108:115–121.

*Imboden JB, Canter A, Cluff LE. Symptomatic recovery from medical disorders. *Journal of the American Medical Association.* 1961;178(13):1182–1184.

Katon W, Kleinman A, Rosen G. Depression and somatization: a review. *American Journal of Medicine.* 1982;72:127–135, 241–247.

*Lipowski ZJ. Somatization: the concept and its clinical application. *American Journal of Psychiatry.* 1988;145(11):1358–1368.

*Lipowksi ZJ. Somatization and depression. *Psychosomatics.* 1990;31(1):13–21.

*Mechanic D. The concept of illness behavior. *Journal of Chronic Diseases.* 1961; 15:189–194.

Mechanic D. Response factors in illness: the study of illness behavior. *Social Psychiatry.* 1966;1(1):11–20.

*Mechanic D, Volkart EH. Illness behavior and medical diagnoses. *Journal of Health and Human Behavior.* 1960;1:86–94.

*Mechanic D, Volkart EH. Stress, illness behavior, and the sick role. *American Sociological Review.* 1961;26:51–58.

Merskey H. The importance of hysteria. *British Journal of Psychiatry.* 1986;149:23–28.

Minc S. Psychological aspects of backache. *Medical Journal of Australia.* 1968;1: 964–965.

Parsons T. Illness and the role of the physician: a sociological perspective. In: Kluckholm C, Murray HA. *Personality in Nature, Society, and Culture.* New York: Alfred A Knopf; 1967:609–617.

*Pilowsky I. Abnormal illness behaviour. *British Journal of Medical Psychology.* 1969; 42:347–351.

*Pilowsky I. A general classification of abnormal illness behaviours. *British Journal of Medical Psychology.* 1978;51:131–137.

*Pilowksy I. *Abnormal Illness Behaviour.* New York: Wiley; 1997.

Rosenbaum JF. Comments on "Chronic Pain as a variant of depressive disease. The pain-prone disorder." *Journal of Nervous and Mental Disease.* 1982;170(7):412–414.

*Ruesch J, Bowman KM. Prolonged post-traumatic syndromes following head injury. *American Journal of Psychiatry.* 1945;102:145–163.

*Shorter E. *From Paralysis to Fatigue.* New York: Maxwell MacMillan; 1992.

*Waddell G, Pilowsky I, Bond MR. Clinical assessment and interpretation of abnormal illness behaviour in low back pain. *Pain.* 1989;39:41–53.

Wooley SC, Blackwell B, Winget C. A learning theory model of chronic illness behavior: theory, treatment, and research. *Psychosomatic Medicine.* 1978;40(5):379–401.

WHIPLASH AND FIBROMYALGIA

Aaron LA, Bradley LA, Alarcon GS, et al. Perceived physical and emotional trauma as precipitating events in fibromyalgia. *Arthritis and Rheumatism.* 1997;40(3):453–460.

Aaron LA, Bradley LA, Alarcon GS, et al. Authors' reply. *Arthritis and Rheumatism.* 1998;41(2):379–380.

Buskila D, Neumann L, Vaisberg G, et al. Increased rates of fibromyalgia following cervical spine injury. *Arthritis and Rheumatism.* 1997;40(3):446–452.

Cohen ML, Quintner JL. Fibromyalgia syndrome, a problem of tautology. *Lancet.* 1993;342:906–909.

Cohen ML, Quintner JL. Altered nociception, but not fibromyalgia, after cervical spine injury: comment on the article by Buskila et al. *Arthritis and Rheumatism.* 1998;41(1): 183–190.

Croft P, Schollum J, Silman A. Population study of tender point counts and pain as evidence of fibromyalgia. *British Medical Journal.* 1994;309:696–699.

Ferrari R, Kwan O. Perceived physical and emotional trauma as precipitating events in fibromyalgia: Comment on article by Aaron et al [letter]. *Arthritis and Rheumatism*. 1999. In press.

Ferrari R, Russell AS. Neck injury and chronic pain syndromes: comment on the article by Buskila et al [letter]. *Arthritis and Rheumatism*. 1998;41(4):758–759.

Smith MD. Relationship of fibromyalgia to site and type of trauma: comment on the articles by Buskila et al and Aaron et al [letter]. *Arthritis and Rheumatism*. 1998;41(2):378.

Wolfe F. The fibromyalgia syndrome: a consensus report on fibromyalgia and disability. *Journal of Rheumatology*. 1996;23(3):534–538.

ASSESSMENT AND TREATMENT

Barnsley L, Lord SM, Bogduk N. Comparative local anaesthetic blocks in the diagnosis of cervical zygapophysial joint pain. *Pain*. 1993;55:99–106.

Barnsley L, Lord SM, Wallis BJ, Bogduk N. False-positive rates of cervical zygapophysial joint blocks. *Clinical Journal of Pain*. 1993;9:124–130.

Barnsley L, Lord SM, Wallis BJ, Bogduk N. Lack of effect of intraarticular corticosteroids for chronic pain in the cervical zygapophyseal joints. *New England Journal of Medicine*. 1994;330:1047–1050.

Barnsley L, Lord SM, Wallis BJ, Bogduk N. The prevalence of chronic cervical zygapophysial joint pain after whiplash. *Spine*. 1995;20(1):20–26.

*Bogduk N. In response [letter]. *Spine*. 1996;21(1):150–151.

Bogduk N, Lord SM. Cervical spine disorders. *Current Opinion in Rheumatology*. 1998; 10:110–115.

Bogduk N, Lord SM, Barnsley L. In response [letter]. *Spine*. 1997;22(12):1420–1421.

*Borchgrevink GE, Kaasa A, McDonagh D, et al. Acute treatment of whiplash neck sprain injuries. A randomized trial of treatment during the first 14 days following car accident. *Spine*. 1998;23(1):25–31.

Brodin H. Cervical pain and mobilization. *Journal of Manual Medicine*. 1985;2:18–22.

Byrn C, Borenstein P, Linder LE. Treatment of neck and shoulder pain in whip-lash syndrome patients with intracutaneous sterile water injections. *Acta Anaesthesiologica Scandinavica*. 1991;35:52–53.

Cassidy JD, Lopes AA, Yong-Hing K. The immediate effect of manipulation versus mobilization on pain and range of motion in the cervical spine: a randomized controlled trial. *Journal of Manipulative and Physiological Therapeutics*. 1992;15(9):570–575.

Cassidy JD, Lopes AA, Yong-Hing K. The immediate effect of manipulation versus mobilization on pain and range of motion in the cervical spine: a randomized controlled trial [letter]. *Journal of Manipulative and Physiological Therapeutics*. 1993;16(4):279–280.

Fattori B, Borsari C, Vannucci G, et al. Acupuncture treatment for balance disorders following whiplash injury. *Acupuncture & Electro-Therapeutics Research International Journal*. 1996;21:207–217.

Ferrari R. Comment on Polatin et al, Predictive value of Waddell's signs [letter]. *Spine*. 1999;24(3):306.

Ferrari R, Kwan O, Russell AS, Schrader H, Pearce JMS. The best approach to the problem of whiplash? One ticket to Lithuania, please. *Clinical and Experimental Rheumatology*. 1999. In press.

Ferrari R, Russell AS. Pain in the neck for a rheumatologist. *Scandinavian Journal of Rheumatology*. 1999. Submission.

Foley-Nolan D, Moore K, Codd M, et al. Low energy high frequency pulsed electromagnetic therapy for acute whiplash injury. *Scandanavian Journal of Rehabilitation Medicine*. 1992;24:51–59.

Fredin Y, Elert J, Britschgi N, et al. A decreased ability to relax between repetitive muscle contractions in patients with chronic symptoms after whiplash trauma of the neck. *Journal of Musculoskeletal Pain*. 1997;5(2):55–70.

Gennis P, Miller L, Gallagher EJ, et al. The effect of soft cervical collars on persistent neck pain in patients with whiplash injury. *Academic Emergency Medicine*. 1996;3(6): 568–573.

Gurumoorthy D, Twomey L. The Quebec task force on whiplash-associated disorders [letter]. *Spine*. 1996;21(7):897–899.

Kent H. BC tackles whiplash-injury problem. *Canadian Medical Association Journal*. 1998;158(8):1003–1005.

Lavin RA. Cervical pain: a comparison of three pillows. *Archives of Physical Medicine and Rehabilitation*. 1997;78:193–198.

Levitt MA. Research can be a pain in the neck. *Academic Emergency Medicine*. 1996; 3(6):563–564.

Lipman FD. Malingering in personal injury cases. *Temple Law Quarterly*. 1962;35: 141–162.

Lord SM, Barnsley L, Bogduk N. The utility of comparative local anaesthetic blocks versus placebo-controlled blocks for the diagnosis of cervical zygapophysial joint pain. *Clinical Journal of Pain*. 1995;11:208–213.

Lord SM, Barnsley L, Wallis BJ, Bogduk N. Chronic cervical zygapophysial joint pain after whiplash. *Spine*. 1996;21:1737–1745.

Lord SM, Barnsley L, Wallis BJ, McDonald GJ, Bogduk N. Percutaneous radio frequency neurotomy for chronic cervical zygapophyseal joint pain. *New England Journal of Medicine*. 1996;335:1721–1726.

Magnússon T, Ragnarsson T, Björnsson A. Occipital nerve release in patients with whiplash trauma and occipital neuralgia. *Headache*. 1996;36:32–36.

Maigne JY. Letter to editor. *Spine*. 1997;22(12):1420.

*McKenzie RA. *The Cervical and Thoracic Spine*. New Zealand: Spinal Publications Ltd; 1990.

*McKinney LA. Early mobilisation and outcome in acute sprains of the neck. *British Medical Journal*. 1989;299:1000–1008.

Mealy K, Brennan H, Fenelon GC. Early mobilization of acute whiplash injuries. *British Medical Journal*. 1986;6:27–33.

Mendelson G. Measurement of conscious symptom exaggeration by questionnaire: a clinical study. *Journal of Psychosomatic Research*. 1987;31(6):703–711.

Moffat M. Letter to editor. *Spine*. 1996;21(1):150.

Neal LA. The pitfalls of making a categorical diagnosis of post-traumatic stress disorder in personal injury litigation. *Medical Sciences and the Law*. 1994;34(2):117–122.

Olson VL. Whiplash-associated chronic headache treated with home cervical traction. *Physical Therapy*. 1997;77:417–424.

Pettersson K, Toolanen G. High-dose methyl-prednisolone prevents extensive sick-leave after whiplash injury. In: Pettersson K, ed. *Whiplash Injury. A Clinical, Radiographic and Psychological Investigation*. Umeå, Sweden; 1996. Umeå University, Thesis.

*Provinciali L, Baroni M, Illuminati L, Ceravolo MG. Multimodal treatment to prevent the late whiplash syndrome. *Scandinavian Journal of Rehabilitation Medicine*. 1996; 28:105–111.

Resnick PJ. The detection of malingered mental illness. *Behavioural Sciences and the Law*. 1984;2(1):21–38.

Sand T, Bovim G, Helde G. Intracutaneous sterile water injections do not relieve pain in cervicogenic headache. *Acta Neurologica Scandinavica*. 1992;86:526–528.

Sbordone RJ, Long CJ, eds. *The Ecological Validity of Neuropsychological Testing*. Florida: St. Lucie Press; 1995.

Smythe HA, Gladman A, Mader R, Peloso P, Abu-Shakra M. Strategies for assessing pain and pain exaggeration: controlled studies. *Journal of Rheumatology*. 1997;24: 1622–1629.

*Spitzer WO, Skovron ML, Salmi LR, et al. Scientific monograph of the Quebec Task Force on Whiplash-Associated Disorders. *Spine*. 1995;20(suppl 8):1S–73S.

Stewart KB, Murray H, Hess RA. Whiplash. *Nursing*. August 1998:33.

Teasell RW, Shapiro AP, Mailis A. Medical management of whiplash injuries: an overview. *Spine: State of the Art Reviews*. 1993;7(3):481–499.

Van Akkerveeken PF, Vendrig AA. Chronic symptoms after whiplash: a cognitive approach. In: Gunzburg R, Szpalski M, eds. *Whiplash Injuries. Current Concepts in Prevention, Diagnosis, and Treatment of the Cervical Whiplash Syndrome*. Philadelphia: Lippincott-Raven; 1998:183–191.

Waddell G, Pilowsky I, Bond MR. Clinical assessment and interpretation of abnormal illness behaviour in low back pain. *Pain*. 1989;39:41–53.

Wallis BJ, Lord SM, Bogduk N. Resolution of psychological distress of whiplash patients following treatment by radiofrequency neurotomy: a randomized, double-blind, placebo-controlled trial. *Pain*. 1997;73:15–22.

Williams MM, Hawley JA, McKenzie RA, van Wijmen PM. A comparison of the effects of two sitting postures on back and referred pain. *Spine*. 1991;16(10):1185–1191.

Woodward MN, Cook JCH, Gargan MF, Bannister GC. Chiropractic treatment of chronic 'whiplash' injuries. *Injury*. 1996;27(9):643–645.

PROGNOSIS

*Balla JI. Report to the Motor Accidents Board of Victoria on whiplash injuries, 1984. In: Hopkins A, ed. *Headache. Problems in Diagnosis and Management*. London: WB Saunders; 1988:268–289.

Braaf MM, Rosner S. Symptomatology and treatment of injuries of the neck. *New York State Journal of Medicine*. 1955;55(1):237–242.

Braaf MM, Rosner S. Whiplash injury of the neck: symptoms, diagnosis, treatment, and prognosis. *New York State Journal of Medicine*. 1958;58:1501–1507.

DeGravelles WD, Kelley JH. *Injuries Following Rear-End Automobile Collisions*. Springfield, IL: Charles C Thomas; 1969:132–165.

Dvorák J, Valach L, Schmid S. Cervical spine injuries in Switzerland. *Journal of Manual Medicine*. 1989;4:7–16.

*Evans RW. Some observations on whiplash injuries. *Neurologic Clinics*. 1992;10(4): 975–997.

Gargan MF, Bannister GC. Long-term prognosis of soft-tissue injuries of the neck. *Journal of Bone and Joint Surgery*. 1990;72-B(5):901–903.

Gargan MF, Bannister GC. The rate of recovery following whiplash injury. *European Spine Journal*. 1994;3:162–164.

Goldney RD. "Not cured by verdict": a re-evaluation of the literature. *Australian Journal of Forensic Science*. 1989;20:295–300.

*Gotten N. Survey of one hundred cases of whiplash injury after settlement of litigation. *Journal of the American Medical Association*. 1956;162(9):865–867.

*Hildingsson C, Toolanen G. Outcome after soft-tissue injury of the cervical spine. *Acta Orthopaedica Scandinavica*. 1990;61(4):357–359.

*Hohl M. Soft-tissue injuries of the neck in automobile accidents. Factors influencing prognosis. *Journal of Bone and Joint Surgery*. 1974;56-A(8):1675–1682.

*Karlsborg M, Smed A, Jespersen H, et al. A prospective study of 39 patients with whiplash injury. *Acta Neurologica Scandinavica*. 1997;95:65–72.

Kelly R. The post-traumatic syndrome. *Pahlavi Medical Journal*. 1972;3:530–547.

Kelly R. The post-traumatic syndrome: an iatrogenic disease. *Forensic Science*. 1975;6: 17–24.

Knight PO, Wheat JD. The whiplash injury—clinical and medico-legal aspects. *Bulletin of the Tulane University Medical Facility*. 1959;18(4):199–214.

MacNab I. The "whiplash syndrome." *Orthopedics Clinics of North America*. 1971;2(2): 389–403.

MacNab I. Acceleration extension injuries of the cervical spine. *Advocates' Quarterly*. 1979–1981;2:77–93.

*Maimaris C, Barnes M, Allen M. Whiplash injuries of the neck: a retrospective study. *Injury*. 1988;19:393–396.

*Mendelson G. Not cured by a verdict. *Medical Journal of Australia*. 1982;2:132–134.

Mendelson G. Follow-up studies of personal injury litigants. *International Journal of Law and Psychiatry*. 1984;7:179–188.

*Miles KA, Maimaris C, Finlay D, Barnes MR. The incidence and prognostic significance of radiological abnormalities in soft tissue injuries to the cervical spine. *Skeletal Radiology*. 1988;17:493–496.

Norris SH, Watt I. The prognosis of neck injuries resulting from rear-end vehicle collisions. *Journal of Bone and Joint Surgery.* 1983;65-B(5):608–611.

Parmar HV, Raymakers R. Neck injuries from rear impact road traffic accidents: prognosis in persons seeking compensation. *Injury.* 1993;24(2):75–78.

Radanov BP, Sturzenegger M. Predicting recovery from common whiplash. *European Neurology.* 1996;36:48–51.

*Radanov BP, Sturzenegger M, Di Stefano GD, Schnidrig A. Relationship between early somatic, radiological, cognitive and psychosocial findings and outcome during a one-year follow-up in 117 patients suffering from common whiplash. *British Journal of Rheumatology.* 1994;33:442–448.

Radanov BP, Sturzenegger M, Di Stefano GD, Schnidrig A, Aljinovic M. Factors influencing recovery from headache after common whiplash. *British Medical Journal.* 1993; 307:652–655.

*Robinson DD, Cassar-Pullicino VN. Acute neck sprain after road traffic accident: a long-term clinical and radiological review. *Injury.* 1993;24(2):79–82.

Ryan GA, Taylor GW, Moore VM, Dolinis J. Neck strain in car occupants: injury status after 6 months and crash-related factors. *Injury.* 1994;25:533–537.

Schrader H, Obelieniene D, Bovim G, et al. Natural evolution of late whiplash syndrome outside the medicolegal context. *Lancet.* 1996;347:1207–1211.

Schutt CH, Dohan FC. Neck injury to women in auto accidents. *Journal of the American Medical Association.* 1968;206:2689–2692.

*Smed A. Cognitive function and distress after common whiplash injury. *Acta Neurologica Scandinavica.* 1997;95:73–80.

*Thiemeyer JS, Duncan GA, Hollins GG Jr. Whip-lash injuries of the cervical spine. *Virginia Medical Monthly.* 1958;85:171–174.

*Watkinson A, Gargan MF, Bannister GC. Prognostic factors in soft-tissue injuries of the cervical spine. *Injury.* 1991;22(4):307–309.

Supplementary Information

Anatomy and Function of the Neck

This section will describe the anatomy and function of the neck so that readers may become familiar with terms or concepts used in the medical literature on whiplash. This chapter is not a detailed discussion of anatomy but rather an attempt to decode the cryptic language of physicians for readers.

The neck comprises many different tissues and organs, and the anatomical relationships among these can be complex. The chief structures to be considered in whiplash patients are the spinal column (composed of the vertebrae, intervertebral discs, facet joints, and ligaments), the spinal cord and nerves, and the muscles. This section will also discuss blood supply to these structures.

VERTEBRAE

A vertebra is a bony structure with a "body" (or main part) at the front (anterior) of the spine. The spine (or spinal column) has 24 separate vertebrae (singular—vertebra), with additional fused vertebrae in the lowest part of the spine. The spinal column extends from the base of the skull to the coccyx (tailbone). The neck has seven—cervical—vertebrae (see Figure 15–1). The first cervical vertebra (the atlas) is a ring of bone that superiorly (above) meets the bony base of the skull and inferiorly (below) meets the second cervical vertebra (the axis). (See Figures 15–2A, 15–2B, and 15–3.) This second vertebra (axis) has an important attachment to the first by strong ligaments and by the close approximation of one part of the axis (called the odontoid process) to the atlas above (see Figure 15–4). These two vertebrae allow for head nodding and some rotation of the head.

From each vertebra, two bony arches (pedicles) reach back (posterior) and meet in the midline to form a ring. This ring is the bony enclosure for the spinal cord. Where the two arches meet, another bony structure (a process) extends directly back (posterior). One can see or feel the spinous processes as humps under the skin of the back. Other bony processes extend to the side (lateral) like wings. They are the transverse processes (see Figures 15–5 and 15–6). The distance from the tip of

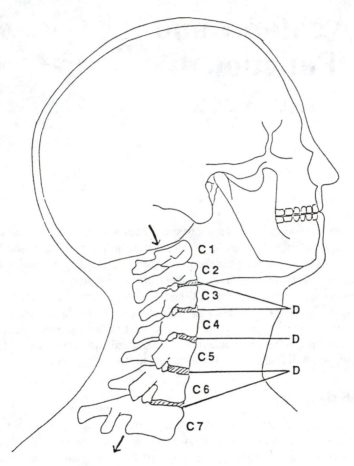

Figure 15–1 The Cervical Spine (Arrows Indicate Entrance and Exit of Spinal Cord through Cervical Spine). *Note:* C1 = first cervical vertebra (also called the atlas), C2 = second cervical vertebra (also called the axis), C3–C7 = third to seventh cervical vertebrae, D = intervertebral disc.

the spinous process that a person can feel under the skin to the front of the vertebra body can be about 2 to 3 inches (5 to 7.5 centimeters). (Thus, individuals who claim they can feel the vertebra and its various parts must be magically able to pass their fingers through skin, muscle, ligaments, and inwards about 2 to 3 inches while doing so.) Finally, facet processes extend from one spinous process to those above and below, forming facet joints. (See discussion below and Figure 15–6.)

Fractures involve the bony structures of the vertebra. Because these bones surround or lie near the spinal cord and nerves, fractures may lead to a piece of bone

Posterior (back)

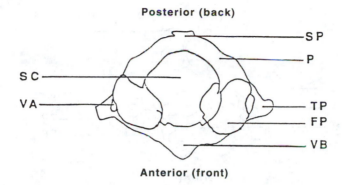

Anterior (front)

Figure 15–2A The Atlas (Seen from Above). *Note:* FP = facet process, which meets skull bone above; SC = spinal (or vertebral) canal, through which spinal cord travels as it descends through cervical spine; VA = foramen (hole), through which vertebral artery (which supplies cervical spine and lower brain) travels; VB = vertebral body; SP = spinous process; TP = transverse process; P = pedicle.

moving and pressing on or cutting the spinal cord. This can lead to paralysis and sudden death. The odontoid process of the second cervical vertebra (the axis) can fracture off and penetrate the spinal cord nearby. This is one of the ways hanging can lead to sudden death, because it suddenly snaps this bony process off and causes it to tear the spinal cord. Most accident victims usually have a neck X-ray because of the threat of fractures of the cervical spine. If a fracture is identified, then there may be further assessments and surgical repair of the fracture. An ambulance attendant may tell an accident victim to keep the neck straight and wear a hard collar until X-rays can be done.

INTERVERTEBRAL DISCS

Intervertebral discs (or just discs) are nearly circular pads of fibrous tissue with a tough ring of fibers on the outside (called annulus fibrosus) and an inner gel-like center called the nucleus pulposus (see Figure 15–7). The gel is capable of absorbing and retaining water and, when surrounded by the annulus, acts as a firm cushion. The discs lie between each adjacent pair of vertebrae and have fibrous attachments to the bone of the vertebra above and below (see Figure 15–8).

The disc can stretch and bulge in different directions to allow the vertebrae above and below to move with respect to each other. When a vertical load (head to toe) is applied to the spine, the disc also acts as a cushion to the spine (see Figure 15–9). Thus, if you jump down from a certain height, the intervertebral discs will prevent the vertebrae from hitting each other. They will absorb the forces by expanding outward when compressed from above or below.

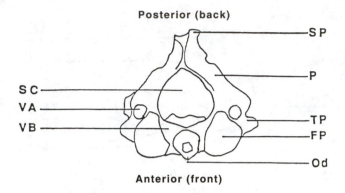

Posterior (back)

S P

P

S C

VA

VB

T P

F P

Od

Anterior (front)

Figure 15–2B The Axis (Seen from Above). *Note:* FP = facet process, which meets skull bone above; SC = spinal (or vertebral) canal, through which spinal cord travels as it descends through cervical spine; Od = odontoid process (of axis), which is attached by ligaments to atlas; VA = foramen (hole), through which vertebral artery (which supplies cervical spine and lower brain) travels; VB = vertebral body; SP = spinous process; TP = transverse process; P = pedicle.

When a disc is described as being ruptured (or slipped), it means that the tough, fibrous annulus has been torn. The inner, gel-like nucleus will protrude back (posterior) through the tear (thus, a bulging or protruding disc). This bulging material may press on a nerve (thus, a pinched nerve) or, if quite large, may press on the nearby spinal cord (see Figures 15–10A and 15–10B). In either case, a physician may be able to detect specific signs of pressure on the nerves or spinal cord by testing reflexes, muscle strength, and skin sensation in the arms and legs.

With increasing age, the disc that was once 90% water loses some of this fluid and will tend toward 70% water content. This may reduce the cushioning capacity of the disc to absorb forces and may make it more likely to tear. Disc degeneration is the label for the result of this process and the accompanying radiologic findings. Other terms for this include spondylosis, spondylitis, osteoarthritis, and arthritis of the spine (the latter two are not very appropriate in that they imply disease).

"Degenerative disc disease" is a misnomer. Disc degeneration is not a disease but a natural consequence of aging. As such, it does not signify disease or injury. Despite the theoretical consideration of increased vulnerability to injury, most people will develop disc degeneration as they age and yet will not have any symptoms. Disc degeneration was labeled as a disease in the 1940s when anatomical dissection of cadavers, usually older individuals, revealed pathologic (abnormal compared to, say, a 20 year old) changes in the cervical spine.

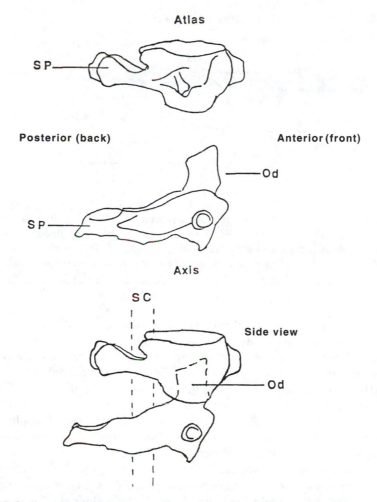

Atlas

S P—

Posterior (back)   **Anterior (front)**

—Od

S P—

Axis

S C

Side view

—Od

Figure 15–3 The Atlas and Axis Separately, and Also as Linked in the Cervical Spine (Seen from the Side). *Note:* SP = spinous process, Od = odontoid process of axis, SC = spinal (or vertebral) canal.

Changes of the discs, in particular, correlated with radiologic changes on X-ray. In other words, the more abnormal the X-ray, the more abnormal the pathologic findings would be on autopsy. Physicians then did not understand, as physicians today do, the natural process of disc degeneration that occurs with aging, beginning generally toward the end of the third decade of life.[1] Everyone develops disc degeneration, and eventually everyone develops abnormal radiologic findings associated with disc degeneration. The original investigators in the 1940s also

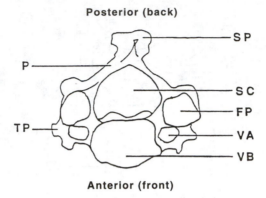

Figure 15–4 Typical Cervical Vertebrae (Seen from Above). *Note:* FP = facet process to form joint with vertebra above; SC = spinal (or vertebral) canal, through which spinal cord travels as it descends through cervical spine; VA = hole for vertebral blood vessels; VB = vertebral body; SP = spinous process; TP = transverse process; P = pedicle.

had no way of knowing if disc degeneration could cause symptoms, but because the discs looked so abnormal they assumed that it did. Unfortunately, the misnomer has persisted in use, even though many would prefer to simply use the phrase "disc degeneration," with no implication that this is a disease.

The question then arose, Is disc degeneration a cause of neck pain? Because disc degeneration is so common in the general population and becomes more common with age, many doubted that there was a true causal relationship between disc degeneration and pain. In 1954, for example, C. Pallis et al stated that "many clinicians are loath to attribute special importance to what is, after all, an extremely common radiological finding."

Nevertheless, it is possible to determine if disc degeneration causes symptoms by establishing a causal relationship. (Causal relationships are discussed further in Chapter 16.) Essentially, to establish such an association, one must first demonstrate a statistical association. The disc degeneration should occur more often in those with neck pain than in those without neck pain. To establish an association of an abnormal X-ray with neck pain, for example, one would first collect a group of individuals who are the same as the study group in age, occupation, overall health, and so on. They would otherwise only differ in one respect—they would have no neck pain. Then, one would examine the neck X-rays of this non–neck pain (control) group. If the group without neck pain has an abnormal X-ray as often as the group with pain, then there is no association between that X-ray result and neck pain. Even if one is able to establish an association, however, this does not, in itself, establish that there is a causal relationship.

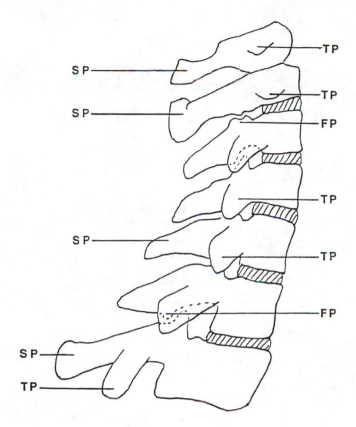

Figure 15–5 The Processes of the Cervical Spine. *Note:* TP = transverse process, SP = spinous process, FP = facet process to form joint with vertebrae above and below (hidden in this view by the transverse process).

To establish a causal relationship requires first an association between one event (disc degeneration) and the second event (neck pain). As explained below, with neck or back pain and no abnormal neurologic findings (eg, no loss of reflexes and no muscle weakness), there is no association between disc degeneration on X-ray and neck or back pain. An association does exist when the patients have both pain and abnormal neurologic findings on examination.[2–4]

Numerous studies deal with the association between abnormal findings on X-ray and the presence of neck pain. Very early, in 1944, A. Oppenheimer's studies led him to doubt that disc degeneration was the cause of isolated neck pain. Addressing the question of correlation between symptoms and either the presence or the severity of X-ray changes, he noted that:

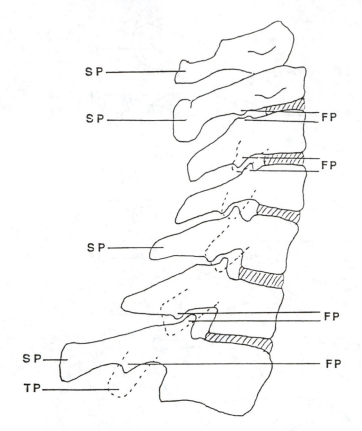

Figure 15–6 The Facet Joints of the Cervical Spine (Transverse Process Has Been Cut Away). *Note:* SP = spinous process, FP = facet process.

Not every disk lesion produces clinical manifestations. In a series of 200 apparently healthy persons not conscious of any symptoms, flattened disks were found in . . . 11 percent.

. . . Clinical manifestations suggestive of disk lesions are due to some other diseases in about 10 percent of the cases, and . . . their connection with a demonstrable disk lesion is questionable in at least another third. From these observations it should be inferred that the [X-ray] demonstration of a diseased disk does not prove the diskogenetic origin of the complaint.

In 1954, Pallis et al studied 50 asymptomatic (no neck pain) patients who had no previous injury: "75 per cent showed narrowing of the spinal canal due to var-

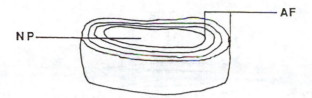

Figure 15–7 The Intervertebral Disc with Its Components (Annulus Fibrosus and the Gel-like Nucleus Pulposus). *Note:* AF = annulus fibrosus, NP = nucleus pulposus.

ious combinations of posterior osteophytosis, subluxation of cervical vertebrae, and [straightening of the normal cervical lordosis]."

The incidence is lower in individuals under age 50 but is still 20% to 30%. Disc degeneration begins, even before it appears on X-ray, around age 20 to 25. In 1963, Z. B. Friedenberg and W. T. Miller compared 160 asymptomatic individuals with an equal number of symptomatic individuals between age 30 and 70. Their "findings cast doubt on the relative value of [X-rays] in determining the clinical significance of degenerative disease of the cervical spine."

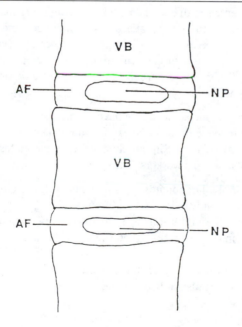

Figure 15–8 The Intervertebral Discs (Anterior View). *Note:* VB = vertebral body, AF = annulus fibrosus, NP = nucleus pulposus.

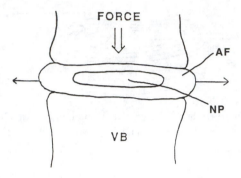

Figure 15–9 The Intervertebral Disc Response to a Vertical—Head to Toe—Load (Anterior View). *Note:* VB = vertebral body, AF = annulus fibrosus, NP = nucleus pulposus.

H. Miller et al (1955) placed matters in perspective.

> First, it must be constantly borne in mind that cervical spondylosis is essentially a radiological diagnosis, depending on physical signs on a radiograph. When we realize that such physical signs are the rule rather than the exception in the x-ray plates of all middle-aged and elderly patients, the significance of such radiological evidence is clearly limited. The radiological changes of cervical spondylosis seem, in fact, to be merely a sign of middle age perhaps somewhat more reliable than the finding of grey hair.
>
> Amongst asymptomatic subjects, we have found that more than 90% of underground miners between the ages of 50 and 55 show radiologically significant spondylosis. . . . Similar changes were encountered in about [70 percent] of sedentary workers in the same age bracket.
>
> It is clear that in the large majority of patients with radiologically significant cervical spondylosis, the condition is quite asymptomatic. . . . It is evident that the ubiquitousness of these x-ray changes calls for special caution in the attribution of etiological significance.

Thus, the presence of neck pain (without neurologic findings) and disc degeneration on X-ray are not statistically associated. (Again, the same is true for back pain.)

Interestingly, studies using more modern radiologic techniques (ones that detect disc degeneration before an X-ray can) also demonstrate the lack of association between neck or back pain and disc degeneration. Using the most sophis-

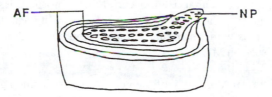

Figure 15–10A Protruding (Bulging) Intervertebral Disc. *Note:* AF = annulus fibrosus, NP = nucleus pulposus.

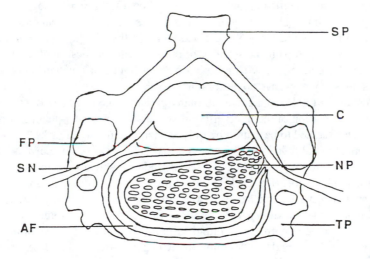

Figure 15–10B Protruding (Bulging) Intervertebral Disc (Seen from Above, Protruding Disc Presses on Spinal Nerve as It Exits the Spine). *Note:* AF = annulus fibrosus, NP = nucleus pulposus, SN = spinal nerve, FP = facet process, TP = transverse process, C = spinal cord, SP = spinous process.

ticated of these techniques—for example, magnetic resonance imaging (MRI)—L. M. Teresi et al (1987) examined 100 asymptomatic (pain-free) patients between 45 and 79 years old. They found that:

> Spinal cord involvement by degenerative disease was observed in a large percentage of patients in this study (23% of patients older than 64 years of age), and produced no symptoms.

> Cord compression also occurred in the absence of symptoms and was secondary to disk protrusion in all cases. These results in our entirely asymptomatic population are compatible with those of an earlier report by Pennin et al. in a study of symptomatic patients.

Our findings indicate that a wide variety of abnormalities may be asymptomatic. . . . The radiologist and referring clinician, therefore, must be cautious with attributing clinical symptoms to structural abnormalities seen on MR images.

Conducting a similar MRI study of the cervical spine, including even younger patients, S. D. Boden et al (1990) found a relatively high incidence of abnormalities in individuals with no symptoms.

It is thus incorrect to attribute patients' neck pain to disc degeneration unless they also had the specific neurologic findings shown to have an association with radiological findings. The fallacy of linking neck pain to disc degeneration on X-ray is even more evident when one considers that there is little correlation between the severity of pain and severity of radiological changes. In other words, a patient can have severe neck pain with a normal X-ray, or a patient with severe changes on X-ray may have no neck pain.

Oppenheimer (1944) found that "in many patients who were free of symptoms complete obliteration of the intervertebral spaces was present, whereas in others severe [pain] seemed to be caused by only moderate thinning of disks."

Friedenberg et al (1960) also discovered that "there was . . . no correlation between the intensity of pain and the degree of [radiographically] visible changes."

For the lumbar spine (low back), with all imaging techniques, the same lack of a clear statistical association exists between the presence of disc degeneration and pain. Studies have shown that 15% to 50% of pain-free (asymptomatic) subjects can have the same abnormalities found in painful subjects. For example, M. T. Modic et al (1984) found that "asymptomatic degenerative disc disease was identified in [30%] of patients under [age] 35."

In addition, studies have shown that there is little correlation between the severity of pain and the severity of disc degeneration in the lumbar spine. Abnormalities may even be found in regions of the spine where the patient is having no pain. As stated by Boden et al (1990):

The finding that an asymptomatic individual has more than a one-in-four chance of having an abnormal magnetic resonance image emphasizes the danger of predicating a decision to operate on the basis of any diagnostic tests in isolation. . . . Images of asymptomatic subjects confirm observations that have been made with computerized tomography and myelography studies that these findings are part of a normal, or at least common, aging process.

Finally, there was an old theory (dating back to 1944 at least) that the finding of disc degeneration in younger individuals was the result of previous injury. In more than 50 years of study, no population-based, controlled study has ever clearly demonstrated this. Instead, a number of the independent studies (cited above) show that normally 5% to 12% of people under the age of 40 should have abnormal neck X-rays (Friedenberg et al 1960, D. R. Gore et al 1986). At least 30% of people under age 35 have disc degeneration on MRI scans even though they have no symptoms (Modic et al 1984). Even larger percentages of young (under age 40) individuals have abnormal radiological changes of the lumbar spine (Boden et al 1990, D. L. Kent et al 1992, Modic et al 1984, H. Paajanen 1989). Studies of "whiplash" patients show that the X-ray at the time of the accident reveals the same rates of radiologic signs of disc degeneration as in asymptomatic populations (see "Radiology of Whiplash" in Chapter 5).

The following points are clear:

1. Without specific neurologic findings, there is a lack of a clear association between neck pain and the presence of disc degeneration. An individual without neck pain is just as likely to have an abnormal X-ray as one with neck pain.
2. The severity of changes on X-ray bears no relationship to the severity of pain.
3. Finding evidence of disc degeneration radiologically at a young age does not imply previous injury and is an expected finding in a certain sizable percentage of healthy subjects.

Rarely, acute neck pain can result from sudden tears of the annulus and bulging of a disc (this happens much more often in the lower spine). The disc may or may not then press on a nerve. Even when it does not, acute pain may occur. Pain is not helpful in distinguishing a pinched nerve from one not pinched. Surgeons have learned that certain signs on examination (like loss of normal reflexes or strength) best distinguish those who truly have a pinched nerve from those who do not. Most other signs are unreliable in making this distinction, and indeed surgery without these important signs usually fails to relieve symptoms.

Finally, it is interesting that J. van der Donk et al (1991) demonstrated that personality traits and a certain psychosocial history were better predictors of whether an individual would have neck pain than were findings of disc degeneration.

FACET JOINTS

As stated above, the intervertebral disc joins the body of each vertebra to the vertebrae above and below it. Each vertebra has bony facet processes that reach above and below to link with these facet processes from adjacent vertebra. These processes form a facet joint. A tough, fibrous capsule surrounds each joint, and lubricant fluid fills the capsule (see Figure 15–11). These joints act with the vertebrae to allow for mobility. Some have argued that damage to these joints (like arthritis) can produce symptoms. Damage to these joints can, however, also exist

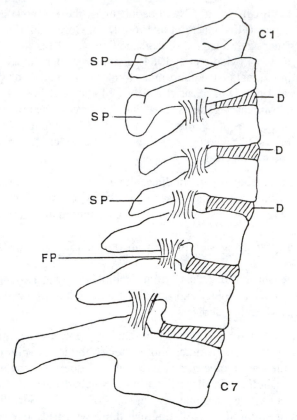

Figure 15–11 Facet Joints of Cervical Spine, Formed by Facet Process of Adjacent Verte-brae, Surrounded by Fibrous Capsule (Transverse Processes Have Been Removed. See Also Figures 15–5 and 15–6). *Note:* C1–C7 = seven cervical vertebrae, FP = facet processes and facet joint formed by these processes, SP = spinous process, D = interver-tebral disc.

without any symptoms. Such damage increases with age, even though there may be no symptoms.

LIGAMENTS

There are many ligaments supporting the bony structures of the spine. The lig-aments have the capacity to stretch enough to allow movement while at the same time remaining tough and protecting from injury. In front (anterior) of the verte-brae there is the anterior longitudinal ligament, which extends down the entire length of the spine. Immediately behind (posterior to) the body of the vertebrae is a posterior longitudinal ligament of similar characteristics (see Figures 15–12A and 15–12B).

There are numerous other ligaments, each running from one vertebra to the adjacent one. Where the two bony arches (pedicles) from the vertebrae meet, there is the ligamentum flavum (which also runs the length of the column). Between the spinous processes there are the interspinous ligaments. Between the transverse processes there are the intertransverse ligaments (see Figure 15–13). Thus, the ligaments offer perhaps the most extensive protection of the spine.

NECK MUSCLES

There are numerous muscles involved in moving and protecting the neck. Figures 15–14A, 15–14B, and 15–15 show some of these. They include, in pairs, the trapezius, sternocleidomastoid, scalene, splenius capitis, semispinalis capitis, semispinalis cervicis, longissimus cervicis, rectus capitis, and interspinalis cervicis.

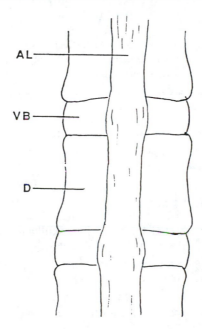

Figure 15–12A Anterior Longitudinal Ligament As It Runs Down Anterior (Front) Surface of Spine, Attaching to Vertebrae and Intervertebral Discs (See Also Figure 15–13). *Note:* AL = anterior longitudinal ligament, VB = vertebral body, D = intervertebral disc.

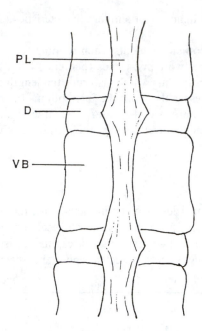

Figure 15–12B Posterior Longitudinal Ligament As It Runs Down Posterior (Back) Surface of Spine, Attaching to Vertebrae and Intervertebral Discs. *Note:* PL = posterior longitudinal ligament, VB = vertebral body, D = intervertebral disc.

These muscles are responsible for the various neck movements and simultaneously offer stability. When muscle strain is being considered in whiplash patients, it is usually in reference to these muscles.

SPINAL CORD AND NERVES

The spinal cord descends through the base of the skull and runs in the cylindrical canal formed by the vertebrae. This space is the spinal canal (see Figures 15–2A and 15–2B). The anterior longitudinal ligament, posterior longitudinal ligament, the vertebral body, and discs protect the spinal cord in front (anterior). The ligamentum flavum, pedicles (or arch), the spinous and transverse processes, their various ligaments, and the muscles protect the spinal cord in back (posterior).

A membrane called the dura wraps around the spinal cord and the beginnings of the nerves. The fluid within the dura bathes the spinal cord. The nerves leave the spinal cord in pairs (right and left) by passing through the hole left between

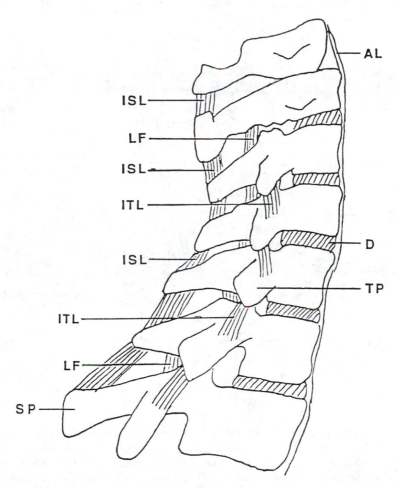

Figure 15–13 Various Ligaments of the Cervical Spine (Viewed from the Side). *Note:* AL = anterior longitudinal ligament, ISL = interspinous ligament, ITL = intertransverse ligament, LF = ligamentum flavum, D = intervertebral disc, TP = transverse process, SP = spinous process.

---

adjacent vertebrae (called the intervertebral foramen—foramina is plural). Fatty tissue surrounds the nerves as they pass through this foramen (see Figures 15–10B, and 15–16).

A bulging disc, spinal cord tumor, or other mass in the spinal canal may press on the nerves before they pass through the foramen. A narrow foramen may also press on nerves while they pass through. This narrowing can occur if one vertebra

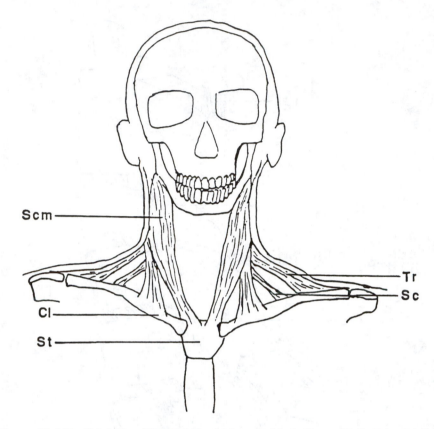

Figure 15–14A Chief Superficial Muscles of Anterior Neck (Occurring in Pairs, Right and Left). *Note:* Scm = sternocleidomastoid muscle (attaches at skull, clavicle, and sternum), Tr = trapezius muscle (attaches at skull, spinous processes, and shoulder bones), Sc = scalene muscle (attaches to neck bones and upper ribs), Cl = clavicle (collarbone), St = sternum (breastbone).

has moved excessively with respect to the adjacent vertebra, narrowing the foramen formed by the two vertebrae. Alternatively, the discs between the vertebrae may become thinner, and this will narrow the foramen because this brings the bones closer together (see Figure 15–17).

Most people with disc degeneration or abnormal position of the vertebrae will not have a pinched nerve. As many as 30% of young people have such changes even though they have no symptoms. (See "Radiology of Whiplash" in Chapter 5.) A pinched nerve can cause pain to travel down the arm or leg, but most individuals with neck or back pain that radiates down their arm or leg do not have a

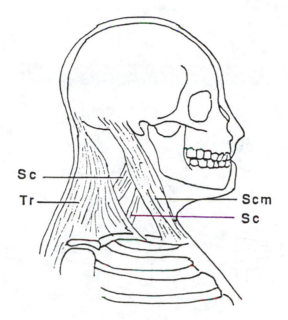

Figure 15–14B Chief Superficial Muscles of Neck (Seen from the Side). *Note:* Scm = sternocleidomastoid muscle, Sc = scalene muscle, Tr = trapezius muscle.

pinched nerve. Surgery to release a pinched nerve in these individuals is often unsuccessful unless specific signs are present on physical examination. Symptoms alone are not reliable enough.

The spinal canal may itself be narrowed. Called spinal stenosis, this condition can be congenital (due to a birth defect), develop as a result of the vertebrae being in abnormal positions, or develop because of excessive bone growth along the canal where the discs have been degenerating. In most cases, however, spinal stenosis does not cause symptoms. When it does cause symptoms, it usually also results in specific neurologic abnormalities on examination.

BLOOD SUPPLY

Blood from the heart flows through the major artery of the body—the aorta. From this, branches called the carotid arteries travel into the neck and supply the brain and face. Specific branches from the aorta, called the vertebral arteries, travel up alongside the cervical spine and supply the bones, discs, and spinal cord with blood.

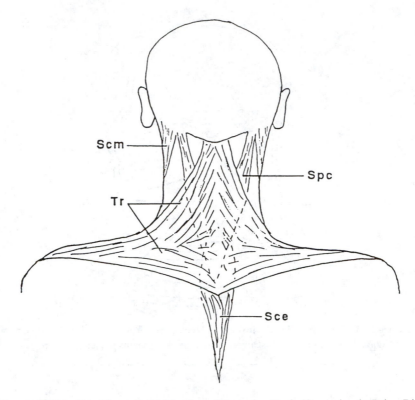

Figure 15–15 Chief Superficial Muscles of Posterior Neck (Occurring in Pairs, Right and Left). (Beneath These Muscles Are the Deeper Muscles Not Shown, including Splenius Capitis, Longissimus Cervicis, Rectus Capitis, Interspinalis Cervicis.) *Note:* Scm = sternocleidomastoid muscle, Tr = trapezius muscle, Spc = semispinalis capitis (attaches to skull and C3–C7 spinous processes), Sce = semispinalis cervicis (attaches to spinous processes of C2–C5 and thoracic vertebrae).

BRACHIAL PLEXUS AND THORACIC OUTLET

The brachial plexus is a group of nerves coming from the spinal cord as it travels through the neck. These nerves come together and travel through the deep structures of the neck, under the collarbone (clavicle), and into the arm. The thoracic outlet is the space nerves travel through in the lower part of the neck and upper part of the chest. It is a triangular space with muscles on two sides and bone on the third side (see Figure 15–18).

It is here that the rare thoracic outlet syndrome originates. In this syndrome, the thoracic outlet is abnormally small, and so it compresses the nerves and the

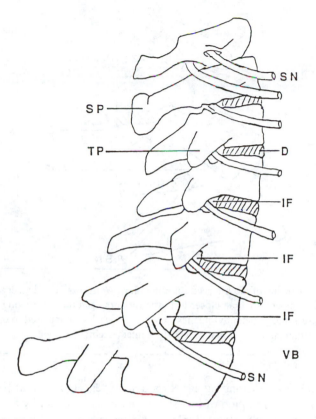

Figure 15–16 Intervertebral Foramina (Singular—Foramen) Formed by Adjacent Vertebrae Above and Below. (The Spinal Nerves Leave the Spinal Cord and Pass in Right and Left Pairs out of the Spine through These Holes.) *Note:* SN = spinal nerve, D = intervertebral disc, TP = transverse process, SP = spinous process, VB = vertebral body, IF = intervertebral foramen.

---

blood vessels in this area. This may cause pain and poor circulation in the arm. This is mentioned here because some believe that whiplash patients have an injury in this region. The thoracic outlet syndrome is discussed further in Chapter 7.

NECK MOVEMENTS

The neck protects the spinal cord while at the same time remaining flexible and mobile. The cardinal neck movements are flexion (bringing chin toward chest), extension (tilting head back to look up at ceiling), rotation (looking over shoul-

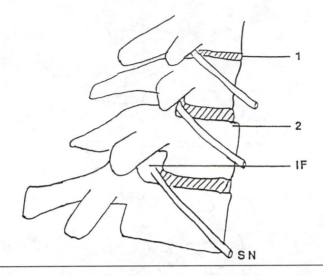

Figure 15–17 Narrowing of the Intervertebral Foramen. *Note:* 1 = disc degeneration and thinning, bringing upper vertebrae closer to lower vertebrae and thus narrowing the foramen; 2 = forward slippage (spondylolisthesis) of lower vertebrae compared to one above, thus narrowing foramen; SN = spinal nerve; IF = intervertebral foramen.

der), and lateral flexion (bringing ear toward shoulder). The normal (common, usual, typical) range of motion of the neck is discussed in detail by S. M. Foreman and A. C. Croft (1988, 1995). Table 15–1 offers some available data.

As the table shows, the range of neck motion in the normal population varies considerably at any given age as well as according to age. Studies that have examined the range of motion of the spine at each vertebral level have found similar variations.

In summary, the neck has a complex, integrated structure with the potential for many abnormalities. Recall, however, that many of these abnormalities either oc-

Table 15–1 Neck Range of Motion According to Age

Movement	Male Age 19 (Degrees)	Male Age 59 (Degrees)	Female Age 19 (Degrees)	Female Age 59 (Degrees)
Flexion	47–81	27–64	47–81	27–64
Extension	62–108	40–80	54–114	33–97
Rotation	60–90	46–78	55–95	43–78
Lateral flexion	33–59	21–48	33–60	23–47

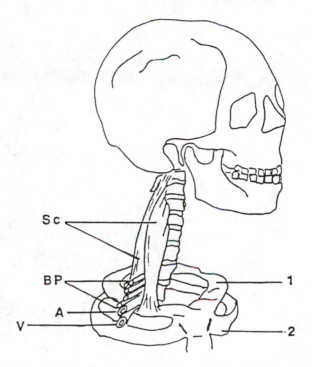

Figure 15–18 The Thoracic Outlet. (The Nerves and Blood Vessels of the Neck Pass through the Thoracic Outlet and Travel into the Arm. The Outlet Is Bordered on the Sides by Scalene Muscles and Below by the First Rib.) *Note:* Sc = scalene muscle, BP = brachial plexus, 1 = first rib, 2 = second rib, A = artery, V = vein.

---

cur as part of the normal aging process or in young, healthy individuals with no symptoms. This is a critical consideration as one reviews the medical literature on whiplash.

TEMPOROMANDIBULAR JOINT

The temporomandibular joint is complex and the subject of much controversy. The lower jaw (mandible) and skull form the joint. It has three chief components: the condyle (or bony process) of the jaw, the articular eminence (part of the skull), and the articular disc, which lies between these two bony processes. Fluid bathes the disc (see Figures 15–19A and 15–19B).

Tough, fibrous tissue makes up the disc. It allows the jaw to move as if on a hinge and to slide forward when one opens the mouth. Muscles attached to the

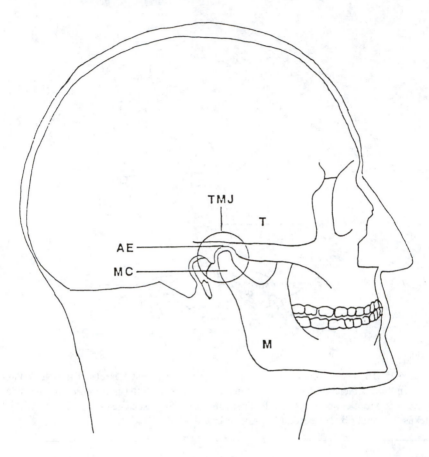

Figure 15–19A The Temporomandibular Joint. *Note:* AE = articular eminence, TMJ = temporomandibular joint, M = mandible (lower jaw), MC = mandibular condyle, T = temporal bone.

skull (temporalis, pterygoids, and masseters) and ligaments hold the lower jaw (mandible) in place.

Some believe that damage to the mandibular condyle, to the ligaments, or to the disc may alter the normal function of this joint and therefore cause pain with normal jaw motion. It is important to know, however, that studies of asymptomatic individuals have demonstrated that many abnormalities exist without causing symptoms. This is analogous to the finding that abnormalities on neck and back X-ray are not necessarily (and indeed unlikely to be) responsible for symptoms.

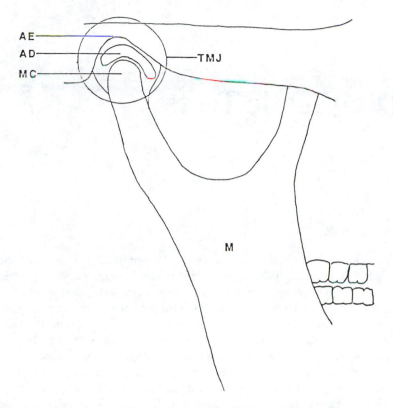

Figure 15–19B Close-up View of Temporomandibular Joint. (The Joint Is Formed by the Articular Eminence from the Skull, the Mandibular Condyle, and the Articular Disc. Muscles and Ligaments Are Not Shown.) *Note:* TMJ = temporomandibular joint, AD = articular disc, M = mandible (lower jaw), MC = mandibular condyle, AE = articular eminence.

REFERENCES

1. Ghosh P. *The Biology of the Intervertebral Disc.* Vol II. Boca Raton, FL: CRC Press; 1988.
2. Wilkinson HA, LeMay ML, Ferris EJ. Clinical-radiographic correlations in cervical spondylosis. *Journal of Neurosurgery.* 1969;30:213–218.
3. Boden SD, Wiesel SW, Laws ER Jr, Rothman RH. *The Aging Spine.* Philadelphia: WB Saunders; 1991.
4. Litt AW. Imaging and the diagnosis of degenerative disease of the cervical spine. In: Cooper PR, ed. *Degenerative Disease of the Cervical Spine.* American Association of Neurological Surgeons; 1992:17.

CHAPTER 16

Diagnostic Tests

INTRODUCTION

This section discusses the diagnostic tests commonly used in the study of whiplash patients, especially the tests involving technical equipment. A diagnostic test is any test that may provide the physician with a diagnosis of some specific injury or disease. Tests can be as simple as asking the patient a set of standard questions or specific maneuvers on physical examination. There are also more elaborate tests on body fluids and tissues and tests that provide images of the body.

Medical researchers have been studying (and learning from experience) which tests provide the best diagnoses. It may seem surprising that many tests being used today have not first been thoroughly evaluated to find out how appropriately or accurately the tests yield a correct diagnosis. In medicine, physicians learn about and understand the value of tests when the tests are used, often over a period of years. After this period, the medical community keeps useful tests and discards the remainder. That means that a test relied on today as evidence for a diagnosis may be deemed poor in the long run. In the meantime, physicians may draw erroneous conclusions using such tests. Misconceptions then propagate through the medical literature. This is an unfortunate process.

ABNORMAL AND NORMAL

Evaluating diagnostic tests involves answering two difficult questions:

1. What is a normal (or abnormal) test result?
2. What does an abnormal test result signify?

In some cases, it is only after years of using a given test that researchers learn the correct answers to these questions.

First, one must define a "normal test result." This is not always simple. Normal is not always equivalent to healthy. Normal, in its strictest sense, means common, usual, or typical. If 70% of the population smoked cigarettes, then smoking would be normal because it is common, usual, and typical, even though we would certainly not consider it healthy. When the general population is studied with a test, most of the people (being common, usual, or typical of the population) have similar test results. These are then called "normal," and most of the people are considered healthy. Thus, one associates a normal test result with being healthy. Does that mean a normal test result will always mean healthy and an abnormal test result will always signify unhealthy? Not always. That depends very much on how "normal test result" is defined.

"Normal" and "healthy" are not equivalent terms, but researchers would like a normal test result to mean "healthy" and an abnormal test result to mean "unhealthy" (diseased or injured). Researchers thus use specific definitions for a normal test result. Ideally, the definition of a normal test result is such that when experts find this result, they conclude the patient is healthy. When they find an abnormal test result, they conclude that the patient is unhealthy. So which definitions of normal and abnormal test results could achieve this?

One might define normal as the result seen in young people. Under this definition, as people age they will become increasingly abnormal. The aging process changes many body tissues. The neck X-ray of a 60 year old looks quite different from that of a 20 year old even though both will insist they are quite healthy and feel well. As people age, more and more abnormal test results will appear in a number of areas.

One has to realize that the aging process is itself considered normal. There is a genetic program, in a simplified sense, for human cells to die, not to live forever unchanged. So one has to consider aging as a normal phenomenon. Otherwise, physicians will have to tell most of the older population that no matter how well they feel, they are severely diseased. One would have to say that a 60 year old's neck X-ray is abnormal because it does not look like a 20 year old's neck X-ray. Indeed, it is normal (common, usual, typical) for a 60 year old to have an X-ray that looks different from a 20 year old's X-ray. For that older age group, such an X-ray is normal, and the majority of individuals in this age group have no neck pain or concerns with their necks. Thus, defining normal test results as those results seen in young people is unsatisfactory. A compromise is the additional comment of "normal for the patient's age," but this still leaves an unclear definition of normal or abnormal test result in many instances.

Thus, experts often use another definition of normal, one that is a statistical observation of what test results occur in a healthy sample of the population. To understand this definition, one uses certain basic statistics.

STATISTICS OF BEING NORMAL

Many measured phenomena have what statisticians call a "normal distribution." This is a distribution where most test results are close to the average for the group. As the result moves further above or below the average, there are fewer numbers of the sample population with those test results.

The normal distribution is the pattern of results for many of the tests used in medicine. When studying an apparently healthy population, one finds the distribution of their test results around the average to have this shape. Most people will have test values at or near the average. Some healthy people will have a result above average, and some will have a result below average. The further the result moves from the average, the fewer the number of healthy people with that test result. They are all healthy, however, no matter how far removed from the average. Researchers observe that there are always a small number of healthy people with test results that appear to be quite far away from the average.

Nevertheless, this distribution can help identify a definition of abnormal that is likely to indicate an individual with disease or injury. The assumption is that as disease or injury develops in individuals, their test results move further and further away from the average for healthy people. This does not mean that an individual with a test result far removed from the average is automatically an individual with disease. The normal distribution of test results in the healthy population shows that there are always a few healthy people whose values are at the outer limits, or far from the average. Identifying individuals with test results far removed from the average simply increases the statistical likelihood that the individual has disease. That is, the farther away from the average, the fewer the number of healthy people with those results.

Thus, one must be careful in choosing the cutoff. If a cutoff for normal is too close to the average, then one will label too many healthy people as diseased. If the cutoff value is too far from the average, then diseased individuals may fall within a range one considers normal.

Arbitrarily, in medicine, one often chooses the range of normal as the range where one finds 95% of healthy people. Researchers realize that 5% of healthy people lie outside this range, so do not immediately label these healthy people as diseased without further study. Experts also realize that some people with disease will have values that are just inside the normal range, and so the disease might be missed. It is not a perfect definition of normal, but it is still helpful in practice.

There are statistical methods that one uses to calculate the range (above and below the average) where one finds 95% of healthy people. When reporting a test result, one cites the normal range as, say, "55 to 90." This means that 95% of healthy people will have test results between 55 and 90. Experts realize that 5% of healthy people will have test results outside this range but expect it to be more likely that these people are diseased (or injured). Researchers assess further anyone with test results outside the normal range to see if they are diseased or just healthy people who happen to have these test results.

So this approach helps answer the first question, What is a normal (or abnormal) test result? The second question, What does an abnormal test result signify?

is also answered. An abnormal test result signifies two possibilities. Either the individual has disease (or injury) or is healthy and just happen to be one of those 5% of healthy people whose values lie far from the average.

For more tests used to study whiplash patients, researchers did not check the normal distribution in the healthy population. Without doing so, one cannot be sure what a normal result is. There is, therefore, a risk of labeling individuals as unhealthy when their test results lie within the normal distribution of healthy people. Medical studies often apply a specific test to a few healthy people, usually young people. The people all have similar results. Then, instead of testing a much larger sample to find the range of values in which 95% of the healthy population lie, the researchers go ahead and study whiplash patients. Some whiplash patients have values near the average of those few healthy, young individuals, but many have values further removed from the average. The researchers consider them abnormal or unhealthy (injured). Eventually, studies examine the normal distribution of test results in the healthy population. These studies reveal a very wide range of results for healthy people, and suddenly whiplash patients are no longer unhealthy as measured by that test.

Assume for a moment, however, that abnormal test results are appearing more often in a group of whiplash patients. What does this mean? The question of the significance of an abnormal finding in whiplash patients concerns the causal relationship (eg, Is the X-ray indicating the cause of the patient's chronic pain?).

CAUSAL RELATIONSHIP

If a patient has neck pain, and a certain test result is abnormal, is that abnormality an indicator of the cause of symptoms? Not necessarily. As explained before, to establish this link, one must first demonstrate the statistical association—the abnormal test result occurs more often in those with neck pain than in those without neck pain. To establish an association of an abnormal X-ray with neck pain, for example, one would first collect a group of individuals who are the same as the study group in age, occupation, overall health, and so on. They should differ in one chief respect—they have no neck pain. Then, one would collect the neck X-rays of this non–neck pain (control) group. If members of the group without neck pain have abnormal X-rays as often as the group with pain, then one cannot establish an association between that X-ray result and the symptom.

The selection of the control group and the study group is critical. Though, ideally, members of the control group will be identical to the study group in all respects but the one under consideration (ie, neck pain), it is impossible to obtain a perfectly matched control group. It is often possible inadvertently to select a study group that just happens to have a higher incidence of the abnormal test result becase of how one selects the group. Selection methods have been designed to minimize these sources of bias. Researchers must try to avoid bias in control groups. It is in this respect that so many studies fail to validate their conclusions. They reach the conclusion that there is an association between a certain test result and a certain symptom, but they fail to have a proper control group. (Indeed, some studies use no control group at all.)

Even with an association between a test result and a symptom, there is not yet an established causal relationship. Instead, one uses specific methods to establish a causal relationship. There are many methods, but some of the common ones include statements of plausibility, identification of temporal relationships, and experimental demonstration of cause and effect.

Plausibility

The simplest, but also the least reliable, way to establish a causal relationship is to show that the causal relationship seems plausible. It is too easy to develop a very plausible chain of events to explain a potential causal relationship. Many such arguments in the scientific literature are later disproven. Yet plausibility may be sufficient in some cases. Consider, for example, individuals who had burns on their arm and who were exposed to hot things. One would establish the causal relationship by first demonstrating an association. That is, one would examine a control group who did not have burns and see how many members of this group had their hands in hot things (like fire or boiling water). One would find that people with burns had their hands in or near hot things more often than those without burns. With the statistical association being demonstrated, one would use some method to establish a causal relationship. One could do this by plausibility: "You play with fire, you get burned." It seems plausible, and most would accept that argument. This is not satisfactory, however, for many other cases, particularly where there are more complex sequences of events. So one uses other methods.

Temporal Relationships

Some consider chronology as sufficient evidence of a causal relationship. If an individual felt well one day, had a car accident the next day, and felt unwell the day after that, one would conclude that the car accident caused the symptoms. The difficulty with such conclusions, however, is that they pay little attention to the mechanism of such a causal relationship. If the symptoms occurred because the accident happened, are they due to injury or fright, or to other factors? So while a temporal relationship may help to establish causation, it may say little about the actual factors involved in causation. Some would prefer to identify the factors in the accident that generated the symptoms to be sure that the symptoms are not arising for other reasons. Using a temporal relationship as the basis for concluding causation by way of the accident is even more problematic when the symptoms occur months or years later. The injured party claims a remote event is the cause. In such cases, it is possible that other intervening events have broken the chain of causation. Trying to prove, for example, that exposure to a given chemical caused lung cancer 30 years later is not a simple task. Although it is true that the exposure preceded the cancer, a multitude of other factors may have intervened to have caused the cancer instead. Thus, in some cases, the chronology of events alone is not useful, and again one must rely on more scientifically rigorous methods of establishing causal relationship.

Experimental Demonstration of Cause and Effect

Perhaps the most reliable (but difficult) method of establishing causal relationship is by experimentation. Here one intentionally invokes the abnormality (detected as an abnormal test result) or event in a controlled environment (one removes or notes other confounding factors). One then determines the effect on outcome. As an example, consider the still-used Koch postulates on germ theory. More than two centuries ago, some postulated that germs (bacteria) caused disease. To establish the causal relationship, Koch suggested that one had first to find the germ more often in those with disease than in those who were healthy. That is, one had first to show the statistical association. Then one would inject the germ from the infected individual into a healthy individual. When the healthy individual became ill, then one had to find the germ in that newly ill individual. One establishes the causal relationship in this way with a high degree of confidence. One can further extend the demonstration of causal relationship by demonstrating resolution of the disease by removing the germ (antibiotics).

Summary

Concepts of abnormal versus normal, the significance of abnormal findings, and the requirements for establishing associations and causal relationships remain complex. In a desire to confirm a causal relationship between an acute whiplash injury and reporting of chronic pain due to chronic damage from that injury, many have undertaken numerous investigations. The next two sections will deal with the radiologic and neurologic tests researchers use to study whiplash patients.

RADIOLOGIC TESTS

X-rays

One may also refer to X-rays as radiographs or roentgenograms. To make an X-ray image, a certain type of energy (X-rays) passes through the subject. The

X-rays then contact a plate behind the subject to develop an image. Materials through which X-rays do not pass easily, such as bone or metal, will appear white on the X-ray. Materials through which X-rays pass easily, like air around subjects (or in their lungs), will appear black.

In the neck, ligaments, intervertebral discs, the spinal cord and nerves, and blood vessels appear black, so that one cannot easily detect damage to them. A fracture in bone appears as a black line across the white image of the bone. The image shows fat and muscle, but these materials appear somewhat translucent.

X-rays are two-dimensional images of a three-dimensional object. If an individual were compressed flat from front to back, many bones and other structures would overlap each other. The bones in the front of the chest appear as if pressed against the spine in back and indeed make the spine impossible to detect in some parts. That is why radiologists use special techniques and views from different angles to cope with the problem of overlapping images. For example, if two bones overlap on an X-ray image taken from the front, then an X-ray taken from the side will show which bone is in front and which is behind.

X-rays of the neck may be necessary in accident victims to look for a fracture that, if the spine becomes excessively mobile or the broken fragment moves, can lead to spinal cord injury.

When one interprets an X-ray as being normal or abnormal, one must realize that an abnormality on X-ray is not necessarily an explanation for a patient's symptoms.

As discussed previously, disc degeneration is a normal phenomenon of aging, even though many use the misnomer "degenerative disc disease." Indirect signs on X-ray of disc degeneration include disc space narrowing, osteophytes, misalignment of the vertebrae, and subluxation. As disc degeneration is a part of the aging process, these findings become more common among older people.

As the disc degenerates, it loses volume, thus appearing as a narrowed disc space on X-ray (the vertebrae above and below the disc appear closer together). Along with this finding, there are bony changes, including thickening of the bone near the discs (sclerosis). In addition, the bone of the vertebrae develops outgrowths near the disc known as osteophytes. In some cases, these outgrowths "pinch" nerves that are leaving the spinal canal, because the outgrowths narrow the width of the nerve exits. Without specific neurologic findings (evidence of a pinched nerve), however, there is no correlation between symptoms and the presence of osteophytes. In fact, there is an unusual condition known as diffuse idiopathic skeletal hyperostosis. This refers simply to bony outgrowths from the vertebrae that may be extremely large compared to osteophytes. These outgrowths may sometimes grow so large as to fuse with the bony outgrowths of vertebrae above and below. Despite th dramatic radiologic appearance of this condition, physicians associate no clinical significance (ie, no symptoms) to it.

With disc degeneration, there may also be facet joint degeneration and ligament degeneration, which may alter the entire spine alignment. Where the spine has an expected curvature (lordosis), it may become straight or even curve in the opposite direction to that expected (kyphosis). Again, despite the dramatic appearance, there is little correlation between the severity of these changes and symptoms unless specific neurologic abnormalities (indicating that there is compression of nerve structures) exist.

Thus, disc degeneration and its resultant radiologic findings are an expected phenomenon in the healthy population. Disc degeneration is a normal part of the aging process and is, unless specific neurologic abnormalities accompany it, not correlated with symptoms, regardless of how dramatic the radiologic appearance may be.

Yet, despite many studies showing that radiologic findings of disc degeneration do not correlate with symptoms, this belief has persisted throughout much of the history of whiplash-related research. Even today, some medical and legal experts have this misconception.

Discography

Though few advocate discography now, it was popular in the 1960s and 1970s, particularly when it was becoming clear that abnormal X-rays of the neck did not necessarily indicate disease or injury. A disc without degeneration has a gel-like center with 90% water content. One can inject only a very little fluid into a disc before it stretches to cause pain. A degenerated disc, however, has only 70% water or may be bulging through the fibrous annulus and therefore has more room to expand. One can inject more fluid before pain occurs. Using this process, physicians could also see if the pain patients experienced was the same they had been having before the procedure. A special dye injected with the fluid shows up on X-ray. If a disc has a tear, then instead of the dye collecting in the center of the disc, some travels away from the center.

The problem found here was that many of the healthy population (people with no neck pain) have very abnormal discograms. So the significance of what one labels an abnormal discogram is unclear; abnormal discograms could occur in people with and without neck pain. Thus, it is not a useful technique.

Bone Scans

Bone scans (or scintigraphy or scintigrams) are useful in detecting many bone diseases as well as disease or injury involving ligaments, tendons, and muscles. When bone or nearby tissue becomes injured or diseased, bone cells that try to heal the injury or disease are activated. These cells take up calcium and other substances from the blood. To perform a bone scan, then, one injects the individual with a special solution containing phosphate (which the bone cells will take up) with a radioactive substance attached to it. This solution travels throughout the body. The radioactive substance emits radiation that a scanner detects. Most bones take up small amounts of the solution, but injured or diseased bone takes up much more of the solution. Damaged muscle may also take up some of this solution.

Using this type of scan, one can detect bone disease or injury, disc degeneration, ligament or muscle tears, and inflammation in any of these parts of the body. One often finds positive bone scans (ones that show excess solution collecting in certain areas) in older individuals because they have disc degeneration, even if they have no symptoms from it. Minor muscle or ligament injury would not generally show up on a bone scan, but more significant injuries would. A bone scan helps to rule out more significant injuries in whiplash patients but would leave minor injuries undetected.

Myelography

Myelography produces myelograms. One forms images with a "dye" injected through the spine from the back into the spinal canal where the spinal cord lies. The dye travels up and down the spinal canal as part of the fluid that normally bathes the cord and its nerves. An X-ray shows where the dye travels. When there is a protruding disc or something pressing against a nerve, this blocks the dye from traveling past that region. This blockage offers indirect evidence of something pressing near the cord or nerves.

Again, however, around 30% of the healthy population (people with no symptoms) have these abnormal findings.

Computed Tomography

Computed tomography (CT) or computer-assisted tomography is essentially a series of special low-dose X-rays that allow one to visualize a cross-section of the body. The initial X-ray beam passes through the individual, front to back, and then the X-ray emitter moves over a few degrees and passes another beam, which comes out at a slightly different angle. The beam keeps moving a few degrees and making an image every time, until it has done a complete circle around the body. A computer then assembles this data and makes an image that looks like a cross-section or slice of the body. The whole process repeats to produce slices from head to toe.

CT scanning produces a picture that is impossible to produce with standard X-ray techniques. The anatomical information is more detailed, and the problem of overlapping structures (a problem of standard X-rays) is avoided.

Because of the detail it offers, CT scanning has shown that even more healthy and young people have disc degeneration.

Magnetic Resonance Imaging

Magnetic resonance imaging (MRI) does not use X-rays as a source of energy. Instead, MRI uses radio waves emitted while the patient is in a powerful magnetic field. The tissues of the body have different electrical and magnetic properties, and through complex data processing techniques, signals of electrical and magnetic activity from these tissues can be used to form an extremely detailed image. Because a tiny blood vessel (even 0.75 millimeters) will have different electrical and magnetic properties than the nerve it lies next to, for instance, the two structures will appear quite different. The image shows each structure to occupy a different shade, from white to gray to black.

As CT does, MRI produces images of slices of the body. Unlike CT, MRI can produce these slices in many different planes. Not surprisingly, MRI can find abnormalities that no other imaging technique can. In fact, 30% of young, healthy people have abnormal MRI scans of the spine, no matter how well they feel.

Temporomandibular Joint Imaging

One can image the temporomandibular joint (TMJ) by X-ray, CT, MRI, and arthrography (injecting dye into joint and taking an X-ray). There have been population studies of healthy individuals to determine how often abnormalities might occur in those with no symptoms. As noted above, finding an abnormality is not equivalent to finding the cause of the patient's symptoms. (There is more discussion about the controversy of TMJ disorders elsewhere in the book.)

Summary

There are many diagnostic tests to study the structures of the head and neck. With each, physicians have had to learn that one cannot necessarily attribute imaging abnormalities to disease or injury since so many healthy people have these abnormalities. The following discussion about the neurologic and psychological tests used to study whiplash patients reiterates this point.

NEUROLOGIC AND PSYCHOLOGICAL TESTS

Electroencephalography

Electroencephalography produces an electrocephalogram (EEG) by observing the electrical signals detected by electrodes placed systematically on the scalp. These readings reveal the electrical activity of the brain.

Many factors, including sleep deprivation, drugs, state of alertness, brain injury, and various brain diseases, alter this electrical activity. EEG is an invaluable tool for working with patients with seizure disorders. A seizure that is occurring or has recently occurred markedly alters the electrical activity of the brain.

There is considerable variation of the EEG in the healthy population, however, and a healthy individual's EEG may vary from time to time. Researchers using EEGs have found some similar abnormalities in healthy people and whiplash patients.

Brainstem Auditory Evoked Responses

Brainstem auditory evoked responses (BAERs) or brainstem auditory evoked potentials are also electrical signals measured on the scalp. One measures them by stimulating the hearing of the subject and then measuring the electrical changes in the part of the brain (the brainstem) that provides the individual with normal equilibrium.

Humans have a complex network of nerve fibers that collect information about sound from the inner ear and then transmit this information to other parts of the brain. This system links the eyes, ears, and limbs. Problems with this system produce ringing in the ears (tinnitus) and sometimes hearing loss. Because the inner ear is also part of one's equilibrium system, problems with balance may also be involved.

One detects numerous diseases causing injury at any site, from the inner ear to the brainstem and brain, by examining the electrical signals during such tests. Unfortunately, the electrical recordings are very complex, and minor changes in the measuring technique can cause variation. Two experimenters can interpret an individual's tracing differently, making it difficult to be sure what the tracing represents. Finally, the tracings can differ between the left and the right side of the brain and on different test dates. Thus, some of the experimental studies on whiplash patients have the common flaw of using a technique in which one can misinterpret the significance of certain abnormalities.

Electronystagmography

Electronystagmography produces an electronystagmogram (ENG) by measuring the electrical activity near the eye in response to various visual or other cues. When a person's head is moving in space, the inner ear detects this motion and allows the person to remain balanced (to maintain equilibrium). Information from a person's limbs and eyes also feeds into the equilibrium system.

Rotating individuals, showing them pictures of their environment in motion, or stimulating their limbs to indicate motion stimulates the equilibrium system. As people respond to these stimuli, there are characteristic eye movements and brain activity that occur. If there is a defect in the system, a person might experience dizziness or vertigo (the sensation that the environment or the individual is spinning). Also, abnormal eye movements (called nystagmus) may occur.

With electronystagmography, as with other tests, there is variation within the healthy population and even when testing the same individual on different occasions, making the significance of some apparent abnormalities unclear.

Electromyography

Electromyography produces electromyograms (EMGs) by measuring the electrical signals of muscle activity during muscle contraction. One also uses electrical impulses to stimulate muscles.

There are some variations in the healthy population that one considers in EMG studies, but there are fewer difficulties with EMG than there are with ENG.

Nerve Conduction Studies

These studies measure the nerve activity with skin stimulation so that a sensation travels up a nerve toward the brain, or one stimulates a nerve and measures its activity. The most common use of nerve conduction studies is in detecting carpal tunnel syndrome, a condition in which there is compression of one of the nerves passing into the hand.

There are, however, a number of abnormalities that can appear in the healthy population, and misinterpretation of the significance of certain findings can lead to the wrong conclusions. Some once thought various abnormalities in nerve conduction studies were proof of the diagnosis of the controversial thoracic outlet syndrome. Many point out that these abnormalities may be useless diagnostically, as there is a wide range of "normal" values in the general population (M. Cherington et al 1986–1989, A. C. Cuetter and D. M. Bartoszek 1989, D. A. Nelson 1990, T. Smith and W. Trojaborg 1987, A. J. Wilbourn 1990). Even in normal subjects, there are differences in test results between the left and right arms. Finding these abnormalities in patients suspected of having thoracic outlet syndrome does not therefore offer any proof at all.

Psychological Tests

Some practitioners use tests such as the Minnesota Multiphasic Personality Inventory (MMPI-2) and the Symptom Check List (SCL-90-R) to study whiplash patients. The tests involve a series of questions designed to distinguish individuals with certain psychological conditions. They do have limited value, however, in that their findings best correlate with more severe kinds of psychological disturbance, and they may fail to characterize milder disturbances well.

To what degree MMPI results measure an effect of the psyche on the expression of chronic pain, rather than the effect of chronic pain on the psyche, is not always easy to distinguish. Also, the use of these tests in the medicolegal setting has not been formally validated.

Another use of psychological testing is obviously in the detection of malingering, as is discussed in Chapter 12.

SUMMARY

There are many neurologic and psychological tests used to study whiplash patients. The tests are of limited diagnostic capability, however, because either abnormalities frequently occur in the healthy population or researchers have not yet studied the healthy population adequately to define the range of normal. In addition, the results may be misinterpreted in an effort to draw meaningful conclusions regarding causal relationships between abnormalities and symptoms.

Dispelling the Myths—Issues for Cross-Examination

It is historical continuity that maintains most assumptions—not a repeated assessment of their validity.

—de Bono E. *Lateral Thinking*. London: Penguin Books; 1990:82.

Many people may be surprised to learn that some statements made by medical experts are not based on tested facts. Authors will often cite references that appear to validate a claim. But sometimes those cited articles themselves do not provide any validation or are very poor studies.

Many myths about whiplash have remained in circulation for years. Listed below are some myths, followed by articles that address them.

Myth: Straightening of the cervical lordosis, cervical kyphosis, subluxation of the vertebral joints, angulation of the spine, and disc degeneration seen on neck X-rays are all signs of chronic damage that persists from the acute injury that is then responsible for reporting of chronic symptoms in whiplash patients.

See Chapter 5. The following articles discuss studies showing that these abnormalities on X-ray are just as commonly found in healthy subjects.

****

Borden AGB, Rechtman AM, Gershon-Cohen J. The normal cervical lordosis. *Radiology*. 1960;74:806–809.

Crowe HE. Whiplash injuries of the cervical spine. In: *Section of Insurance, Negligence, and Compensation Law, Proceedings*. American Bar Association; 1958:176–184.

Elias F. Roentgen findings in the asymptomatic cervical spine. *New York State Journal of Medicine*. 1958;58:3300–3303.

Fineman S, Borrelli FJ, Rubinstein BM, Epstein H, Jacobson HG. The cervical spine: transformation of the normal lordotic pattern into a linear pattern in the neutral posture. *Journal of Bone and Joint Surgery.* 1963;45-A(6):1179–1206.

Gore DR, Sepic SB, Gardner GM. Roentgenographic findings of the cervical spine in asymptomatic people. *Spine* 1986;11(6):521–524.

Gore DR, Sepic SB, Gardner GM, Murray MP. Neck pain: a long-term follow-up of 205 patients. *Spine.* 1987;12(1):1–5.

Helliwell PS, Evans PF, Wright V. The straight cervical spine: does it indicate muscle spasm? *Journal of Bone and Joint Surgery [British].* 1994;76-B:103–106.

Juhl JH, Miller SM, Roberts GW. Roentgenographic variations in the normal cervical spine. *Radiology.* 1962;78:591–597.

Lottes JO, Luh AM, Leydig SM, Fries JW, Burst DO. Whiplash injuries of the neck. *Missouri Medicine.* 1959;56(6):645–650.

Miles KA, Maimaris C, Finlay D, Barnes MR. The incidence and prognostic significance of radiological abnormalities in soft tissue injuries to the cervical spine. *Skeletal Radiology.* 1988;17:493–496.

Rechtman AM, Borden AGB, Gershon-Cohen J. The lordotic curve of the cervical spine. *Clinical Orthopedics.* 1961;20:208–215.

Zatzkin HR, Kveton FW. Evaluation of the cervical spine in whiplash injuries. *Radiology.* 1960;75:577–583.

Myth: Whiplash causes or accelerates disc degeneration, as seen on X-ray.

See Chapter 5. There is no good evidence that being a whiplash victim causes or accelerates disc degeneration. The following studies looked at whiplash patients and compared them to healthy subjects to see who showed more disc degeneration over time. Other articles review this issue. The few studies or authors that have tried to maintain this myth are critiqued and mentioned in Chapter 5.

****

Hildingsson C, Toolanen G. Outcome after soft-tissue injury of the cervical spine. *Acta Orthopaedica Scandinavica.* 1990; 61(4):357–359.

Jónsson H Jr, Cesarini K, Sahlstedt B, Rauschning W. Findings and outcome in whiplash-type neck distortions. *Spine.* 1994;19(24): 2733–2743.

Miles KA, Maimaris C, Finlay D, Barnes MR. The incidence and prognostic significance of radiological abnormalities in soft tissue injuries to the cervical spine. *Skeletal Radiology.* 1988;17:493–496.

Munro D. Relation between spondylosis cervicalis and injury of the cervical spine and its contents. *New England Journal of Medicine.* 1960;262(17):839–846.

Parmar HV, Raymakers R. Neck injuries from rear impact road traffic accidents: prognosis in persons seeking compensation. *Injury.* 1993; 24(2):75–78.

Pearce JMS. Whiplash injury: a reappraisal. *Journal of Neurology, Neurosurgery, and Psychiatry.* 1989;52:1329–1331.

Pearce JMS. Whiplash injury: fact or fiction? *Headache Quarterly, Current Treatment and Research.* 1993;3:45–49.

Redmond AD. Prognostic factors in soft tissue injuries of the cervical spine [letter]. *Injury.* 1992;23(1):71.

Robinson DD, Cassar-Pullicino VN. Acute neck sprain after road traffic accident: a long-term clinical and radiological review. *Injury.* 1993; 24(2):79–82.

Myth: Patients with disc degeneration on X-ray at the time of the rear-end collision will have a poor outcome because of those changes.

See Chapter 5. Studies that follow the outcomes of whiplash patients find no difference in outcome in regards to what the X-ray looked like at the beginning. Again, the few studies that argue otherwise are highly flawed; these are addressed in Chapter 5 as well as in Chapter 13. (See comments under M. Hohl 1974, S. H. Norris and I. Watt 1983, and B. P. Radanov et al 1996 in Chapter 13.)

****

Balla JI. Report to the Motor Accidents Board of Victoria on whiplash injuries, 1984. In: Hopkins A, ed. *Headache. Problems in Diagnosis and Management.* London: WB Saunders; 1988:256–289.

DeGravelles WD, Kelley JH. *Injuries Following Rear-End Automobile Collisions.* Springfield, IL: Charles C Thomas; 1969.

Hildingsson C, Toolanen G. Outcome after soft-tissue injury of the cervical spine. *Acta Orthopaedica Scandinavica.* 1990;61(4):357–359.

Pearce JMS. Whiplash injury: a reappraisal. *Journal of Neurology, Neurosurgery, and Psychiatry.* 1989;52:1329–1331.

Pearce JMS. Whiplash injury: fact or fiction? *Headache Quarterly, Current Treatment and Research.* 1993;3:45–49.

Myth: Abnormalities on cervical spine X-ray explain the reporting of chronic symptoms by whiplash patients.

See Chapter 5. Whiplash patients have no more changes on neck X-ray than do healthy subjects. As well, there is no correlation between the pain reported and the X-ray findings. Whiplash patients report pain whether they have a normal X-ray or not.

****

Balla JI. Report to the Motor Accidents Board of Victoria on whiplash injuries, 1984. In: Hopkins A, ed. *Headache. Problems in Diagnosis and Management.* London: WB Saunders; 1988: 256–289.

Balla JI, Iansek R. Headaches arising from disorders of the cervical spine. In: Hopkins A, ed. *Headache. Problems in Diagnosis and Management.* London: WB Saunders; 1988:243–267.

Friedenberg ZB, Broder HA, Edeiken JE, Spencer HN. Degenerative disk disease of cervical spine. *Journal of the American Medical Association.* 1960;174(4):375–380.

Friedenberg ZB, Miller WT. Degenerative disc disease of the cervical spine. A comparative study of asymptomatic and symptomatic patients. *Journal of Bone and Joint Surgery.* 1963;45-A(6):1171–1178.

Gore DR, Sepic SB, Gardner GM. Roentgenographic findings of the cervical spine in asymptomatic people. *Spine.* 1986;11(6): 521–524.

Gore DR, Sepic SB, Gardner GM, Murray MP. Neck pain: a long-term follow-up of 205 patients. *Spine.* 1987;12(1):1–5.

Jensen OK, Justesen T, Nielsen FF, Brixen K. Functional radiographic examination of the cervical spine in patients with post-traumatic headache. *Cephalalgia.* 1990;10:295–303.

Juhl JH, Miller SM, Roberts GW. Roentgenographic variations in the normal cervical spine. *Radiology*. 1962;78:591–597.

Miller H, Brain R, Russell WR, O'Connell JEA. Discussion on cervical spondylosis. *Proceedings of the Royal Society of Medicine*. 1955;49: 197–208.

Oppenheimer A. Pathology, clinical manifestations and treatment of lesions of the intervertebral disks. *New England Journal of Medicine*. 1944;230(4):95–105.

Pallis C, Jones AM, Spillane JD. Cervical spondylosis. *Brain*. 1954;77: 274–289.

Pearce JMS. Whiplash injury: fact or fiction? *Headache Quarterly, Current Treatment and Research*. 1992;3:45–49.

Robinson DD, Cassar-Pullicino VN. Acute neck sprain after road traffic accident: a long-term clinical and radiological review. *Injury*. 1993; 24(2):79–82.

See also "Radiology of Whiplash" in Chapter 5.

Myth: Abnormalities detected by myelography explain the reporting of chronic symptoms by whiplash patients.

See Chapter 5. These two studies show that healthy subjects very often have the same myelogram abnormalities that are claimed to be causing pain in whiplash patients.

****

Hitselberger WE, Witten RM. Abnormal myelograms in asymptomatic patients. *Journal of Neurosurgery*. 1968;28:204–206.

Odom GL, Finney W, Woodhall B. Cervical disk lesions. *Journal of the American Medical Association*. 1958;166(1):23–28.

Myth: Abnormalities detected by discography explain the reporting of chronic symptoms by whiplash patients.

See Chapter 5. These studies show that healthy subjects very often have the same discography abnormalities that are claimed to be causing pain in whiplash patients.

****

Holt EP Jr. Fallacy of cervical discography. *Journal of the American Medical Association.* 1966;188(9):799–801.

Holt EP Jr. Further reflections on cervical discography. *Journal of the American Medical Association.* 1975;231(6):613–614.

Sneider SE, Winslow OP Jr, Pryor TH. Cervical diskography: is it relevant? *Journal of the American Medical Association.* 1963;185(3): 163–165.

Myth: Soft tissue injury such as ligament injury is undetectable by X-rays, so one cannot rule out significant ligament injury in whiplash patients as the cause of acute or chronic pain.

See Chapter 5. This is false because bone scans and magnetic resonance imaging are able to detect such injuries if they are significant, and the studies below found no evidence of such injury in whiplash patients reporting chronic pain.

****

Barton D, Allen M, Finlay D, Belton I. Evaluation of whiplash injuries by technetium 99^m isotope scanning. *Archives of Emergency Medicine.* 1993;10:197–202.

Hildingsson C, Hietala SO, Toolanen G. Scintigraphic findings in acute whiplash injury of the cervical spine. *Injury.* 1989;20:265–266.

Ronnen HR, de Korte PJ, Brink PRG, et al. Acute whiplash injury: is there a role for MR imaging? A prospective study of 100 patients. *Radiology.* 1996;201:93–96.

Myth: Abnormalities detected by magnetic resonance imaging explain the reporting of chronic symptoms by whiplash patients.

See Chapter 5. These magnetic resonance imaging studies show that abnormalities are no more common in whiplash patients than in healthy subjects.

****

Borchgrevink GE, Smevik O, Haave I, Lereim I, Haraldseth O. MRI of cerebrum and cervical column within two days after "whiplash" neck sprain injury. In: *Proceedings of the Society of Magnetic Resonance Third Scientific Meeting and Exhibition, 1995, August 19–25, Nice, France*. 1995:243.

Borchgrevink GE, Smevik O, Nordby A, et al. MR imaging and radiography of patients with cervical hyperextension-flexion injuries after car accidents. *Acta Radiologica*. 1995;36:425–428.

Fagerlund M, Björnebrink J, Pettersson K, Hildingsson C. MRI in acute phase of whiplash injury. *European Radiology*. 1995;5:297–301.

Karlsborg M, Smed A, Jespersen H, et al. A prospective study of 39 patients with whiplash injury. *Acta Neurologica Scandinavica*. 1997;95: 65–72.

Maimaris C. Neck sprains after car accidents [letter]. *British Medical Journal*. 1989;299:123.

Pearce JMS. Subtle cerebral lesions in "chronic whiplash syndrome"? [letter]. *Journal of Neurology, Neurosurgery, and Psychiatry*. 1993; 56(12):1328–1329.

Pettersson K, Hildingsson C, Toolanen G, Fagerlund M, Björnebrink J. MRI and neurology in acute whiplash trauma. No correlation in prospective examination of 39 cases. *Acta Orthopedica Scandinavica*. 1994;65(5):525–528.

Pettersson K, Hildingsson C, Toolanen G, Fagerlund M, Björnebrink J. Disc pathology after whiplash injury. A prospective magnetic resonance imaging clinical investigation. *Spine*. 1997;22:283–288.

Ronnen HR, de Korte PJ, Brink PRG, et al. Acute whiplash injury: is there a role for MR imaging? A prospective study of 100 patients. *Radiology*. 1996;201:93–96.

Teresi LM, Lufkin RB, Reicher MA, et al. Asymptomatic degenerative disk disease and spondylosis of the cervical spine: MR imaging. *Radiology*. 1987;164:83–88.

Yarnell PR, Rossie GV. Minor whiplash head injury with major debilitation. *Brain Injury*. 1988;2(3):255–258.

Myth: The abnormalities found on temporomandibular joint imaging are definitely signs of injury in whiplash patients and are always associated with pain.

See Chapter 6. Virtually all the abnormalities often claimed to be the source of temporomandibular disorder (TMD) in whiplash patients are found in healthy subjects quite often. Most of those patients with TMD claims had these abnormalities before the accident.

Some might argue that the accident "activates" a silent lesion, but then so too would chewing steak (the forces are the same, according to Howard et al). As well, it is quite likely that Lithuanians also have these abnormalities, yet they do not seem to have TMD after suffering acute neck sprain.

****

Ferrari R, Leonard M. Whiplash and temporomandibular disorders. *Journal of the American Dental Association*. 1998;129:1739–1745.

Muir CB, Goss AN. The radiologic morphology of asymptomatic temporomandibular joints. *Oral Surgery, Oral Medicine, Oral Pathology*. 1990;70:349–354.

Muir CB, Goss AN. The radiologic morphology of painful temporomandibular joints. *Oral Surgery, Oral Medicine, Oral Pathology*. 1990; 70:355–359.

Tasaki MM, Westesson PL, Isberg AM, Ren YF, Tallents RH. Classification and prevalence of temporomandibular joint disk displacement in patients and symptom-free volunteers. *American Journal of Orthodontics and Dentofacial Orthopedics*. 1996;109:249–262.

Westesson PL. Reliability and validity of imaging diagnosis of temporomandibular joint disorder. *Advances in Dental Research*. 1993; 7(2):137–151.

Westesson P, Eriksson L, Kurita K. Reliability of a negative clinical temporomandibular joint examination: prevalence of disk displacement in asymptomatic temporomandibular joints. *Oral Surgery, Oral Medicine, Oral Pathology*. 1989;68:551–554.

Westesson P, Eriksson L, Kurita K. Temporomandibular joint: variation of normal arthrographic anatomy. *Oral Surgery, Oral Medicine, Oral Pathology*. 1990;69:514–519.

Myth: Abnormalities detected by thermography explain the reporting of chronic symptoms by whiplash patients.

****

Awerbuch MS. Thermography—its current diagnostic status in musculoskeletal medicine. *Medical Journal of Australia.* 1991; 154:441–444.

Awerbuch MS. Thermography—wither the niche? *Medical Journal of Australia.* 1991;154:444–447.

Myth: Abnormalities detected by electroencephalography explain the reporting of chronic symptoms by whiplash patients.

See Chapter 7.

****

Ferrari R, Russell AS. Development of persistent neurological symptoms in patients with simple neck sprain. *Arthritis Care & Research.* 1999;12(1)70–76.

Gurdjian ES, Thomas LM, eds. *Neckache and Backache.* Springfield, IL: Charles C Thomas; 1970.

Jacome DE. EEG in whiplash: a reappraisal. *Clinical Electroencephalography.* 1987;18(1):41–45.

Jacome DE, Risko M. EEG features in post-traumatic syndrome. *Clinical Electroencephalography.* 1984;15(4):214–221.

Rowe MJ. Normal variability of the brain-stem auditory evoked response in young and old adult subjects. *Electroencephalography and Clinical Neurophysiology.* 1978;44:459–470.

Myth: Abnormalities on hearing, eye, and balance testing are evidence of nervous system injury in whiplash patients.

See Chapter 7.

****

Ferrari R, Russell AS. Development of persistent neurological symptoms in patients with simple neck sprain. *Arthritis Care & Research.* 1999;12(1)70–76.

Noseworthy JH, Miller J, Murray TJ, Regan D. Auditory brainstem response in postconcussion syndrome. *Archives of Neurology.* 1981;38: 275–278.

Pearce JMS. Subtle cerebral lesions in "chronic whiplash syndrome"? [letter]. *Journal of Neurology, Neurosurgery, and Psychiatry*. 1993; 56(12):1328–1329.

Stockard JJ, Stockard JE, Sharbrough FW. Nonpathologic factors influencing brainstem auditory evoked potentials. *American Journal of EEG Technology*. 1978;18:177–209.

Yarnell PR, Rossie GV. Minor whiplash head injury with major debilitation. *Brain Injury*. 1988;2(3):255–258.

Myth: Whiplash patients have a mild form of brain injury.

See Chapter 7 and the two reviews below.

****

Alexander MP. In the pursuit of proof of brain damage after whiplash injury. *Neurology*. 1998;51:336–340.

Ferrari R, Russell AS. Development of persistent neurological symptoms in patients with simple neck sprain. *Arthritis Care & Research*. 1999;12(1)70–76.

Myth: Whiplash patients have thoracic outlet syndrome or nerve compression in the neck and arm.

See Chapter 7.

****

Cherington M. A conservative point of view of the thoracic outlet syndrome. *American Journal of Surgery*. 1989;158:394–395.

Cherington M, Cherington C. Thoracic outlet syndrome: reimbursement patterns and patient profiles. *Neurology*. 1992;42:943–945.

Cuetter AC, Bartoszek DM. The thoracic outlet syndrome: controversies, overdiagnosis, overtreatment, and recommendations for management. *Muscle and Nerve*. 1989;12:410–419.

Daube JR. Nerve conduction studies in the thoracic outlet syndrome. *Neurology*. 1975;25:347.

Ferrari R, Russell AS. Development of persistent neurological symptoms in patients with simple neck sprain. *Arthritis Care & Research.* 1999;12(1)70–76.

Hachinski V. The thoracic outlet syndrome. *Archives of Neurology.* 1990;47:330.

Nelson DA. Thoracic outlet syndrome and dysfunction of the temporomandibular joint: proved pathology or pseudosyndromes? *Perspectives in Biology and Medicine.* 1990;33(4): 567–576.

Sanders RJ, Monsour JW, Gerber WF, Adams WR, Thompson N. Scalenectomy versus first rib resection for treatment of the thoracic outlet syndrome. *Surgery.* 1979;85(1):109–121.

Smith T, Trojaborg W. Diagnosis of thoracic outlet syndrome. *Archives of Neurology.* 1987;44:1161–1163.

Wilbourn AJ. Thoracic outlet syndrome surgery causing severe brachial plexopathy. *Muscle and Nerve.* 1988;11:66–74.

Wilbourn AJ. The thoracic outlet syndrome is overdiagnosed. *Archives of Neurology.* 1990;47:328–330.

Youmans JR. *Neurological Surgery.* Vol 4. 3rd ed. Philadelphia: WB Saunders; 1990.

Myth: The neck frequently undergoes hyperextension in low-velocity rear-end collisions.

The acute injury in low-velocity collisions, if there is one, does not appear to be through neck hyperextension. In many cases, one does not expect any injury at all.

****

Bailey M. Assessment of impact severity in minor motor vehicle collisions. *Journal of Musculoskeletal Pain.* 1996;4(4):21–38.

DuBois RA, McNally BF, DiGregorio JS, Phillips GJ. Low velocity car-to-bus test impacts. *Accident Reconstruction Journal.* 1996;8(5): 44–51.

Geigl BC, Steffan H, Leinzinger P, Roll, Mühlbauer M, Bauer G. The movement of head and cervical spine during rearend impact. In: *Pro-*

ceedings of the International IRCOBI Conference on the Biomechanics of Impact, 1994, Lyon, France. 127–137.

Gough JP. Human occupant dynamics in low-speed rear end collisions: an engineering perspective. *Journal of Musculoskeletal Pain.* 1996; 4(4):11–19.

Howard RP, Bowles AP, Guzman HM, Krenrich SW. Head, neck, and mandible dynamics generated by "whiplash." *Accident Prevention and Analysis.* 1998;30(4):525–534.

Matsushita T, Sato TB, Hirabayashi K, et al. X-ray study of the human neck motion due to head inertia loading. In: *Proceedings of the Thirty Eighth Stapp Car Crash Conference.* Paper #942208. Warrendale, PA: Society of Automotive Engineers; 1994:55–64.

McConnell WE, Howard RP, Guzman HM, et al. Analysis of human test subject kinematic responses to low velocity rear end impacts. In: *Proceedings of the Thirty Seventh Stapp Car Crash Conference.* Paper #930889. Warrendale, PA: Society of Automotive Engineers; 1993: 21–30.

McConnell WE, Howard RP, Van Poppel J, et al. Human head and neck kinematics after low velocity rear-end impacts—understanding "whiplash." In: *Proceedings of the Thirty Ninth Stapp Car Crash Conference.* Paper #952724. Warrendale, PA: Society of Automotive Engineers; 1995:215–238.

Nielsen GP, Gough JP, Little DM, West DH, Baker VT. Human subject responses to repeated low speed impacts using utility vehicles. In: *Proceedings of the Forty First Stapp Car Crash Conference.* Paper #970394. Warrendale, PA: Society of Automotive Engineers; 1997: 189–212.

Ono K, Kanno M. Influences of the physical parameters on the risk to neck injuries in low impact speed rear-end collisions. In: *Proceedings of the International IRCOBI Conference on the Biomechanics of Impacts, September 8–10, 1993, Eindhoven, Netherlands.* 1993:201–212.

Ono K, Kanno M. Influences of the physical parameters on the risk to neck injuries in low impact speed rear-end collisions. *Accident Analysis and Prevention.* 1996;28(4):493–499.

Rosenbluth W, Hicks L. Evaluating low-speed rear-end impact severity and resultant occupant stress parameters. *Journal of Forensics Sciences.* 1994;39(6):1393–1424.

Scott MW, McConnell WE, Guzman HM, et al. Comparison of human and ATD head kinematics during low-speed rearend impacts. In: *Proceedings of the Thirty Seventh Stapp Car Crash Conference.* Paper #930094. Warrendale, PA: Society of Automotive Engineers; 1993:1–8.

Siegmund GP, Bailey MN, King DJ. Characteristics of specific automobile bumpers in low-velocity impacts. In: *Proceedings of the Thirty Eighth Stapp Car Crash Conference.* Paper #940916. Warrendale, PA: Society of Automotive Engineers; 1994.

Siegmund GP, Williamson PB. Speed change (ΔV) of amusement park bumper cars. In: *Proceedings of the Canadian Multidisciplinary Road Safety Conference VIII, June 14–16, 1993, Saskatoon, Saskatchewan.* 1993:299–308.

Szabo TJ, Welcher J. Dynamics of low speed crash tests with energy absorbing bumpers. In: *Proceedings of the Thirty Sixth Stapp Car Crash Conference.* Paper #921573. Warrendale, PA: Society of Automotive Engineers; 1992:1367–1375.

Szabo TJ, Welcher JB, Anderson RD. Human occupant kinematic response to low speed rear-end impacts. In: *Proceedings of the Thirty Eighth Stapp Car Crash Conference.* Paper #940532. Warrendale, PA: Society of Automotive Engineers; 1994:23–35.

West DH, Gough JP, Harper GTK. Low speed rear-end collision testing using human subjects. *Accident Reconstruction Journal.* 1993;5(3): 22–26.

Myth: There is experimental evidence to show that rear-end collisions without direct jaw impact cause injury to the temporomandibular joint (TMJ).

See Chapter 6. When there is no blunt jaw impact, the forces on the TMJ are no greater than those in normal daily jaw activities.

****

Christensen LV, McKay DC. Reflex jaw motions and jaw stiffness pertaining to whiplash injury of the neck. *Journal of Craniomandibular Practice.* 1997;15(3):242–260.

Ferrari R, Leonard M. Whiplash and temporomandibular disorders. *Journal of the American Dental Association.* 1998;129:1739–1745.

Goldberg HL. Trauma and the improbable anterior displacement. *Journal of Craniomandibular Disorders: Facial and Oral Pain*. 1990;4(2): 131–134.

Heise AP, Laskin DM, Gervin AS. Incidence of temporomandibular joint symptoms following whiplash injury. *Journal of Oral and Maxillofacial Surgery*. 1992;50:825–828.

Howard RP, Benedict JV, Raddin JH, Smith HL. Assessing neck extension-flexion as a basis for temporomandibular joint dysfunction. *Journal of Oral and Maxillofacial Surgery*. 1991;49:1210–1213.

Howard RP, Bowles AP, Guzman HM, Krenrich SW. Head, neck, and mandible dynamics generated by "whiplash." *Accident Prevention and Analysis*. 1998;30(4):525–534.

Howard RP, Hatsell CP, Guzman HM. Temporomandibular joint injury potential imposed by the low-velocity extension-flexion maneuver. *Journal of Oral and Maxillofacial Surgery*. 1995;53:256–262.

Kirk WS Jr. Whiplash as a basis for TMJ dysfunction. *Journal of Oral and Maxillofacial Surgery*. 1992;50:427–428.

Kupperman A. Whiplash and disc derangement [letter]. *Journal of Oral and Maxillofacial Surgery*. 1988;46(6):519.

Olin M. Components of complex TM disorders. *Journal of Craniomandibular Disorders: Facial and Oral Pain*. 1990;4(3):193–196.

Roydhouse RH. Whiplash and temporomandibular dysfunction [letter]. *Lancet*. June 1973:1394–1395.

Small EW. An investigation into the psychogenic bases of the temporomandibular joint myofascial pain dysfunction syndrome. *Advances in Pain Research and Therapy*. 1976;1:889–894.

Szabo TJ, Welcher JB, Anderson RD. Human occupant kinematic response to low speed rear-end impacts. In: *Proceedings of the Thirty Eighth Stapp Car Crash Conference*. Paper #940532. Warrendale, PA: Society of Automotive Engineers; 1994:23–35.

West DH, Gough JP, Harper GTK. Low speed rear-end collision testing using human subjects. *Accident Reconstruction Journal*. 1993;5(3): 22–26.

Myth: Women get whiplash more often than men because they have longer necks, thinner necks, and weaker neck muscles.

This has never been proven, and a study by C. J. Kahane (1982) showed that evidence exists that head restraints should offer even more protection for women than they do for men. Head restraints, even in the down position, would be high enough for most women, as they are actually designed for men.

****

Kahane CJ. *Evaluation of Head Restraints: Federal Motor Vehicle Safety Standard 202*. Washington, DC: National Highway Traffic Safety Administration, Office of Program Evaluation; 1982.

O'Neill B, Haddon W Jr, Kelley AB, Sorenson WW. Automobile head restraints—frequency of neck injury claims in relation to the presence of head restraints. *American Journal of Public Health*. March 1972: 399–406.

West DH, Gough JP, Harper GTK. Low speed rear-end collision testing using human subjects. *Accident Reconstruction Journal*. 1993;5(3): 22–26.

Myth: Head restraints will prevent reporting of chronic symptoms only if users adjust them to the appropriate height.

****

Kahane CJ. *Evaluation of Head Restraints: Federal Motor Vehicle Safety Standard 202*. Washington, DC: National Highway Traffic Safety Administration, Office of Program Evaluation; 1982.

Lövsund P, Nygren A, Salen B, Tingvall C. Neck injuries in rear end collisions among front and rear seat occupants. In: *Proceedings of the International IRCOBI Conference on the Biomechanics of Impacts, 1988, September 14–16, Bergisch, Gladbach, Germany, Bron, France*. 1988:319–325.

Schrader H, Obelieniene D, Bovim G, et al. Natural evolution of late whiplash syndrome outside the medicolegal context. *Lancet*. 1996; 347:1207–1211.

Thomas C, Faverjon G, Hartemann F, et al. Protection against rear-end accidents. In: *Proceedings of the International Research Council on the Biomechanics of Impacts (IRCOBI) Conference, Bron, France*. 1982: 17–29.

See also Chapter 22.

Myth: Experiments using human volunteers reproduce the reporting of chronic symptoms following acute whiplash injury.

See Chapter 5 and any article reporting whiplash experiments. All have failed to produce a subject reporting chronic symptoms, even though subjects frequently suffer the acute injury.

Myth: The head accelerations encountered in typical collisions that produce whiplash patients are sufficient to cause significant muscle, ligament, and disc damage.

See Chapter 5. Actually, in virtually all cases of Grade 1 or 2 whiplash-associated disorder, the injury must necessarily be a minor muscle or ligament sprain. Otherwise, the available studies would have detected more damage than this. Recall also that in Germany, Greece, and Lithuania, the whiplash injury must be a minor injury to have such a good outcome. There is no reason to conclude that most whiplash patients in those countries somehow avoid the more severe injuries.

The studies below (summarized in Chapter 20) show that volunteers do not have serious injury despite experiencing the same or higher accelerations than most whiplash patients. These volunteers suffer from days to weeks of symptoms.

****

Gadd CW, Culver CC. A study of responses and tolerances of the neck. In: *Proceedings of the Fifteenth Stapp Car Crash Conference.* Warrendale, PA: Society of Automotive Engineers; 1971:256.

Kallieris D, Schmidt G. Neck response and injury assessment using cadavers and the US-SID for far-side lateral impacts of rear seat occupants with inboard-anchored shoulder belts. In: *Proceedings of the Thirty Fourth Stapp Car Crash Conference.* Paper #902313. Warrendale, PA: Society of Automotive Engineers; 1990:93–99.

Lange W. Mechanical and physiological response of the human cervical vertebral column to severe impacts applied to the torso. In: *Symposium on Biodynamic Models and Their Applications, Wright-Patterson Air Force Base, Ohio.* 1970:141.

McElhaney JH, Myers BS. Biomechanical aspects of cervical trauma. In: Nahum AM, Melvin JW, eds. *Accidental Injury. Biomechanics and Prevention.* New York: Springer-Verlag; 1993:323–325.

Patrick LM. Studies of hyperextension and hyperflexion injury in volunteers and human cadavers. In: Gurdjian ES, Thomas LM, eds. *Neckache and Backache.* Springfield, IL: Charles C Thomas; 1970:92–119.

Sances A Jr, Myklebust J, Cusick JF, et al. Experimental studies of brain and neck injuries. In: *Proceedings of the Twenty Fifth Stapp Car Crash Conference.* Paper #811032. Warrendale, PA: Society of Automotive Engineers; 1981:149–194.

Sances A Jr, Myklebust J, Kostreva D, et al. Pathophysiology of cervical injuries. In: *Proceedings of the Twenty Sixth Stapp Car Crash Conference.* Paper #821153. Warrendale, PA: Society of Automotive Engineers; 1982:41–90.

Sances A Jr, Weber RC, Larson SJ, et al. Bioengineering analysis of head and spine injuries. *Critical Reviews in Biomedical Engineering.* 1981;5:79–118.

Szabo TJ, Welcher J. Dynamics of low speed crash tests with energy absorbing bumpers. In: *Proceedings of the Thirty Sixth Stapp Car Crash Conference.* Paper #921573. Warrendale, PA: Society of Automotive Engineers; 1992:1367–1375.

Myth: One can expect a physical injury in rear-end collisions that are associated with velocity changes in the struck vehicle of 8 to 10 km/h (4.8–6.0 mph) or less, or frontal or lateral collisions that are associated with velocity changes in the struck vehicle of 16 to 20 km/h (10–12 mph) or less.

No. These are the rock-bottom threshold levels. Even in such cases, the symptoms in volunteers are so minor they last for only a few hours. The probability of actual injury below these thresholds is very low, and other explanations for symptoms become much more probable. See Chapter 5 and Chapter 20.

****

Bailey M. Assessment of impact severity in minor motor vehicle collisions. *Journal of Musculoskeletal Pain.* 1996;4(4):21–38.

Gough JP. Human occupant dynamics in low-speed rear end collisions: an engineering perspective. *Journal of Musculoskeletal Pain.* 1996; 4(4):11–19.

Myth(?): Seat belts increase the risk of reporting chronic symptoms after an accident.

See Chapter 22.

Myth: The mechanism of neck injury due to seat belts is by increased forces of neck flexion. These forces have been shown to produce serious neck injury in human experiments.

Numerous studies below have shown that these forces produce only minor injury with weeks of symptoms or no symptoms at all, even though the volunteers are subjected to extreme neck flexion. Also see Chapter 22.

****

Ewing CL, Thomas DJ, Beeler GW Jr, et al. Dynamic response of the head and neck of the living human to -Gx impact acceleration. In: *Proceedings of the Twelfth Stapp Car Crash Conference.* Paper #680792. Warrendale, PA: Society of Automotive Engineers; 1968:424–439.

Ewing CL, Thomas DJ, Patrick LM, Beeler GW Jr, Smith MJ. Dynamic response of the head and neck of the living human to -Gx impact acceleration—II. In: *Proceedings of the Thirteenth Stapp Car Crash Conference.* Paper #690817. Warrendale, PA: Society of Automotive Engineers; 1969:400–415.

Grunsten RC, Gilbert NS, Mawn SV. The mechanical effects of impact acceleration on the unconstrained human head and neck complex. *Contemporary Orthopaedics.* 1989;18(2):199–202.

Lange W. Mechanical and physiological response of the human cervical vertebral column to severe impacts applied to the torso. In: *Symposium on Biodynamic Models and Their Applications, Wright-Patterson Air Force Base, Ohio.* 1970:141.

Mertz HJ, Patrick LM. Strength and response of the human neck. In: *Proceedings of the Fifteenth Stapp Car Crash Conference.* Paper

#710855. Warrendale, PA: Society of Automotive Engineers; 1971: 2903–2928.

Patrick LM. Studies of hyperextension and hyperflexion injury in volunteers and human cadavers. In: Gurdjian ES, Thomas LM, eds. *Neckache and Backache.* Springfield, IL: Charles C Thomas; 1970:92–119.

Tarriere C, Sapin C. Biokinetic study of the head to thorax linkage. In: *Proceedings of the Thirteenth Stapp Car Crash Conference.* Warrendale, PA: Society of Automotive Engineers; 1969:365.

Myth: It is impossible for peer copying, cultural factors, patient expectation, and public attention to create an environment where accident victims attribute chronic symptoms to an acute injury.

****

Aubrey JB, Dobbs AR, Rule BG. Laypersons' knowledge about the sequelae of minor head injury and whiplash. *Journal of Neurology, Neurosurgery, and Psychiatry.* 1989;52:842–846.

Champion GD. Whiplash in Australia: illness or injury? [letter]. *Medical Journal of Australia.* 1992;157:574.

Ford CV. *The Somatizing Disorders. Illness as a Way of Life.* New York: Elsevier Biomedical; 1983.

Livingston M. Whiplash injury: misconceptions and remedies. *Australian Family Physician.* 1992;21(11):1642–1644.

Mittenberg W, DiGiulio DV, Perrin S, Bass AE. Symptoms following mild head injury: expectation as aetiology. *Journal of Neurology, Neurosurgery, and Psychiatry.* 1992;55:200–204.

Myth: Whiplash is commonly seen in all parts of the world where automobile accidents are common.

****

Balla JI. The late whiplash syndrome: a study of an illness in Australia and Singapore. *Culture, Medicine and Psychiatry.* 1982;6:191–210.

Bonk A, Giebel GD, Edelmann M, Huser R. Whiplash outcome in Germany. *Journal of Rheumatology*. 1999. In press.

Ferrari R, Russell AS. Epidemiology of whiplash—an international dilemma. *Annals of Rheumatic Diseases*. 1999;58:1–5.

Livingston M. Whiplash injury: misconceptions and remedies. *Australian Family Physician*. 1992;21(11):1642–1644.

Mills H, Horne G. Whiplash—manmade disease. *New Zealand Medical Journal*. 1986;99:373–374.

Obelieniene D, Schrader H, Bovim G, et al. Pain after whiplash—a prospective controlled inception cohort study. *Journal of Neurology, Neurosurgery, and Psychiatry*. 1999;66:279–284.

Partheni M, Miliaras G, Constantoyannis C, Voulgaris S, Spiropoulou P, Papadakis P. Whiplash rate of recovery in Greece. *Journal of Rheumatology*. 1999. In press.

Schrader H, Obelieniene D, Bovim G, et al. Natural evolution of late whiplash syndrome outside the medicolegal context. *Lancet*. 1996; 347:1207–1211.

Myth: Other forms of trauma to soft tissues of the neck often lead to reporting of chronic pain.

The first two articles below are from a surgical point of view, wherein the surgeon does a great deal that injures soft tissues during surgery, yet chronic pain is not a result. Why? The third article is an example of how neck movements and sprains outside the medicolegal context do not result in chronic neck pain.

****

Dinning TAR. Whiplash in Australia: illness or injury? [letter]. *Medical Journal of Australia*. 1993;158:138, 140.

Fleming JFR. The neurosurgeon's responsibility in "whiplash" injuries. *Clinical Neurosurgery*. 1973;20:242–252.

Kassirer MR, Manon N. Head banger's whiplash. *Clinical Journal of Pain*. 1993;9:138–141.

CHAPTER 18

Whiplash Timelines

How did the whiplash dilemma evolve over the years? In reality, its evolution was in part determined by events many years ago and only accelerated in the last part of the twentieth century.

HISTORIC TIMELINE

1866 J. E. Erichsen gives lectures on railway spine as an injury and publishes his famous text in the following year.

1886 J. E. Erichsen publishes his theory of spinal concussion as the cause of railway spine, with no evidence to support his theory.

1888 A. Strümpell explains railway spine as a traumatic neurosis rather than a physical injury.

1900–1930 Traumatic neurosis replaces railway spine as the diagnostic term.

1928 H. E. Crowe coins the term "whiplash injury" for automobile accident victims reporting chronic neck pain. Medical community apparently unaware of history lesson from railway spine.

1943 Article by H. W. Smith and H. C. Solomon to attempt to resolve the issue of compensation for traumatic neurosis.

1945 A. G. Davis publishes article explaining whiplash and its cause, with no evidence provided. He is also the first to state that a straight cervical spine on neck X-ray is the sign of injury, again with no proof.

1946–1998 More than 100 articles propose theories about the source of chronic damage after the acute injury that is supposedly responsible for whiplash patients' reporting of chronic symptoms. In these articles, authors consider many sources of the damage, including everything between the head and the buttocks.

1955–1998 There are hundreds of experimental collisions, none of which lead to a subject reporting chronic symptoms after the acute injury.

1996, 1999   German, Greek, and Lithuanian accident victims behave exactly like volunteers in experimental collisions, suffering acute injury but not reporting chronic pain thereafter.

RADIOLOGIC TIMELINE

1953   J. R. Gay and K. H. Abbott proclaim that neck X-rays show the whiplash injury.

1953   A. Myers states the belief that whiplash injury can cause degenerative disc disease.

1955–1998   Several studies show that whiplash does not cause disc degeneration or accelerate the changes of disc degeneration as seen on X-rays. Also, several studies show poor correlation between symptoms and changes on neck X-rays.

1958   G. L. Odom et al show poor correlation between myelogram findings and symptoms.

1958–1962   A number of studies prove that findings on neck X-ray of changes in cervical lordosis are not a sign of whiplash injury.

1963   S. E. Sneider et al show that discography does not reveal any chronic neck damage that arises from the acute injury to be responsible for chronic symptom reporting.

1966   E. P. Holt Jr also shows that discography does not reveal any chronic neck damage that arises from the acute injury to be responsible for chronic symptom reporting.

1968   W. E. Hitselberger and R. M. Witten show that myelography does not reveal any chronic neck damage that arises from the acute injury to be responsible for chronic symptom reporting.

1987–1998   A number of studies show that magnetic resonance imaging does not reveal any chronic neck damage that arises from the acute injury to be responsible for chronic symptom reporting.

1989, 1993   C. Hildingsson et al and then D. Barton et al show that bone scans do not reveal any chronic neck damage that arises from the acute injury to be responsible for chronic symptom reporting.

1995–1998   A. Otte et al show that positron emission tomography (PET) and single photon emission tomography (SPECT) scans do not reveal evidence of brain injury in whiplash patients.

NEUROLOGIC TIMELINE

1960   S. K. Shapiro and F. Torres find abnormal electroencephalograms (EEGs) in whiplash patients.

1970	E. S. Gurdjian and L. M. Thomas find normal EEGs in whiplash patients.
1971	F. A. Gibbs explains that such abnormalities are mild and commonly found in the general population.
1978	M. J. Rowe shows that brainstem auditory evoked potentials (BAEPs) frequently have mild abnormalities in the general population.
1979	K. H. Chappa et al show that BAEPs are not useful in finding the "whiplash injury."
1982	P. Benna et al reach similar conclusions as above.
1984	D. E. Jacome and M. Risko find normal EEGs in whiplash patients.
1988–1997	A number of clinical studies fail to find evidence of brain injury in whiplash patients.
1990	J. R. Youmans explains why nerve conduction studies do not reveal any chronic neck damage that supposedly arises from the acute injury and is responsible for chronic symptom reporting.
1992	T. M. Ettlin et al find normal EEGs in whiplash patients.
1995–1998	A. Otte et al show that PET and SPECT scans do not reveal evidence of brain injury in whiplash patients.

TIMELINE OF EXPERIMENTS

1955	D. M. Severy et al show that a dummy head hyperextends in rear-end collisions, but the study cannot produce chronic symptom reporting in the human volunteer.
1963	J. Wickstrom et al kill hares using head accelerations about 10 to 50 times greater than those in collisions producing whiplash patients.
1964	I. MacNab conducts his monkey-dropping experiments.
1967	H. J. Mertz and L. M. Patrick show that head restraints eliminate neck hyperextension. They also show that even in experiments with no head restraints, human volunteers report no chronic symptoms.
1968	A. K. Ommaya et al cause brain damage in monkeys with accelerations 10 times greater than those in collisions producing whiplash patients.
1971–1998	Decades of experimental collisions with human volunteers fail to produce a subject reporting chronic symptoms after the acute injury.

1993–1998   A number of experiments with low-velocity collisions fail to produce even acute injury when the change in velocity of the struck vehicle is less than 8 km/h.

1992–1998   L. V. Christensen and D. C. McKay, R. P. Howard et al, T. J. Szabo et al, and D. H. West et al demonstrate that temporomandibular joint forces in rear-end collisions with no direct jaw impact are insufficient to cause injury.

1994   M. E. Allen et al show that everyday events (eg, sneezing or plopping into a chair) involve forces on the head and neck that are as great as the forces in low-velocity collisions reportedly producing whiplash patients.

In Search of the Whiplash Injury

1945	posterior intervertebral joints
1953	cervical ligaments
1953	intervertebral discs
1956	anterior cervical ligaments
1956	autonomic nervous system
1956	fibrous neck tissue
1956	sympathetic nervous system
1957	frontal lobe of brain
1958	cervical nerve roots
1958	deep fascia of neck
1958	vertebral nerve
1962	brainstem
1962	vertebral artery
1964	osteopathic greater lesion complex
1965	thoracic outlet
1994	facet (or zygapophysial) joints

Over the years since, authors have considered the following other sites:

- any aspect of the spinal cord
- auditory ossicles
- basilar artery
- facet joints of the spine
- labyrinth of the inner ear
- lumbar spine discs and nerves
- neck muscles
- occipital lobe of brain
- occiptial nerve
- oculomotor nerve

- ophthalmic artery
- parietal lobe of brain
- petrosal nerve
- temporomandibular joints
- thoracic spine discs and nerves
- trigeminal nerve

CHAPTER 20

Whiplash Experiments

Human experiments into whiplash began in 1955. D. M. Severy et al placed dummies (and humans) in cars being struck at velocities up to 27 mph. Accelerometers documented accelerations up to $7g$ to the car and up to $12g$ for the human and dummy heads. The cars had no head restraints, and engineers used specialized photography to document the head movements. Severy et al were able to confirm by high-speed photography that extension of the neck did indeed occur first, then flexion.

The greater degree of extension of the neck that they demonstrated, however, was only in the dummy, whose neck structure is not at all similar to a human neck, other than being attached to the head at one end and the torso at the other. As well, Severy noted that the dummy could slide up the seat back and then extend its neck. Some claim this is why head restraints may not be preventing whiplash. As later whiplash experiments would show, for many of the typical collision severities that produce whiplash claimants, this type of movement does not occur, especially with seat belt use. One can thus see the danger of using data from a nonhuman study to support a theoretical argument. One cannot expect the results of whiplash experiments with dummies to override those done with humans. One should not apply data from one population (dummies) to another population (humans).

Severy's data also gave an index of the maximum accelerations to the head and neck for impact velocities up to 8.2 mph (13.0 km/h): accelerations of $2.0g$ on the struck car at this velocity caused acceleration of $5.0g$ of the head in hyperextension. No symptoms occurred at the accelerations of 2.9 to $8.0g$ experienced by the volunteer.

Then, in 1967, H. J. Mertz Jr and L. M. Patrick conducted a series of controlled automobile rear-end collisions done with a human volunteer to measure the actual head acceleration. Patrick himself was the volunteer subject of their experiments.

Patrick summarized the results in a text (E. S. Gurdjian and L. M. Thomas 1970), beginning with hyperflexion.

> The subjects used for the dynamic flexion test were a human volunteer . . . and four human cadavers. . . . The kinematics of the head of each subject were obtained from accelerometers which were attached to their heads . . . [a] bite plate . . . [and] the first thoracic vertebra. . . . The volunteer . . . was subjected to 46 . . . runs of various degrees of severity. . . . During these tests, the volunteer attempted to achieve two different degrees of initial muscle tenseness: relaxed and tense. For the relaxed condition, the volunteer relaxed all of his muscles insofar as he was able to do so. . . . For the runs with his muscles tensed, the volunteer tensed his muscles as completely as possible during the entire run.
>
> With his muscles tensed, the volunteer was subjected to sled rides from 1.9–6.8 g . . . 9.6 g level [peak of 14.0 g, for] his most severe exposure. This run . . . resulted in a pain in the neck and back which lasted for several days [only].

Researchers conducted a total of 132 hyperflexion runs with human cadavers. To cause noticeable ligamentous or muscle damage in cadaver cervical spines, the required flexion forces from head accelerations were in excess of 20g.

Researchers then subjected human volunteers and cadavers to hyperextension experiments with head restraints in place. The human volunteer underwent 10 mph (17 km/h), 23 mph (38 km/h), and 44 mph (73 km/h) collisions. The volunteer experienced no symptoms with peak head accelerations of 7, 12, and 28g, respectively. Researchers also subjected the human volunteer to the 10 mph collision without symptoms despite not using a head restraint.

Additional studies in 1971 by Mertz and Patrick also failed to produce symptoms or injury in either hyperflexion or hyperextension using similar forces to those above. In 1979, D. J. Thomas et al reviewed the largest collection of such experiments in humans. They reviewed 1,621 experimental collisions with 62 humans resulting in head accelerations of greater than 16g (greater than some of the collisions producing whiplash patients), with no head restraints. Researchers used a variety of impact directions.

Adding to this, the experiments by C. L. Ewing et al, C. W. Gadd and C. C. Culver, W. Lange, C. Tarriere and C. Sapin, and J. Wismans et al show clearly that symptoms from injury are unlikely to occur with collisions that involve head accelerations of less than 12g.

Another theory that some have considered, however, is that the whiplash injury is not due necessarily to forces from neck hyperflexion or hyperextension but possibly from lateral (side-to-side) flexion (bending the neck with the ear reaching toward the shoulder), or a combination of such forces. Several researchers have, however, ruled out this possibility. The lateral forces experienced in typical rear-end collisions producing whiplash patients are much smaller than those from the rear. Yet one considers that they could still produce injury, because the neck may be more vulnerable from that direction.

The magnitude of such lateral accelerations involved in typical rear-end or frontal collisions producing whiplash patients may be quite low (less than 3g). Ewing et al (1977) conducted their own experiment and cite others (R. C. Grunsten et al 1989, E. B. Weis et al 1963, J. P. Stapp et al 1964 and 1971, A. V. Zaborowski et al 1966) using accelerations of 5 to 10 times this amount, applied fully on the head and neck from the side, forcing lateral flexion to occur. Despite these very high accelerations, no experiment with animals or humans has resulted in evidence of injury. In 1987, F. Bendjellal et al noted the same findings. One would expect high lateral head accelerations only if the impact is from the side when the accident victim is looking forward, or looking to the side and hit from the rear. In any case, experiments simulating these higher forces in living humans did not lead to an individual reporting chronic pain.

ACCELERATIONS AND FORCES

Tables 20–1 through 20–4 compare the accelerations and forces experienced by vehicle occupants or animals in whiplash experiments to those accelerations and forces experienced by whiplash patients. The accelerations are those affecting the head and/or neck complex.

One requires a number of calculations and extraction of data for some of these articles, since not all authors report their results in the same units or manner. The references to each study below the tables deal with this in part. Some articles do not give all the information needed to fill all sections of the tables.

A full treatment of the physics involved in collisions and tissue injury cannot take place here. Some understanding is useful because it is too easy for others to mislead or be misunderstood when quoting the literature of whiplash experiments. Some misuse the data to impress everyone about how great the forces were, whereas others may try to minimize this impression. Insurance companies frequently look at how big the dent is on the car and feel that the patient's pain should be comparable. The relationship between what happens to the vehicle occupant and the amount of car damage is very complex. The injuries sustained depend on many more variables than the size of the dent.

The discussion below may help to make this complex matter more easily understood.

First, the head acceleration may occur along three axes—the X, Y, and Z axes. In plain terms, when the subject is upright, the X axis is along a horizontal line passing from the subject's nose to the back of the skull. Some also call this an an-

TABLES 20–1 TO 20–4 NOTATIONS

N/A Not applicable. This refers to the fact that some experiments were not studying events that required a head restraint or in which a head restraint would affect outcome.

* The velocity, in km/h, is that of the *striking vehicle* only. For vehicles of relatively similar mass, the resultant velocity and accelerations of the *struck vehicle* are always less than the velocity of the *striking vehicle*. Many articles do not quote ΔV, but they do quote the head acceleration, which still allows one to appreciate the collision severity in relation to known thresholds in human volunteers. Striking vehicle velocity was converted to km/h in some cases. Multiply by 0.6 to convert km/h to mph. There is no linear relationship between collision velocity and head acceleration. When collision velocities increase beyond a certain level, the head and neck acceleration may actually decrease.

** One can estimate the head and neck accelerations (and, subsequently, the forces) from many of these articles, depending on the type of vehicle and velocity in question. D. M. Severy et al, for example, found typical collisions produced accelerations of 5.0 to 8.0g. Thus, the value of 20g represents the higher range of head and neck acceleration for collisions producing whiplash patients and may exceed that experienced by most whiplash patients.

† The acceleration reported is for the vehicle occupant's head, measured at various sites in the head and neck complex. The acceleration comes from the information in the articles quoted. Striking vehicle velocities are not available or not applicable in some of the entries below. The tables show peak accelerations.

+ In the animal experiments, the table shows forces to appreciate comparisons between animals and whiplash patients. That is, the same head acceleration leads to lower force in animals, as they have lower head masses. One derives forces by multiplying the head mass by the acceleration, then multiplying this by 9.8 to obtain a force in N.

++ The study gives 26g accelerations for the sled, which means the head and neck acceleration may be higher than 26g.

†† The researchers detected and defined the extent of damage in cadaver and animal studies in varied ways, from detailed dissection to gross assessment of ligament laxity by bone position on X-ray.

  The tables divide the whiplash experiments into those using animals, those using cadavers, and those using living humans. The experiments are arranged in chronological order in the tables and in the legend below. For each experiment, comparison figures for collisions that produce whiplash patients are shown.

Table 20–1 Whiplash Experiments—Animals

Study	Impact Velocity (km/h)*	Impact Direction	Acceleration (gs)†	Head and Neck Mass (kg)+	Head and Neck Forces (N)+	Results††	Head Restraint
Collisions producing whiplash patients	3–60	Varied	2.0–20**	5.5	108–1,078	Whiplash patients	Varied
Wickstrom et al[1]		Rear	153–218	1.0	1,499–2,136	No evidence of injury on autopsy	No
Wickstrom et al[2]	58–108	Rear	17–46	3.0	500–1,352	Injury only at the higher range of forces	No
Wickstrom et al[3]	58–108	Rear	17–46	3.0	500–1,352	No injury on autopsy	Yes
Unterharnscheidt[4]		Front	10–63	1.0	98–617	No injury on autopsy	No
Liu et al[5]		Rear and front	50–70	1.0	490–686	Minimal injury	No

[1]Wickstrom J, Martinez JL, Johnston D, Tappen NC. Acceleration-deceleration injuries of the cervical spine in animals. In: *Proceedings of the Seventh Stapp Car Crash Conference*; Warrendale, PA: Charles C Thomas; 1963:284–301.
Researchers subjected the hares to hyperextension forces and performed autopsy at various times for different hares. See pages 294–296 for forces.

[2]Wickstrom JK, Martinez JL, Rodriguez R Jr, Haines DM. Hyperextension and hyperflexion injuries to the head and neck of primates. In: Gurdjian ES, Thomas LM, eds. *Neckache and Backache*. Springfield, IL: Charles C Thomas; 1970:108–117.
Nonhuman primates undergo hyperextension. The collision velocity is an estimate by the authors of this article.

continues

Table 20-1 continued

[3]Wickstrom JK, Martinez JL, Rodriguez R Jr, Haines DM, 110.
Researchers tested the benefit of head restraints on these primates to see if any injury could be produced. The authors in this article estimate the collision velocity to be between 35 and 65 mph (58 to 108 km/h).

[4]Unterharnscheidt F. Traumatic alterations in the rhesus monkey undergoing -Gx impact acceleration. *Neurotraumatology*, 1983;6:151–167.
This study showed that no injury could be produced in frontal collision unless head and neck accelerations exceed 64g.

[5]Liu YK, Chandran KB, Heath RG, Unterharnscheidt F. Subcortical EEG changes in rhesus monkeys following experimental hyperextension-hyperflexion (whiplash). *Spine*. 1984;9(4):329–338.
This study of monkeys undergoing hyperextension and hyperflexion reveals that only 33% developed some minor electroencephalogram (EEG) abnormality despite forces of up to 686 N on the head and neck. Such forces may be much higher than those in typical collisions producing whiplash patients. Nevertheless, the abnormalities were minor and short-lived.
One assumes the head and neck mass to be approximately 1.0 kg, and the sled acceleration of 35g may correspond to a higher value for the head and neck of up to 60g.

Table 20–2 Whiplash Experiments—Cadavers

Study	Impact Velocity (km/h)*	Impact Direction	Acceleration (g)†	Results††	Head Restraint
Collisions producing whiplash patients	3–60	Varied	2.0–20**	Whiplash patients	Varied
Tarriere and Sapin[1]		Front	Up to 20	No injury	No
Tarriere and Sapin[2]	17–38	Rear		No injury, except at highest velocity	No
Lange[3]		Rear	26++	Significant ligament injury	No
Lange[4]		Rear	19	Minor disc injury	No
Lange[5]		Front	>40	Significant disc and ligament injury	No
Lange[6]		Front	39	No evidence of injury	No
Lange[7]		Rear	12	No evidence of injury	No
Gadd and Culver[8]		Side		Minimal injury	No
Clemens and Burow[9]		Rear and front	50–100	Injury	No
	19–25		20–36	Injury	No
Hu et al[10]	51	Rear	455	Fractures	No
Wismans et al[11]	61	Front	30	No symptoms in living humans	No
Kallieris and Schmidt[12]	50	Side	18	Muscle injury with minor symptoms in living humans	No

continues

Table 20-2 continued

Kallieris et al[13]	50	Front and side	18.5–20.9	Muscle injury	No
Panjabi et al[14]		Rear	10.5	Minor ligament sprain	No

[1]Tarriere C, Sapin C. Biokinetic study of the head to thorax linkage. In: *Proceedings of the Thirteenth Stapp Car Crash Conference.* Society of Automotive Engineers; 1969:365.
Hyperflexion studies in cadavers show that ligament damage does not occur until accelerations greater than 20g are used.

[2]Tarriere C, Sapin C, 102.
The cadavers undergo hyperextension without head restraint. One cadaver underwent 23 mph (38 km/h) collisions with no injury, and the other underwent the same collision but had minor ligamentous injury.
The authors of the article make the important note that the cadavers had no muscle resistance to the forces and were elderly, so that the experiment results underestimate the tolerable forces for a younger, living human.

[3]Lange W. Mechanical and physiological response of the human cervical vertebral column to severe impacts applied to the torso. In: *Symposium on Biodynamic Models and Their Applications, Wright-Patterson Air Force Base, Ohio.* 1970:141.
Hyperextension studies with cadavers show that head and neck accelerations greater than 30g are necessary to cause ligament damage without head restraints and that no damage will occur at this acceleration with head restraints.

[4]Lange W.
Hyperextension studies with cadavers.

[5]Lange W.
Hyperflexion studies with cadavers show that disk and ligament damage occurs with accelerations greater than 50g.

[6]Lange W, 2924.
This study used four cadavers in a total of 132 runs to try to discover the upper limit of tolerable forces in neck hyperflexion. None of the hyperflexion studies produce any observable neck damage at accelerations as high as 30g.

[7]Lange W, 2927.

[8]Gadd CW, Culver CC. A study of responses and tolerances of the neck. In: *Proceedings of the Fifteenth Stapp Car Crash Conference.* Warrendale, PA: Society of Automotive Engineers; 1971:256.

456

In lateral flexion studies, there is no damage to the head and neck with accelerations up to 5g in cadavers. Recall that lateral accelerations (that is, along the Y axis) are usually less than 3g in typical rear-end collisions producing whiplash claimants.

[9]Clemens HJ, Burow K. Experimental investigation on injury mechanisms of cervical spine at frontal and rear-front vehicle impacts. In: *Proceedings of the Sixteenth Stapp Car Crash Conference.* Paper #720960. Warrendale, PA: Society of Automotive Engineers; 1972:76–102.
Using cadavers and subjecting them to front- and rear-end collisions, researchers cause damage with accelerations of 50 to 100g (page 81) in front-end collisions and 20 to 36g in rear-end collisions.
These accelerations generally exceed those in typical collisions producing whiplash patients.

[10]Hu AS, Bean SP, Zimmerman RM. Response of belted dummy and cadaver to rear impact. In: *Proceedings of the Twenty First Stapp Car Crash Conference.* Paper #770929. Warrendale, PA: Society of Automotive Engineers; 1977:589–625.
This study subjects human cadavers to extreme accelerations of up to 400g (pages 604 and 619). This produced fractures in some cases.

[11]Wismans J, Philippens M, van Oorschot E, Kallieris D, Mattern R. Comparison of human volunteer and cadaver head-neck response in frontal flexion. In: *Proceedings of the Thirty First Stapp Car Crash Conference.* Paper #872194. Warrendale, PA: Society of Automotive Engineers; 1987:1–11.

[12]Kallieris D, Schmidt G. Neck response and injury assessment using cadavers and the US-SID for far-side lateral impacts of rear seat occupants with inboard-anchored shoulder belts. In: *Proceedings of the Thirty Fourth Stapp Car Crash Conference.* Paper #902313. Warrendale, PA: Society of Automotive Engineers; 1990:93–99.
Cadavers undergo lateral (side) impacts, with accelerations of 18.0g causing muscle damage.
Note, however, that these accelerations are along the Y axis and not the X axis, as occurs in rear-end collisions producing whiplash claimants. There were high accelerations from side impacts, accelerations that whiplash patients cannot experience in the same magnitude, unless the collision is a side impact. In rear-end collisions producing whiplash patients, the Y axis accelerations are only a small fraction of the X axis accelerations (ie, <1.0g along the Y axis for an X axis acceleration of 5.0g). Thus, the extremely high values for the cadaver subjects may be 20 times that in whiplash claimants who have rear-end or front-end collisions but may be appropriate for side collisions.

[13]Kallieris D, Mattern R, Miltner E, Schmidt G, Stein K. Considerations for a neck injury criterion. In: *Proceedings of the Thirty Fifth Stapp Car Crash Conference.* Paper #912916. Warrendale, PA: Society of Automotive Engineers; 1991:401–417.
Similar experiments to those described in note 12, with frontal and side collision confirming that for anything more than minor muscle damage, one requires accelerations to the head of greater than 21g.

[14]Panjabi MM, Cholewicki J, Nibu K, Grauer J, Vahldiek M. Capsular ligament stretches during in vitro whiplash simulations. *Journal of Spinal Disorders.* 1998;11(3):227–232.
Cadaver spines undergo the equivalent of a rear-end collision with a head acceleration of 10.5g. Minor ligament damage begins at this level of acceleration.

Table 20-3 Whiplash Experiments—Cadavers

Study	Impact Velocity (km/h)*	Impact Direction	Acceleration (g)†	Results††	Head Restraint
Collisions producing whiplash patients	3–60	Varied	2.0–20**	Whiplash patients	Varied
Ewing et al[1]		Frontal	7.6	No symptoms	No
Ewing et al[2]		Frontal	4.5–47.8	No symptoms	No
Mertz and Patrick[3]		N/A		No symptoms	No
Patrick[4]		N/A		No symptoms	N/A
Patrick[5]	17–38	Rear		No symptoms and no injury in cadavers, except at 132 lbs	No
Patrick[6]	17,38,73	Rear		No symptoms and no injury in cadavers	Yes
Patrick[7]	12.1–16.6	Front	2.9–9.6	Minor symptoms at highest forces	No
Mertz and Patrick[8]		Frontal	17.4	No symptoms	No
Ewing[9]		Rear	12	No evidence of injury	No
Ewing and Thomas[10]		Rear and frontal	11	No symptoms	No
Ewing et al[11]		Frontal	13.0–28.4	No symptoms	No
Ewing et al[12]		Frontal	14.5–37.0	No symptoms	No
Patrick and Chou[13]		Side	11	No symptoms	No

Ewing et al[14]	50	Frontal	3.3–11.0	No symptoms	No
Wagner[15]	61	Frontal	6.0–10.0	No symptoms	Yes
Wismans et al[16]	66	Frontal	3.0	No symptoms	No
Grunsten et al[17]		Frontal	15	No symptoms	No
Allen et al[18]	N/A	N/A	5.6	No symptoms	N/A

While most of these experiments failed to generate symptoms, some human volunteers have experienced minor and short-lived symptoms. See the following:

Thomas DJ, Ewing CL, Majewski PL, et al. Clinical medical effects of head and neck response during biodynamic stress experiments. In: *Advisory Group for Aerospace Research and Development (AGARD) Conference #267, Lisbon, Portugal.* 1979:15.1–15.15.

Kallieris D, Mattern R, Miltner E, Schmidt G, Stein K. Considerations for a neck injury criterion. In: *Proceedings of the Thirty Fifth Stapp Car Crash Conference.* Paper #912916. Warrendale, PA: Society of Automotive Engineers; 1991:401–417.

[1]Ewing CL, Thomas DJ, Beeler GW Jr, et al. Dynamic response of the head and neck of the living human to -Gx impact acceleration. In: *Proceedings of the Twelfth Stapp Car Crash Conference.* Paper #680792. Warrendale, PA: Society of Automotive Engineers; 1968:424–439.
Human volunteers undergo impacts causing neck hyperflexion.
See page 438 for acceleration values.

[2]Ewing CL, Thomas DJ, Patrick LM, Beeler GW Jr, Smith MJ. Dynamic response of the head and neck of the living human to -Gx impact acceleration—II. In: *Proceedings of the Thirteenth Stapp Car Crash Conference.* Paper #690817. Warrendale, PA: Society of Automotive Engineers; 1969:400–415.
Human volunteers undergo impacts causing neck hyperflexion but with much higher accelerations than in the study in note 1.

[3]Mertz HJ Jr, Patrick LM. Investigation of the kinematics and kinetics of whiplash. In: *Proceedings of the Eleventh Stapp Car Crash Conference.* Paper #670919. Warrendale, PA: Society of Automotive Engineers; 1967:175–206.
and
Patrick LM. Studies of hyperextension and hyperflexion injury in volunteers and human cadavers. In: Gurdjian ES, Thomas LM, eds. *Neckache and Backache.* Springfield, IL: Charles C Thomas; 1970:92–119.
See page 99 of Patrick 1970 article for the various static forces. In this case, the subject underwent the greatest strain of the neck, that is, in a hanging position with the neck extended. Patrick himself was subjected to a stretching force (1469 N) with no symptoms.

continues

Table 20–3 continued

[4]Patrick LM, 99.
The human volunteer undergoes static forces pulling with the head in the neutral, extended, and flexed position. H. J. Mertz and L. M. Patrick (see note 8) point out that the tolerable static forces on the neck are lower than those in dynamic situations (as in rear-end collision).

[5]Patrick LM, 102.
The human volunteer undergoes hyperextension without head restraint. The volunteer experienced a 10 mph (17 km/h) collision, with no symptoms.

[6]Patrick LM, 103–104.
The human volunteer undergoes hyperextension experiments with head restraints in place. The human volunteer underwent 10 mph (17 km/h), 23 mph (38 km/h), and 44 mph (73 km/h) collisions. He experienced no symptoms.

[7]Patrick LM, 105.
Hyperflexion studies with the human volunteer, who developed a few days of neck pain only after multiple runs, but no chronic symptoms.

[8]Mertz HJ, Patrick LM. Strength and response of the human neck. In: *Proceedings of the Fifteenth Stapp Car Crash Conference.* Paper #710855. Warrendale, PA: Society of Automotive Engineers; 1971:2903–2928.
The human volunteer undergoes hyperflexion experiments. Patrick himself underwent 46 runs at different velocities in this experiment. On page 2914, the authors give the values of one of his runs in which he experienced a peak of 17.5g at the forehead and 13.2g at the mouth without any symptoms produced. The runs include occasions with his neck muscles relaxed and then with muscles tensed, again with no symptoms in either case.

[9]Ewing CL, 2927.

[10]Ewing CL, Thomas DJ. Torque versus angular displacement response of human head to -Gx impact acceleration. In: *Proceedings of the Seventeenth Stapp Car Crash Conference.* Paper #730976. Warrendale, PA: Society of Automotive Engineers; 1973:309–342.
Twelve volunteers tolerated head and neck hyperflexion accelerations of 11g and hyperextension accelerations of 20g with no symptoms.

[11]Ewing CL, Thomas DJ, Lustick L, et al. The effect of the initial position of the head and neck on the dynamic response of the human head and neck to -Gx impact acceleration. In: *Proceedings of the Nineteenth Stapp Car Crash Conference.* Paper #751157. Warrendale, PA: Society of Automotive Engineers; 1975:487–512.
Thirteen human volunteers undergo repeated frontal impacts (causing hyperflexion). The head and neck accelerations range from 13.0 to 28.4g (page 509) with no symptoms or injury. More important, the volunteers had a variety of head positions to see if injury would occur not just due to the forces but perhaps only when the head was in a certain position. Regardless of position, in this study, there was no injury produced.

[12]Ewing CL, Thomas DJ, Lustick L, et al. The effect of duration, rate of onset, and peak sled acceleration on the dynamic response of the human head and neck. In: *Proceedings of the Twentieth Stapp Car Crash Conference.* Paper #760800. Warrendale, PA: Society of Automotive Engineers; 1976:3–41. In an attempt to see if accelerations in different directions could cause injury with hyperflexion (frontal impact), the researchers used varied rates and onset of collisions. There was no injury in 10 human volunteers in repeated collisions with accelerations of 14.5 to 37.0g (page 9).

[13]Patrick LM, Chou CC. Response of the human neck in flexion, extension and lateral flexion. In: *Vehicle Research Institute Report VRI 7.3.* New York: Society of Automotive Engineers; 1976. There was no injury in studies of lateral flexion with head and neck forces of 20g.

[14]Ewing CL, Thomas DJ, Majewski PL, et al. Measurement of head, T1, and pelvic response to -Gx impact acceleration. In: *Proceedings of the Twenty First Stapp Car Crash Conference.* Paper #770927. Warrendale, PA: Society of Automotive Engineers; 1977:509–545. A single volunteer underwent repeated frontal collisions causing hyperflexion. There was no injury despite accelerations of the head and neck at 3.3 to 11.0g (page 530).

[15]Wagner R. A 30 mph front/rear crash with human test persons. In: *Proceedings of the Twenty Third Stapp Car Crash Conference.* Paper #791030. Warrendale, PA: Society of Automotive Engineers; 1979:827–840. In this study, 3 volunteers underwent a sled test and were the drivers of a vehicle that would strike another in a rear-end collision at 30 mph (50 km/h). They suffered no injury.

[16]Wismans J, Philippens M, van Oorschot E, Kallieris D, Mattern R. Comparison of human volunteer and cadaver head-neck response in frontal flexion. In: *Proceedings of the Thirty First Stapp Car Crash Conference.* Paper #872194. Warrendale, PA: Society of Automotive Engineers; 1987:1–11.

[17]Grunsten RC, Gilbert NS, Mawn SV. The mechanical effects of impact acceleration on the unconstrained human head and neck complex. *Contemporary Orthopaedics.* 1989;18(2):199–202. Forty-five volunteers underwent impacts causing neck hyperflexion. The researchers used sled accelerations of 15g, meaning that the head and neck accelerations were potentially higher than this.

[18]Allen ME, Weir-Jones I, Motiuk DR, et al. Acceleration perturbations of daily living. *Spine.* 1994;19(11):1285–1290. These researchers measured the accelerations in everyday life. They include sneezing, coughing, plopping into a chair, and other activities. The accelerations in these events are, surprisingly, as high as those some whiplash patients experience. The authors of this article note that the X-axis (flexion-extension) accelerations were 5.6g, with maximum acceleration (in combined axes) of 18g.

Table 20-4 Whiplash Experiments—Low Velocity

Study	Impact Velocity (km/h)*	Impact Direction	Acceleration (g)†	Change in Struck Vehicle Velocity (km/h)—ΔV	Results††	Head Restraint
Collisions producing whiplash patients	3–60	Varied	2.0–20**	Varied	Whiplash patients	Varied
Szabo and Welcher[1]	16	Rear	10.1–13.7	8.0	Minimal (<1 day) or no symptoms	Yes
McConnell et al[2]	7–16***	Rear	4.3	3.0–8.1	Minimal or no symptoms	No
Ono and Kanno[3]	2.0–4.3	Rear and frontal		4–8	No symptoms	
Scott et al[4]		Rear	2.0–6.0	3.9–7.8	Neck pain for 1 day	Yes
Siegmund and Williamson[5]	7.5–9.4	Rear and frontal		6.1–7.63	No symptoms	No
West et al[6]	2.9–19.6	Rear	1.5–18.6	1.7–16.5	Minor symptoms at highest forces	No for all
Allen et al[7]	N/A	N/A	5.6		No symptoms	N/A
Geigl et al[8]		Rear		6.0–12.0	No symptoms	Yes

Study		Direction			Symptoms	
Matsushita et al[9]		Rear, frontal, and lateral	1.4–6.3	2.5–5.8	Minor symptoms for 2–4 days in a few volunteers	Yes
Rosenbluth and Hicks[10]	3–13	Rear	2.8–8.6	3.3–7.8	No symptoms	No
Szabo et al[11]	16	Rear	10.1–13.7	8.0	1 volunteer had minimal neck stiffening for 1 day	Yes
Bailey et al[12]		Lateral		15.0–17.5	Neck, back pain for hours to days	No
McConnell et al[13]		Rear		5.8–10.9	Few had symptoms lasting hours to days	Varied
Dubois et al[14]	2.4–14	Rear	1.0–10	0.29–1.91	Absolutely no injury to bus occupants	No
Castro et al[15]	16–26.4	Rear	8.7–14.2	8.7–14.2	Few had pain for a few days	Some
Nielsen et al[16]		Rear and frontal		1.7–11.0	Few had symptoms lasting for hours	Yes
Brault et al[17]	4.9–10	Rear		4–8	Neck pain for maximum of 2 days	Yes
Howard et al[18]		Rear	3.0–6.0	3.9–10.9	Neck pain for 3 days	Yes

continues

Table 20–4 continued

These experiments confirm that low-velocity collisions produce either no injury or minimal symptoms lasting hours to days, particularly when the change in the struck vehicle's velocity is less than 8 km/h, which is often the case. Despite these low velocities, many whiplash patients appear to be reporting chronic and widespread symptoms. There is no physical mechanism to explain this.

[1]Szabo TJ, Welcher J. Dynamics of low speed crash tests with energy absorbing bumpers. In: *Proceedings of the Thirty Sixth Stapp Car Crash Conference.* Paper #921573. Warrendale, PA: Society of Automotive Engineers; 1992:1367–1375.
This study included 5 volunteers who were nonmilitary personnel, including 3 men and 2 women. The researchers examined rear-end collisions and also did magnetic resonance imaging scans before and after the impacts. Symptoms lasted either just for minutes or until the next day, in one case.

[2]McConnell WE, Howard RP, Guzman HM, et al. Analysis of human test subject kinematic responses to low velocity rear end impacts. In: *Proceedings of the Thirty Seventh Stapp Car Crash Conference.* Paper #930889. Warrendale, PA: Society of Automotive Engineers; 1993:21–30.
Volunteers (4 males aged 25 to 43) underwent impacts causing neck extension. See page 26 for acceleration values. The velocity of the striking vehicle ranged from as low as 1.8 km/h to 19.6 km/h in a variety of impacts. There were no symptoms.

[3]Ono K, Kanno M. Influences of the physical parameters on the risk to neck injuries in low impact speed rear-end collisions. In: *Proceedings of the International IRCOBI Conference on the Biomechanics of Impacts, September 8–10, 1993, Eindhoven, Netherlands.* 1993:201–212.
There were both rear and frontal collisions, with 3 men between the ages of 22 and 43. They developed no symptoms.

[4]Scott MW, McConnell WE, Guzman HM, et al. Comparison of human and ATD head kinematics during low-speed rearend impacts. In: *Proceedings of the Thirty Seventh Stapp Car Crash Conference.* Paper #930094. Warrendale, PA: Society of Automotive Engineers; 1993:1–8.
These researchers demonstrated that a dummy is a poor surrogate for predicting whiplash injury in low-velocity collisions. A male volunteer (age 50) underwent 7 rear-end collisions, producing neck pain for 1 day.

[5]Siegmund GP, Williamson PB. Speed change (ΔV) of amusement park bumper cars. In: *Proceedings of the Canadian Multidisciplinary Road Safety Conference VIII, June 14–16, 1993, Saskatoon, Saskatchewan.* 1993:299–308.
There were 2 men in rear and frontal impacts. There were no symptoms reported.

[6]West DH, Gough JP, Harper GTK. Low speed rear-end collision testing using human subjects. *Accident Reconstruction Journal.* 1993;5(3):22–26.
This detailed study gives indications of the relationship between impact speed and ΔV for some vehicle systems and confirms that below a ΔV of 8.0 km/h, the possibility of injury is remote. The researchers used 5 men aged 25 to 43.

7. Allen ME, Weir-Jones I, Motiuk DR, et al. Acceleration perturbations of daily living. *Spine*. 1994;19(11):1285–1290.

These researchers measured the accelerations in everyday life. They include sneezing, coughing, plopping into a chair, and other activities. The accelerations in these events are, surprisingly, as high as those some whiplash patients experience. The authors of this article note that the X axis (flexion-extension) accelerations were 5.6g, with maximum acceleration (in combined axes) of 18g.

8. Geigl BC, Steffan H, Leinzinger P, Roll, Mühlbauer M, Bauer G. The movement of head and cervical spine during rearend impact. In: *Proceedings of the International IRCOBI Conference on the Biomechanics of Impact, 1994, Lyon, France*. 1994:127–137.

Using a sled system, 25 volunteers (2 female) of ages 20 to 60 underwent impacts with a ΔV of 6.0–12.0 km/h and had no symptoms. They had also included experiments with a variety of initial head rotations forward and distances from the head restraint. None of these variations produced symptoms.

9. Matsushita T, Sato TB, Hirabayashi K, et al. X-ray study of the human neck motion due to head inertia loading. In: *Proceedings of the Thirty Eighth Stapp Car Crash Conference*. Paper #942208. Warrendale, PA: Society of Automotive Engineers; 1994:55–64.

The researchers used 4 women and 22 men in low-velocity collisions (rear-end, frontal, and lateral), with X-ray analysis of the neck motion during the collision. Each volunteer had an MRI study of the neck prior to the tests. The researchers used relaxed and tensed muscle states and different seated postures. Symptoms lasted for 2 to 4 days in a few volunteers.

10. Rosenbluth W, Hicks L. Evaluating low-speed rear-end impact severity and resultant occupant stress parameters. *Journal of Forensics Sciences*. 1994;39(6):1393–1424.

One man (age 63) and one woman (age 55) underwent impact velocities of 3 to 13 km/h resulting in a ΔV of 3.3 to 7.8 km/h. They had no symptoms.

11. Szabo TJ, Welcher JB, Anderson RD. Human occupant kinematic response to low speed rear-end impacts. In: *Proceedings of the Thirty Eighth Stapp Car Crash Conference*. Paper #940532. Warrendale, PA: Society of Automotive Engineers; 1994:23–25.

Two women and 3 men, with ages of 27 to 58, participated. Some had been identified as having disc degeneration (cervical or lumbar) by magnetic resonance imaging (MRI) scan. No symptoms occurred except minor neck stiffness the next day in 1 volunteer. There were no changes to MRI findings 3 months after the collision.

12. Bailey MN, Wong BC, Lawrence JM. Data and methods for estimating the severity of minor impacts. In: *Proceedings of the Thirty Ninth Stapp Car Crash Conference*. Paper #950352. Warrendale, PA: Society of Automotive Engineers; 1995:139–173.

These authors give the data for lateral collisions conducted by A. Zaborowski in 1964. For more recent data for lateral collisions, see G. P. Nielsen et al. The researchers report that the threshold for minor injury in a lateral collision is a ΔV of about 16 km/h. The striking vehicle (of equal mass) would have to be travelling at 24 to 32 km/h to generate this threshold. The symptoms reported include neck and back pain for hours to days, as well as hip pain.

13. McConnell WE, Howard RP, Van Poppel J, et al. Human head and neck kinematics after low velocity rear-end impacts—understanding "whiplash." In: *Proceedings of the Thirty Ninth Stapp Car Crash Conference*. Paper #952724. Warrendale, PA: Society of Automotive Engineers; 1995:215–238.

continues

Table 20–4 continued

[14]DuBois RA, McNally BF, DiGregorio JS, Phillips GJ. Low velocity car-to-bus test impacts. *Accident Reconstruction Journal.* 1996;8(5):44–51.
This study demonstrates that when a car hits a bus in a rear-end collision, for the bus occupants to have a whiplash injury, the velocity of impact would likely be fatal for the car occupant. Thus, one does not expect whiplash injury in bus occupants with most rear-end collisions. A detailed discussion is worthwhile to understand why they may have come to this conclusion. See Chapter 21.

[15]Castro WHM, Schilgen M, Meyer S, et al. Do "whiplash injuries" occur in low-speed rear impacts? *European Spine Journal.* 1997;6:366–375. The researchers used a group of 19 men and women in multiple car and bumper car collisions. They found that only a few reported symptoms, and these lasted for a few days. They cite the threshold for injury as being around a ΔV of 10 km/h.

[16]Nielsen GP, Gough JP, Little DM, West DH, Baker VT. Human subject responses to repeated low speed impacts using utility vehicles. In: *Proceedings of the Forty First Stapp Car Crash Conference.* Paper #970394. Warrendale, PA: Society of Automotive Engineers; 1997:189–212. Seven men were involved in rear and frontal impacts. After repeated exposures, only two individuals experienced any symptoms, and these lasted just hours. The researchers demonstrated that the threshold for injury in frontal impacts is at least a ΔV of the struck vehicle of 12 to 20 km/h.

[17]Brault JR, Wheeler JB, Siegmund GP, Brault EJ. Clinical response of human subjects to rear-end automobile collisions. *Archives of Physical Medicine and Rehabilitation.* 1998;79:72–80.
This study appears to be anomalous with respect to the threshold for reporting acute symptoms after rear-end collision. The authors suggest that a rear-end collision with a ΔV of 4 km/h can be expected to lead to acute neck pain or headache.

[18]Howard RP, Bowles AP, Guzman HM, Krenrich SW. Head, neck, and mandible dynamics generated by "whiplash." *Accident Prevention and Analysis.* 1998;30(4):525–534.
A study with 7 men (aged 32 to 59) in experimental rear-end collisions found that acute neck pain, lasting for 3 days, occurred. There was no jaw pain or other symptoms commonly said to be part of the so-called "TMJ injury." They also found that seated height and head position relative to the head restraint were irrelevant to injury in these collisions.

466

teroposterior, or front-to-back, direction. The Y axis is along a horizontal line passing between the subject's two ears, that is, from one ear to the other. The Z axis is along a vertical line passing from the top of the skull down along the length of the spine. (See Figure 20–1 below.)

The acceleration along the axis can be positive acceleration (usually just called acceleration) or negative acceleration (sometimes called deceleration). For example, when one strikes an occupant from behind and his or her neck extends, this is positive (+) acceleration. When one strikes the occupant from in front (so the oc-

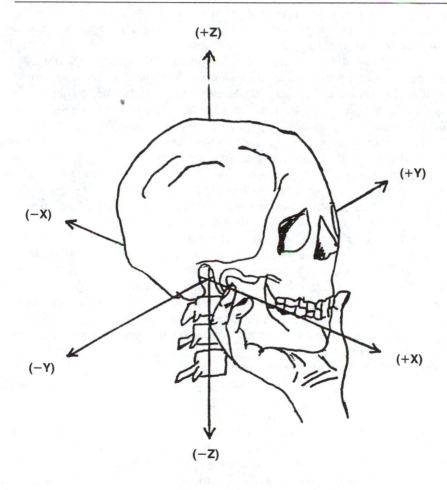

Alas, poor Yorick!

Figure 20–1 The X-Y-Z Coordinate System (as Viewed by Hamlet)

cupant is facing the force that he or she collides with) and the neck flexes, this is negative ($-$) acceleration.

Researchers commonly use this system, but one must always be careful to ensure, when comparing data from different sources, that the axis system is the same. For instance, S. M. Foreman and A. C. Croft illustrate a system where the X axis, in the system above, is in the position of the Z axis. One could very easily make the mistake of reading an article that discusses Z axis forces and believe that the authors were referring to the front-to-back X axis other authors use. This would then lead to false conclusions regarding the forces whiplash patients experience in neck flexion and extension. Although some prefer one system or another, the relevant issue is that all comparisons and application of data to whiplash patients must be through an equivalent system.

Accelerations of the head (and, therefore, the forces experienced) along the three axes could conceivably each be responsible for injury. The amount of acceleration one needs to cause injury may be different depending on how much one applies along a given axis. For instance, an acceleration of 40g along the Y axis may not cause injury, but 20g along the Z axis might cause injury.

In the typical types and velocities of front-end or rear-end collisions producing whiplash patients, the greatest accelerations are along the X axis, and lesser accelerations are along the other axes. The head acceleration experienced in whiplash patients is about 2.0 to 20.0g in the X axis direction in most cases. The tables show the X axis direction to allow comparison between the experience of whiplash patients and the experience of subjects of experimental studies.

The data most often available are along the X axis, and so the tables consider experiments mostly dealing with this direction. Again, one must always be careful that one is comparing accelerations and forces along the same axes. If one experiment shows, for instance, that a 5.0g acceleration along the Z axis causes injury, this does not mean that a 5.0g acceleration along the X axis is sufficient to cause injury. One can compare the accelerations only along the same axes (making sure the labeling systems are not different) because equal accelerations may cause different results.

Finally, for cadaver experiments, one must also bear in mind that the force at which tissue damage occurs may be lower than one needs in the living human, since protection from damage is, in part, a quality of living tissue. In some cadaver experiments, there is considerable dissection that removes supporting tissues, so that the remaining structures damage more easily. Finally, most cadavers tend to be older than typical whiplash patients, and the effect of aging on supporting structures may be a factor in determining capacity to resist muscle injury. Wismans et al, for example, showed that living humans were not injured and cadavers showed no significant damage even though they were experiencing the same forces. In addition, J. R. Cromack and H. H. Ziperman conducted a study in 1975 to compare real-world injuries (6,221 collisions) with damage seen in experimental cadaver collisions. They found that under the same conditions (velocity of collision, type of car, direction of impact, etc) they were producing serious damage in cadavers, whereas such damage was extremely uncommon in the real-world accident victims under similar conditions. They underline the dangers of applying data from cadaver experiments to living humans: "The injuries produced in cadavers in laboratory tests have no counterpart in the real world. One concludes, therefore, that . . . no comparison exists between these laboratory surrogates and live humans with respect to injury production in car crashes."

ADDITIONAL NOTES

It is always worthwhile to review whiplash experiments carefully and to get assistance, if needed, in doing so. Otherwise, it is easy to reach the wrong conclusion. On occasion, authors quote the forces of injury necessary to cause ligament injury in cadaver experiments and compare this to predicted forces in whiplash patients.

Consider quoting force magnitudes from:

> Pintar FA, Mykebust JB, Yoganadan N, et al. Biomechanics of human spinal ligaments. In: Sances A et al, eds. *Mechanisms of Head and Spine Trauma*. New York: Goshen; 1986:518.

This article provides data on the forces required to damage the ligaments of the human cadaver cervical spine. The study showed that forces in the range of 108 to 450 N can injure various ligaments in the cadaver neck. One might notice that these values are similar to those in the tables above and conclude that this is proof that ligament injury occurs in whiplash patients.

Wrong. The forces in Pintar et al's experiments are in either compression or tension on the spine, which is along the Z axis (vertical). The force of 162 to 270 N for whiplash patients is along the X axis. The force along the Z axis in typical rear-end collisions producing whiplash patients is actually less than this, typically 50% to 60% or less of the X axis force. This Z axis range for whiplash patients is less than the range of forces that caused ligament damage in Pintar et al's cadavers. This fact, and the fact that elderly cadavers may not resist forces of injury as well as living humans, means that one cannot apply Pintar et al's work to whiplash studies.

SUMMARY OF WHIPLASH EXPERIMENTS

The chief observation from review of the tables above is obvious. The likely minimum acceleration experienced by the human head to produce an injury is certainly at least 10g. In rear-end collisions, the threshold for injury is a change in the struck vehicle velocity of more than 8.0 km/h (5 mph) and probably double this in lateral or frontal collisions. Moreover, even when accelerations or velocity changes do exceed these levels, acute pain may occur in the whiplash experiments, but never chronic pain. Something else must happen to the whiplash patient besides the acute injury to explain chronic symptoms. Experiments with living humans have not been able to reproduce the chronic symptoms of whiplash patients. No matter the direction of the impact—rear, frontal, or lateral (side)—living human experiments do not result in individuals reporting chronic symptoms. This is further emphasized by the fact that the human volunteers often underwent several runs in an attempt to induce injury and yet tolerated each attempt without developing chronic symptoms, even if they did develop acute symptoms. Moreover, there are some daily activities (see M. E. Allen et al) that subject the head and neck to the same forces facing whiplash patients but do not cause injury.

Thus, although the acute injury is relatively easy to reproduce, the chronic symptoms have never been reproduced.

Some have argued that there is an inherent limitation in the human volunteer experiments: occupants may be tensed because they know a collision is coming. Some argue that this protects volunteers from some sort of injury that leads to chronic pain and that is why experiment volunteers develop only acute pain. The corollary of this, however, is that whiplash patients who state that they "saw the collision coming" (and instinctively tensed) should also receive an injury that causes only acute pain. On the other hand, some theorized that tense muscles that occur in the occupant prior to collision could be injured in a way that causes chronic pain. In that case, it should be easy to reproduce the chronic symptoms of whiplash in human volunteers. J. P. Gough (1996) has reviewed the literature in low-speed collisions and noted that many of the experiments had a range of muscle conditions, from relaxed to tensed. According to Gough, these studies found that subjects who were relaxed had the same head acceleration as subjects who were tensed.

And even if one believes that whiplash patients more readily develop a muscle or ligament sprain than experimental volunteers do, it does not matter. Developing a sprain, even a severe sprain, is not an explanation for chronic pain reporting. The great majority of whiplash patients reporting chronic symptoms have an injury no more severe than a sprain.

A Closer Look at a Very Low Velocity Study

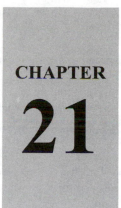

CHAPTER

21

Brault JR, Wheeler JB, Siegmund GP, Brault EJ. Clinical response of human subjects to rear-end automobile collisions. *Archives of Physical Medicine and Rehabilitation*. 1998;79: 72–80.

This section will critique this Brault et al study, which was published in 1998. This study looked at the impact of very low velocity collisions on subjects. In 1998, J. R. Brault et al subjected 42 volunteers to low-velocity rear-end collision. About 30% of the subjects reported minor symptoms, even with a ΔV of as little as 4 km/h. This is contrary to all prior experiments, and one wonders if the collisions caused the symptoms by way of injury.

There are other explanations for these symptoms to be considered and more research needed before concluding that an injury mechanism is likely.

FIRST CONSIDERATION—SYMPTOM AMPLIFICATION

Brault et al sought to use randomly selected subjects "off the street" because the researchers considered these subjects more appropriate than the subjects used in other studies. Why would subjects off the street be more appropriate? As stated by Brault et al, other studies of low-velocity collisions used subjects that were part of the research team, secretaries working for the company, and so on. Brault et al suggested that using these subjects may have altered symptom reporting. This is not to say these other subjects would have falsely reported their symptoms (many research groups, using different individuals, in different countries, find the threshold for symptoms is a change in velocity of 8 km/h).[1] Asserting such widespread conspiracy would be tantamount to accusing all whiplash claimants of malingering.

The subjects of earlier studies had been through dozens of these collisions. They knew there would be no serious injury and did not worry about what pain they might feel. They also set the accident severity limit with which they were comfortable. In other words, they were comfortable with the idea of experiencing a rear-end collision. They had a low level of precollision "nervousness."

Brault et al selected subjects who may not have had the same view of these minor collisions. The subjects had not been through dozens of these minor collisions, may not have known the outcome well in advance, and so forth. Brault et al were attempting to study a more "typical" accident victim.

But as so often happens in science, researchers sometimes, by the way they measure, alter the phenomenon that they wish to measure. Brault et al's subjects cannot have been as familiar with or as knowledgeable about rear-end collisions, as, say, G. P. Nielsen et al's[2] subjects would have been. Brault et al's subjects cannot have had the same psychological preparedness as Nielsen et al's subjects. Thus, Brault et al's subjects must necessarily have been more nervous about the collision that was about to happen. Brault et al thereby introduced a new element into the phenomenon they were trying to measure.

Actual accident victims cannot be nervous specifically about a collision before it happens. Brault et al's subjects may have been. The result is predictable, if one considers what factors affect pain thresholds and symptom amplification.

More than 2,000 studies deal with the physiological correlates to anxiety or "nervousness." Contraction of voluntary muscle is a common physiological correlate that relates to somatic (bodily) symptoms in the setting of altered emotional states.[3] Pain experiments demonstrate that nervousness or attentional focus tends to lower the pain threshold. Under states of nervousness or increased attention to the imminent pain stimulus, pain reporting occurs at a lower threshold of stimulus severity. Studies show, for example, that instructions that may increase nervousness about the imminent pain stimulus will lower the pain threshold and increase the heart rate in response to the stimulus.[4] This phenomenon has been most notable when the pain stimulus is near the head[5] and is more prevalent in females than in males.[5,6] Drawing attention to the imminent pain stimulus (attentional focus) itself predicts lowering of the pain threshold even when one controls for levels of nervousness.[7] Obviously, Brault et al's subjects had their attention drawn to the possibility of an impending pain stimulus. Nielsen et al's subjects may likely have overcome this because they had so little concern about such matters. They had been through many similar events and remembered them as benign.

Symptom amplification occurs in concert with lowering of the pain threshold. A. J. Barsky et al indicated that symptoms intensify when they are attributed to a serious disease.[8] After perceiving the stimulus as painful (at whatever threshold), a person may rate the severity of pain thereafter depending on the circumstances. The Nielsen et al subjects viewed the event they had just experienced, even if it caused pain, as benign. They had experienced it many times with no long-lasting effects. It was almost routine. The Brault et al subjects were likely to be less confident than this and thus to be at risk for symptom amplification, which would have influenced pain reporting from the stimulus onward. Barsky noted that when symptom amplification exists, individuals become hypervigilant for symptoms. They register normal bodily sensations as abnormal and react to bodily sensations with affect and thoughts that intensify the sensations, making them more disturbing.[9]

In this sense, Brault et al have confirmed that different precollision psychological states generate different outcomes. A large body of literature that relates to lowering of pain thresholds and symptom amplification supports this explanation for the study results.

SECOND CONSIDERATION—SYMPTOM ATTRIBUTION

About 30% of Brault et al's subjects reported symptoms. These minor aches and pains lasting 2 to 24 hours are common in daily life, yet most people would not be able to recall when and how often these episodes occur. The symptoms that Brault et al's subjects report may simply reflect spontaneous episodes of headache or neck pain.

To sort this out, the subjects could have completed a daily diary of all aches and pains for, say, a 6-week period before participating in the experiment. Knowing the documented rather than simply the recalled history of minor neck pain and headache before the experiment could have revealed intermittent and mild headache or neck pain episodes.

Brault et al could have used a placebo collision with a control population. The researchers indicated that they tried to make the occupant unaware of the imminent collision. They could have conducted the study so that in some cases occupants would not be in a collision but would be told that they had been in a 4 km/h collision, even if they did not feel it. It would be interesting to see how many of this control group would then later report symptoms.

Researchers conducting other whiplash experiments have learned that the collision severity is likely on a par with sneezing. It is of note that Brault et al do not quote acceleration data, which could then be compared to acceleration data for everyday life experiences cited by M. E. Allen et al (see Chapters 5 and 20).

The significance of results from Brault et al's study are unclear without a control population, particularly when the results disagree with all previous studies.

REFERENCES

1. Gough JP. Human occupant dynamics in low-speed rear end collisions: an engineering perspective. *Journal of Musculoskeletal Pain.* 1996;4(4):11–19.

2. Nielsen GP, Gough JP, Little DM, West DH, Baker VT. Human subject responses to repeated low speed impacts using utility vehicles. In: *Proceedings of the Forty First Stapp Car Crash Conference.* Paper #970394. Warrendale, PA: Society of Automotive Engineers; 1997:189–212.

3. Kellner R. *Psychosomatic Syndromes and Somatic Symptoms.* Washington, DC: American Psychiatric Press; 1991.

4. Cornwall A, Donderi DC. The effect of experimentally induced anxiety on the experience of pressure pain. *Pain.* 1988;35(1):105–113.

5. Buchanan HM, Midgley JA. Evaluation of pain threshold using a simple algometer. *Clinical Rheumatology.* 1987;6(4):510–517.

6. Robin O, Vinard H, Vernet-Maury E, Saumet JL. Influence of sex and anxiety on pain threshold and tolerance. *Functional Neurology.* 1987;2(2):173–179.

7. Arntz A, de Jong P. Anxiety, attention and pain. *Journal of Psychosomatic Research.* 1993;37(4):423–432.

8. Barksy AJ, Goodson JD, Lane RS, Cleary PD. The amplification of somatic symptoms. *Psychosomatic Medicine.* 1988;50:510–519.

9. Barsky AJ. Amplification, somatization, and the somatoform disorders. *Psychosomatics.* 1992;33(1):28–34.

Head Restraints, Seat Belts, and Whiplash

HEAD RESTRAINTS

Despite the widespread consensus supporting the introduction of head restraints, in 1968 and 1969 C. L. Ewing et al considered it important to document head restraints' capacity to prevent whiplash injury. They conducted studies with human volunteers of varying heights to see if height had any relationship to the risk of injury in a rear-end collision. The volunteers had no head restraints. The subjects were all young, healthy males. The volunteers underwent peak head accelerations of more than 47g, with no symptoms produced. The researchers also found that it did not matter at what height above the seat the head rested, since the amount of extension of the neck did not vary with sitting height. Further, there was no evidence of electroencephalogram abnormalities in the subjects in almost 200 test runs. This was an interesting result, as one would have expected some of the volunteers to have developed whiplash, especially without head restraints. It may be that these volunteers were physically more capable of resisting injury, and perhaps they needed to experience even higher forces.

In 1972, J. D. States et al examined the effectiveness of head restraints in rear-end collisions. Looking at all reported rear-end collisions, they found that:

> Head restraints reduce the frequency of whiplash injury by 14%. This disappointing finding is attributable in part to the failure of users to adjust their head restraints. . . .
>
> Head restraints decreased whiplash injury frequency for women . . . more than for men.

Yet using a head restraint improperly was not a sufficient explanation. As emphasized in the study conducted by C. Thomas et al in 1982, "The mispositioning of adjustable [head] restraint is not a sufficient explanation because the injured whose cars are equipped with 'integral' seats still suffered from cervical pains."

In addition, C. J. Kahane examined this argument with an evaluation of head restraints and protection from whiplash. Many had proposed that the mechanism of whiplash was hyperextension of the neck. If this were indeed the correct mechanism, head restraints should reduce whiplash. Kahane found that 75% of head restraints are in the down position and that head restraints reduced the frequency of whiplash symptoms by 10% to 15%. Presumably, the improper use of the restraints explained why their effectiveness was not greater. The author noted, however, that this was not explanation enough.

> The problem of adjustment, however, is not quite as severe as it would appear. . . . Many occupants are short enough that they can obtain adequate protection from a restraint in the "down" position, even if the height is well under 27.5 inches.

> An extensive study by Stowell and Bryant in 1978 showed that 51 percent of the adjustable restraints, whatever their position, reached at least to the base of the occupant's skull, providing full protection for the neck.

Kahane added that most head restraints are designed for a man who is larger than average. Therefore, head restraints, even in the down position, should be sufficiently protective for most women. Yet more women than men report chronic symptoms after acute whiplash injury.

The notion that some occupants involved in a rear-end collision are lifted up the seat back (as described in MacNab's diagrams) is false. W. E. McConnell et al and D. H. West et al (see below) showed this by detailed video analysis. No one has shown that tall occupants involved in rear-end collisions develop whiplash symptoms more frequently than shorter occupants. In fact, in 1969, J. K. Kihlberg showed that the incidence of whiplash was not at all related to occupant height. P. Lövsund et al (1988), in a study of several thousand occupants, also found that occupant height does not predict injury risk, contradicting the findings of a much smaller study by G. Carlsson et al (1985). Further confounding the theory that improperly positioned head restraints lead to whiplash injury are the data of S. Lubin and J. Sehmer (1993): "Only 30.2% of male drivers had correctly positioned head restraints, compared with 67.6% of female drivers."

Continuing to examine the value of head restraints, B. O'Neill et al studied the frequency of whiplash injury insurance claims as a function of head restraint use since 1969. To their surprise, they found that "in only two cases were the observed differences statistically significant between the claimed injury rates for drivers of cars with head restraints . . . and for drivers of cars without head restraints." This was difficult to explain. It meant that either drivers were not using their head restraints properly or that there were other reasons for ongoing claims of whiplash injury.

Further, the frequently quoted concept that women get whiplash more often because of the difference between the male and female neck has not been proven, as explained by O'Neill et al: "There are no well-documented medical explanations for these differences. . . . None of [the] various possibilities has been sufficiently investigated, and most have not been touched scientifically."

In addition, D. B. Olney and A. K. Marsden (1986) found that head restraints had no effect on the incidence of whiplash claims.

So why are claims of acute whiplash injury so prevalent? There are some obvious explanations. Head restraints do not prevent insurance fraud, for example. Whatever percentage reduction in acute injury that head restraints might render, insurance fraud may remove.

Head restraints cannot prevent all problems. First, those who report symptoms following a rear-end collision may be reporting the symptom onset more than, say, 24 hours after the event. The more delayed the symptom, the more likely that it is not from acute injury. Second, emotional reaction from the accident, not physical injury, may produce symptoms such as headache. Finally, when there is acute injury, neck hyperextension may not always be the mechanism.

In 1993, W. E. McConnell et al conducted one of the most revealing studies of neck motion in a rear-end collision. Their work brought doubt to the long-held belief that the neck was forcibly hyperextended in all rear-end collisions. They made a careful analysis with elaborate photography of low-velocity (less than 13 km/h) rear-end collisions. Even with an inappropriately positioned head restraint (too low), there was actually very little extension of the neck at all. As they noted, "Test subject cervical extension and flexion angles . . . were always found to fall within the subject's voluntary physiological limits. Hyperextension or hyperflexion did not occur during any of the test runs, the maximum of about 40 to 45 degrees, even for test runs using the van, which had no headrests."

McConnell et al went on to explain the flaws in previous conceptions of what happens in most rear-end collisions:

> In reviewing the voluminous literature on [whiplash] . . . one must be careful about making the assumption that the conclusions about human head and neck kinematics reached in these studies necessarily apply to low and very low velocity rearend collisions involving "real people." The majority of these studies have been primarily based on higher speed, 24 to 80 km/h (15 to 50 mph) or more, rearend collisions utilizing dummies, cadavers, animals, computer models and very few live volunteers.

Since exaggerated neck motion beyond tolerable human limits had been frequently observed in dummies and cadavers during high speed testing, it has been commonly assumed that cervical hyperextension and hyperflexion would also occur during low and very low velocity collisions. It has been conjectured by many that the forced movement of the neck beyond physiologic limits was the injury mechanism causing the "whiplash" syndrome, especially in thin necked, unprepared people.

The work of R. C. Grunsten et al (1989) supports this. They observed naval volunteers for 12 years after participation in experimental collisions. Volunteers did not use head restraints in these experiments, with accelerations up to 30g (15g when using a sled). No symptoms occurred, and the researchers found that:

> The head remains momentarily upright, followed by rapid tilting toward the energy source. After a brief delay, the head tends to accelerate along a horizontal track similar to that of the trunk. . . . There is no evidence to indicate that the head and neck whip back and forth. . . . The chin does not impact the chest . . . and the muscular recoil brings the head back to approximately the initial neutral position.

> Rebound of the head appears to be constrained by a muscular stretch response and protective muscular contraction, which prevent the head from going significantly beyond the initial position. Thus far, long-term (two to 12 years) clinical and radiographic follow-up has revealed no injury.

As well, in 1993, West et al conducted an important and illustrative study, using vehicles with velocities up to 20 km/h for some of the experiments. A tow truck struck the vehicles (1979 models) along the rear end. The researchers removed rearview mirrors to help keep the drivers unaware of an impending impact, all cars struck were in gear, and the occupants applied the brakes. Regarding the protective effect (if there is a need for one) of head restraints in low-velocity rear-end collisions, West et al noted:

> The forces experienced by vehicle occupants for impacts with [speeds] of less than 5 km/h (3 mph) are generally not sufficient to cause the heads of the vehicle occupants to be displaced rearward far enough to contact the head support. The maximum recorded levels of head acceleration for impacts of this magnitude were less than 3 g. Since no head contact to the head support is expected as a result of impacts of this magnitude, the presence or absence of adequate head support is of no significance. . . . A recent study by Allen et al [showed that] to "plop"

into a chair . . . recorded levels . . . in excess of those which were measured with a 5 km/h impact.

For impacts . . . between 5 and 8 km/h (3 and 5 mph), the forces experienced by the vehicle occupants were sufficient to cause their heads to be displaced rearward into contact with their head supports. No significant rebound from the head supports occurred. . . . Neither the level of cervical bending nor the level of cervical torque measured in these tests reached the level at which injury to the vehicle occupant would be expected.

. . . With properly . . . utilized head restraints, impacts with [speeds] in excess of 8 km/h (5 mph) can be tolerated without injury. . . . The range of motion which females can tolerate without injury is . . . generally greater than for males.

Thus, it seems that head restraints do not significantly reduce claims of acute whiplash injury, even though their use should reduce the incidence of acute injury. If one considers the contributions of insurance fraud, symptom attribution, symptoms from emotional factors, and the possibility of mechanism other than hyperextension for injury, one may understand why. Although head restraints fail to prevent reporting of acute symptoms, are seat belts contributing to increased reporting?

SEAT BELTS

The idea that seat belts contribute to neck injury deserves separate consideration. Some researchers have claimed that seat belts are a risk factor for developing neck injuries, although others question this contention. It is a moot point in the sense that even if seat belts increase the risk of acute neck injury, this does not mean that chronic pain reporting should be an expected result.

Seat belts reduce the incidence of serious injuries and save lives. At the same time, they are likely responsible for other injuries of the chest and abdomen as well as certain fractures.

There are many theories regarding neck injury and seat belts. According to one, the torso begins to decelerate faster than the free head and neck because of the shoulder strap. This causes flexion of the neck and thus injury. S. M. Foreman and A. C. Croft (1988) explain their theory:

The primary reason that neck injuries are accentuated by restraint systems is that the shoulder harness abruptly restrains the decelerating trunk of the occupant while the head's inertia carries it forward unrestrained. This results in a tremendous bending moment at the cervi cothoracic region and is one of the primary reasons why today the flexion injury is often more significant than the extension injury.

In 1972, I. W. Caldwell wrote that:

> The . . . wearing of a seat belt, will, by preventing any significant forward thrust of the passenger, fail to absorb much of the energy engendered and, by that amount, the "whiplash" effect will be doubled or trebled with more disastrous effects on the cervical spine up to a total dislocation and quadriplegia, if not death—unless a head rest is there to prevent this.

There are potential flaws with this reasoning. First, it is conjectural in estimating that in some way a "whiplash" effect doubles or trebles because the subject is wearing a seat belt (there is no experimental data from which to calculate this). Second, the injuries described are often complications of motor vehicle accidents regardless of whether the occupant was wearing a seat belt.

In 1976, M. S. Christian attempted to determine, in part, whether there was a causal relationship between wearing a seat belt and reporting chronic symptoms. Before discussing this and other studies of similar design, it is worthwhile to discuss what the proper way of studying this question would be. First, if the aim is to find out if wearing a seat belt in a collision places the occupant at more risk for reporting acute symptoms, then one should examine all occupants involved in collisions. One should include all, regardless of whether they had symptoms after the collision. Then one should ask who wore seat belts and who did not. One then would compare the total number of occupants who report acute neck pain in each group. If there was a difference between the groups, an association between wearing seat belts and reporting chronic symptoms would have been established.

It is important to include individuals who had no symptoms after an accident because they too may have been wearing seat belts. If they were, then they would, when added to the number of occupants wearing seat belts who had symptoms, dilute the incidence of seat belt–related symptoms. If the occupants who had no symptoms were not wearing seat belts, then this would skew the results in the opposite direction. One cannot assume that occupants who left the collision with no symptoms equally wore or did not wear seat belts.

To date, no one has done such a study. All the studies so far have failed to include every car occupant in the collision (even those who had no injury).

Christian examined 969 occupants, all of whom had some symptoms after an accident. What happened to those who had no symptoms after the accident? Were they wearing seat belts? If they were not, then this would mean less neck pain occurs when people do not wear seat belts. If they were wearing seat belts, however, and did not have neck pain after the accident, then this argues against a neck injury from seat belts. One cannot assume that the group of uninjured occupants in the accidents had equal numbers of belted and unbelted occupants. There may be some real effect of seat belt usage that either protected or increased their risk for neck injury, or there may be no effect at all. The only way to know is to have these other occupants included in the study. Without them, one cannot accurately determine the possible relationship between neck injury and seat belt usage.

There are also a number of other sources of concern in the study.

- The occupants had either minor, moderate, or severe injury, and each occupant went into one of the groups. Does that mean that no subjects had both a leg fracture and neck pain, since one would have had to include them in both the minor and moderate injury groups? Did forcing a patient into this classification scheme add to or take away from the total neck pain cases for seat belt users and nonusers?
- If occupants hit their face against a windshield because they were not wearing a seat belt, yet had no neck pain, to what group would they have been assigned? (If one included them as having not a neck injury but rather a moderate facial injury, then this would bias the number of recorded neck injuries in occupants not wearing seat belts.)
- The researchers compared average velocities of impact for those wearing seat belts to average velocities of impact for those not wearing seat belts. If a vehicle has 4 occupants, 3 of whom are wearing seat belts and 1 who is not, how does the collision velocity for those occupants become divided among seat belt users and nonusers?
- Were the ages of the occupants in each group the same?
- Were the types of collision (eg, front impact, rear impact, side impact, vehicle rolling; velocity is not the only factor important in determining injury risk) the same for seat belt users and nonusers? Certain impact directions may be more likely to lead to neck injury via seat belts.
- Were all occupants wearing the same type of seat belt? Were there just as many front seat occupants using seat belts as rear seat occupants using seat belts? A disparity between the two groups on this variable could also bias the results.
- Are patients who develop symptoms after an accident more or less likely to report them if they are planning a lawsuit against the driver who caused the accident? Since this may influence reporting, it is necessary to know whether there was an equal number of litigation cases in the belted and unbelted groups.
- Are accident victims, particularly those not at fault, likely to say they had their seat belt on or that they did not? There is no benefit to admitting one did not use a seat belt, but there may be a benefit to admitting that one did indeed take all precautions.

Christian has not reported this data (or accounted for it). As well, the average velocity in accidents where occupants were not wearing seat belts was 61.3 km/h and in the group wearing seat belts, 58.4 km/h. These velocities are much higher than the typical velocities in collisions that whiplash patients have. One must always be careful not to apply the results of studies using such a population to collisions involving whiplash patients, since the results may not be applicable at lower velocities. Finally, Christian shows that the difference in neck pain was 12% incidence in those wearing seat belts and 8% in those not wearing seat belts. How significant is this difference? He does not report a statistical measure of the likelihood that these differences occurred by chance alone.

In 1977, C. P. De Fonseka realized these potential sources for bias or confusion. De Fonseka added, quite rightly, "Since the relationships of the occurrence of soft-tissue neck injuries to frontal and rear-end collision respectively are not known it is not possible to attribute injury to flexion or extension and hence to deduce the role of the seatbelt, when worn."

Yet, in 1985, further potentially erroneous statements would arrive. F. Lesoin et al stated that "in a frontal impact, the body is held down in the seat by the safety belt, while the head is thrown violently backwards, thus hyperextending the cervical spine, and causing the same type of injury as hanging."

Indeed! They had it backwards, because in a frontal impact the head and trunk initially move forward. It is in rear impacts that the head moves backward.

Also in 1985, R. H. Roydhouse stated that a shoulder strap belt may cause neck torsion and damage even without neck hyperextension. Roydhouse had absolutely no experimental data to prove that this event could occur and cause a serious neck injury.

In 1984, A. Nygren tabulated the number of neck injuries in patients injured in various types of accidents. The study provokes the same concerns that Christian's study does. While it provides information on the number of neck injuries in belted and unbelted passengers, it is missing much data that could alter conclusions about the risk of neck injury due to use of seat belts. The most important problem with the study, that it did not include uninjured car occupants in the study of who wore seat belts and who did not, is admitted by the author, who said, "The belt usage among uninjured persons was unknown." As well, more than 40% of the injured drivers and passengers could not have their seat belt usage documented.

In 1987, G. T. Deans et al studied a small group of patients (137) in a manner similar to Christian's. They stated that there were more sprains of the neck among the belted than the unbelted.

The statistical difference between the two groups is not great ($p = 0.05$); this difference is close to the difference that would be found if the findings occurred by chance alone.[1] In addition, the researchers base these results on patients' reporting their symptoms and on a select group. The authors needed to examine all individuals involved in collisions and then determine whether being belted meant a higher risk of neck pain.

Similarly, in 1989, N. Yoganandan et al quoted the incidence of whiplash patients among belted and nonbelted occupants who had injuries. Yoganandan et al did not include occupants involved in accidents but without symptoms, and did not document the belt usage of this group; thus, the study provokes concerns similar to those provoked by the above studies. In 1990, U. Maag et al repeated this approach, as did R. Bourbeau et al in 1993.

Thus, no one has established the link between seat belt use and acute neck injury. Yet the effect of seat belt use is not the key issue in whiplash research anyway—the key issue is the cause of chronic pain reports.

REFERENCE

1. Norman GR, Streiner DL. *PDQ Statistics*. Toronto: BC Decker Inc; 1986.

Control of Illness Behavior

This section is part of a work in progress I have undertaken with Dr. Oliver Kwan and Dr. Jon Friel on disability syndromes in general. Setting the stage for future research efforts, we have begun with developing pragmatic conceptual frameworks about the control of illness behavior. The concepts here seem potentially useful in whiplash as well. Some of this material is also dealt with in Chapters 10 and 11.

I think; thereby I secondarily exist.

I learn; thereby I secondarily gain.

INTRODUCTION

This section delves into the thought processes that control the behavior of patients adopting the sick role. They are not necessarily malingering; that is, they are not planning out each step. Yet they are in control. To understand this, it is important to understand how people process information and how this processing affects their behavior.

First, we will discuss a model of the consciousness states, focusing on behavior as thoughts arise and interact in these varied states. Then we will examine how the various forms of gain associated with illness interact within these consciousness states.

STATES OF CONSCIOUSNESS

Models of states of consciousness have been considered from a variety of perspectives. It is beyond the scope of this section to address each of these or fully explain the sometimes confusing terminology in this broad body of literature. Instead, this section will focus on thought processing and goal-oriented behaviors, specifically the illness behavior determined by psychological factors, and how the information processing in different consciousness states ultimately produces that illness behavior.

Such models have relevance in therapy (understanding the underlying thought processes and beliefs patients hold may lead to understanding their illness behavior and altering that behavior) and legal matters. This section will specifically consider accident victims with chronic pain and disability where the illness is thought to be mediated chiefly by psychological factors.

Conscious State

The conscious state is equivalent to awareness and thus appears to be the state where thought processing is most amenable to control. Volition is synonymous with a capacity to control (volition is a matter of free will). Control or volition does not necessarily require conscious awareness of every behavior. It merely entails the availability of choices or alternatives. As long as people are aware of alternatives (or it is judged that they have the capacity to be aware of alternatives), then they have volition.[1]

Unconscious State

The unconscious state has the special property of being entirely outside awareness and control. According to the Freudian model, unconscious thoughts are deep within our psyche and not readily accessible. The unconscious holds those thoughts and thought processes that cannot be brought to awareness because of the operation of a counterforce. Such thoughts are kept in the unconscious state by psychic defenses, for example: they are repressed, at least for a time. Were they suddenly released, psychotic behavior would likely ensue.

Unconscious thoughts are potentially expressed over time through a neurosis. The neurosis evolves when the unconscious thoughts result in excessive intrapsychic disturbance (ie, anxiety and tension) that threatens to undermine the integrity of personality and ego functioning. This intrapsychic tension can be reduced by forming certain symptoms (so-called "neurotic symptoms") and makes it possible to preserve the greater part of one's integration. The preservation of integrity is termed "primary gain," a gain that lies in the mastery of otherwise overwhelming tension or anxiety, albeit at the cost of reduction of function and psychological effectiveness. Further, the development of a neurosis has the primary gain that the unconscious thoughts can be released nonpsychotically, in a way that is more gradual (often over months to years) and that is now amenable to eventual insight and adjustment. Otherwise, given their nature, unconscious thought processes are not generally accessible, except through psychoanalysis, including dream analysis and hypnosis.

If one cannot access one's unconscious thoughts or control the events of primary gain, the neurosis must be, at least in large part, nonvolitional.

The courts have for years been dealing with these two states (conscious and unconscious) within a narrow version of the Freudian model. For them, thought processing is either conscious or unconscious. This dichotomy (two-state model) is insufficient. Indeed, when Freud introduced the concept of the unconscious, it was not in terms of such a dichotomy.[2] A third state—the preconscious—was considered essential. It was thought to function as an intermediary.

Preconscious State

Freud first conceived of the preconscious as merely a passageway from the unconscious to the conscious. Today, cognitive and experimental psychologists view the preconscious state in a more complex and yet practicable way. Thus, if the first step is abandoning the two-state model of conscious/unconscious, and recognizing the preconscious state, the second is viewing the preconscious state as evidenced by experimental psychology. Currently, the preconscious state of thought processing is characterized by unattended (unaware or unnoticed) information processing, that is the initial immediate analysis of one's environment (both external and internal).

The preconscious state of thought processing is characterized by unattended (unaware or unnoticed) information processing, until its output has a mental representation (propositional or nonpropositional) of which people are immediately aware.[3] Whereas the aforementioned unconscious state is the unnoticeable (unaware), which is repressed and cannot be brought to immediate awareness, the preconscious state instead contains all that we know that is not repressed and that can potentially be brought into consciousness without special effort (ie, without psychoanalysis, hypnosis, etc).[2]

Velmans and Dorpat have discussed how preconscious information processing may operate.[4,5] Information may be processed by focusing or not focusing attention on that information, the act of which may then bring a propositional representation to awareness (conscious). In denial, the preconscious information processing shifts attention away from, for example, disturbing stimuli emanating either from oneself or from the environment, to focus instead on less disturbing stimuli. This shifting of focus may occur at the preconscious level and may further allow thoughts that are disturbing to be repressed and placed in the unconscious state, psychic defenses maintaining them where they are unnoticeable and no longer accessible. How information processing leads to attention is determined by a person's prior experiences, value system, goals, and capacity to give sufficient attention to the information at a given time, as well as the overall significance or relevance a person attaches to the information received or being processed.[4]

A pertinent stimulus outside the focus of attention can yet attract attention. If people could not determine the significance of stimuli outside the focus of attention, it would be difficult for them to know when to switch their attention. People must have knowledge of the output of their information processing even though it takes place at a preconscious level. Learning allows for this process, state-dependent learning notwithstanding. Thus, a preliminary analysis of meaning can take place outside the focus of attention, without reportable consciousness.[4]

The preconscious information processing is thus monitored for propositional representations, which are then compared to a person's informational constraints, and attentional capacity, which in turn determines further how that information should be processed (that is one way people exert control, not so much over the information processing but over the evaluation and further processing of that output). Thus, automatic information processing itself is not within awareness, but the propositional representations are monitored and within awareness. This is the efficiency of the processing system, to allow for an apparent automaticity, the output of which can be monitored and allows for input of control or constraints for further processing.

It seems clear that preconscious information processing is essential to certain aspects of illness behavior. For, in the main, illness behavior includes receiving and processing information both from within (perceiving symptoms as painful, for example) and from without (information from one's culture, including the health care and social institutions, and the response of others to one's symptoms reporting). Some aspect of this information processing is likely preconscious. To what extent this information processing is automatic will be discussed later.

Subconscious State

The subconscious state is in one sense a fourth element entwined with the conscious, unconscious, and preconscious states. Following Freud, preconscious information processing is nonaware (nonconscious) processing that may produce or "return" a mental representation of an object or event. When the representation is propositional, people are immediately aware of it. The preconscious processing in itself has no declarative knowledge associated with it; the declarative knowledge arises only as people further process the output of a propositional representation.[3]

There are unusual circumstances, however, in which a thought process leads to declarative knowledge even though the processing is nonconscious (nonaware), with no output of a propositional representation to be aware of. This may occur in hypnosis states, where individuals declare knowledge or behaviors for which they have no conscious representation before or after hypnosis. Another such circumstance is conversion disorder, in which an individual declares paralysis, for example, but has no conscious awareness of the information processing output (mental representation) underlying that declaration. Information processing in which nonconscious procedural knowledge produces no mental representation (phenomenal awareness) but can act on declarative knowledge is referred to as subconscious processing.[6] The origin of the mental events may be in the unconscious Freudian state but does not lead to a mental representation (to enter consciousness), even though it finally involves declarative knowledge. Such phenomena (eg, conversion disorder) have not as yet included chronic pain as the declarative knowledge, because the primary gain achieved via the interaction between unconscious thoughts and further processing of those thoughts to declarative knowledge is not expected to be achieved by chronic pain.

Recall that primary gain is the result of mental processing that renders a reduction in psychic conflicts stemming from unconscious thoughts. The neuroses arise as a manifestation of that primary gain. These neuroses are not produced for the pursuit of secondary gain and are not a result of the availability of secondary gain. Secondary gain comes from without, and primary gain comes from within. Secondary gain arises from the action of others acknowledging the legitimacy of the illness behavior (the sick role contract), while primary gain arises from one's own actions and does not require others to condone the illness behavior. Thus, the subconscious state will not be further dealt with here as it is not relevant to secondary gain and chronic pain.

Summary

Through a long history of clinical observation; experimentation; simultaneous exploration of behavioral, physiological, and biochemical facets of mental activities; and clinical success in psychotherapy, a useful model has emerged. It divides consciousness into the trilogy: conscious, preconscious, and unconscious, with the potential for inclusion of a subconscious processing state that interacts with these. This broader and more approximate model has been largely ignored by the courts, and a large body of research has addressed it.[2,4,6] This model is depicted in Figure 23–1.

SECONDARY GAIN

As stated above, secondary gain, unlike primary gain, is not formed by the individual. Over time, secondary gain has become largely a legal concept. It currently can be understood as arising out of a social construct—the sick role. Parsons was among the first to examine the social construct of the sick role as a partially and conditionally legitimate state that an individual may be granted.[7] Thus, society has decided that an ill individual shall hold this distinct role. The role entails the obligation to cooperate with others for the purpose of "getting well" as soon as possible.

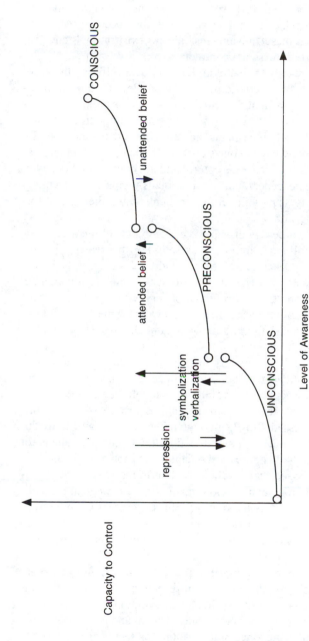

Figure 23–1 States of Consciousness—Quantized, Discontinuous Spectrum. The trilogy of consciousness states may be represented as a spectrum of awareness and capacity to change by free will. The spectrum is discontinuous. That is, internal and external cues engage cerebral processes that gradually (the curved slope) build in intensity and distribution, until a threshold is reached, upon which the thought enters a different level of consciousness. This change in level of consciousness if instantaneous and renders a different capacity for the thought. This instantaneous and quantum level change thus reflects an infinite slope, hence the representation as a quantum level change and the discontinuity.

The change in quantum level is achieved by energy input, for example, via symbolization when changing from unconscious to preconscious or conscious. Equally, attending or unattending beliefs in response to internal or environmental cues (focusing or distracting attention, respectively) will precipitate a quantum level change.

In addition, special rights and privileges are granted to individuals who become ill. They may be relieved from work, social obligations, and civic duties. To the extent that these are advantageous to the individual, they become secondary gains. It should be noted that these "advantages" always exist in one's environment and are awarded as part of the social contract.

Hence, secondary gain is readily available to the individual fulfilling the criteria for the sick role. What are the criteria for the sick role? Because most psychological illnesses involve the stigma that the individual is "at fault," the sick role is most readily granted when the criteria of "no fault" are met. Implicit in this no-fault system, as Ferrari and Kwan[8] describe, is the belief that a disease potentially influences one's behavior largely beyond one's control. If one has knee inflammation, one has knee pain. It is not under one's control and not one's fault. Society in general, many health care gatekeepers, and often patients themselves view psychological illness or disability as partially at least patients' fault: their moral fortitude is often called into question.

The appearance of organic illness (a disease) is certainly one of the most readily available forms of no-fault entry into the sick role. For this reason, debates rage over whether fibromyalgia, chronic fatigue syndrome, late whiplash syndrome, and other conditions are diseases or nondiseases, organic or nonorganic. If society would as readily grant the sick role to a patient with psychological illness as to a patient with organic illness, then fibromyalgia patients would not have to fight constantly to establish their illness as organic disease. They could be granted the sick role as easily as anyone else.

But people do not want freely and readily to grant the sick role to those with psychological illness. No matter how much biochemical evidence exists for depression, for example, depressed patients would prefer to tell their employers and their friends that they are unable to meet their obligations because of their arthritis, not because they are depressed. Why? Although others do not blame individuals for their arthritis, fatigue, or severe pain, they do often blame individuals for their depression. People simply do not readily accept depression as a disease.

Even when it is acknowledged that psychological suffering is genuine suffering, labeling illnesses like fibromyalgia as nonorganic or psychological disqualifies them as no-fault entries into the sick role. This bias is evident in both physicians and insurance companies. No matter the symptoms or their severity, when the origin of symptoms is considered to be emotional, disability is far less likely to be granted by the parties involved.[7]

So the sick role has this implicit requirement: present with a condition that appears to have a no-fault basis, usually a condition resembling a disease. Patients are obligated to minimize reporting of psychological symptoms or disturbances and maximize reporting of physical symptoms such as pain and numbness. If patients admit to psychological disturbance, it is attributed as secondary to the pain, just as a patient with rheumatoid arthritis can develop depression secondary to chronic pain. Society accepts that the pain in rheumatoid arthritis is something beyond one's control, and so it is also beyond one's control if depression follows. Depression is likely beyond one's control, but if a "disease" is not there, society treats the depression differently.

Once one meets the requirements for the sick role, the sick role is granted. But note again, as mentioned earlier, that the sick role is a social contract as well, for there is the proviso that the patient must cooperate with others for the purpose of "getting well" as soon as possible.[8] Thus, the individual must be fully motivated to become well. Once the individual shows any motivation not to get well, then the contract is broken. Society labels the lack of motivation to get well (or motivation to remain ill), in its most extreme form, malingering. In malingering, one consciously plots and carries out one's conscious motivations to remain ill and is fully in control of doing so. Is there another way to carry out one's motivations to maintain the sick role? There may be other ways indeed, and yet it seems odd that anyone would wish to be genuinely ill. It is understandable why malingerers choose to appear ill; they do not lose or suffer as a result.

ECONOMY OF SECONDARY GAIN

Most people believe that being ill is not desirable, and although there are gains to being ill (in this instance, secondary gains), there clearly are losses. But why would anyone pursue secondary gain in the first place if illness also brings losses? What is the net gain if illness brings losses? Illness brings the greatest losses to individuals not otherwise distressed or already suffering. What if individuals are distressed, overburdened, and suffering in a way that gives them no option for a socially acceptable reprieve? What if the losses that most people experience (loss of income, enjoyment of family life, opportunity and hope of achieving one's goals) are already present or relatively unimportant before the illness? What if people's circumstances become so intolerable that abandoning them all might be a viable alternative for psychological survival? Does the illness really bring so much loss that it is inconceivable to adopt this sick role? Perhaps not, and besides, the sick role comes with secondary gains. Perhaps it is this balance that determines whether a person will adopt the sick role. Most people find the balance is too heavily weighed by losses; for some, there are greater gains.

Some individuals who are suffering psychologically before they are known to be sick may hide their symptoms, perhaps even from themselves. They may have suffered many miseries and disappointments, and yet they may have to continue to cope because society will not grant them freedom to do otherwise. They are forced to continue in their miserable lives. Why suffer and not be given the sick role when one can suffer (just change the presentation of symptoms from that of apparent psychological origin to that of apparent disease origin) and get the sick role?

The steps to pursuing secondary gain may be as follows:

1. The sick role has criteria. Those criteria are presumably overlearned in our society.
2. The secondary gains, also presumably overlearned, are available to those with the sick role.
3. The sick role is available to those with no-fault entry (a no-fault illness).
4. The no-fault entry is thus available to those presenting with specified types of symptoms and syndromes.
5. One presents with those symptoms that may lead to a no-fault diagnosis (and minimizes any symptom that might lead to an at-fault diagnosis).
6. One maintains that behavior.

Can this pursuit be achieved by means other than frank malingering—a largely conscious maneuver? Given the dynamics of the model of consciousness states considered above, it is clear that this is possible.

ENACTING OF MOTIVATIONS AND AUTOMATICITY

Motivations are a form of readiness and are goal oriented.[9] Motivation means preparedness for action; an individual is merely waiting for an opportunity. Motivations reach into the individual's environment.[9] A motivation leads one to have an ever-present readiness to identify and further process environmental information that suggests enactment of the motivation is possible. Clearly, for motivations to be enacted, they must lie within the realm of the preconscious and conscious, not the unconscious.

Automaticity may help enact motivations for desired goals in daily life. The preconscious state may thus be very important for processing information within this more automatic realm. Automaticity is, however, vastly misunderstood, for it is often thought to mean that something does not require conscious input.[10]

If one imagines that adoption of the sick role initially at least involves the access to overlearned knowledge, a preconscious processing of gains versus losses, of attention to one's pain rather than to one's recovery, one wonders if the processing could remain beyond one's awareness. In remaining at a preconscious level of processing, would individuals be aware of this behavior? As we discussed above, for goal-oriented behavior, it is more than likely they would.

In most societies, children learn quickly that secondary gain is part of the sick role. This knowledge is held though not always attended to. In this sense, such knowledge is said to be in people's preconscious state. The weighing of secondary gains and losses from illness may be a preconscious process.

Most people do not realize they are weighing gains and losses as they begin to recover from acute injury or illness. Yet most people would have no trouble making a list of secondary gains and losses from having chronic back pain. They could then explain why they prefer health and why they would be motivated to become healthy after injury or illness. The knowledge is within people. Yet they are not consciously aware of going through this decision-making process after every acute back pain episode. To some extent, whoever granted them the sick role following acute injury is prepared to ensure access to secondary gains. Secondary gain is always there under such circumstances. How do people make that initial balance of gains and losses without being aware of it? Our own experience suggests that people do not initially process such information consciously, but they may process it consciously later if they have a goal to reach and maintain.

Control of Goal-Oriented Behavior

Is the adoption of the sick role, as a social behavior, a choice, under one's control, or can it happen automatically, and be truly beyond one's control? For many years, just as there has been a perceived dichotomy of conscious-unconscious thought processes, there has been the misperception that these processes are either automatic or controlled.

The axiomatic definition of automaticity has long been that the thought process be unintentional, involuntary (lack of control), autonomous, and occurring outside awareness. In fact, most cognitive psychologists argue that the term automaticity should be abandoned in favor of the "horsemen" of automaticity: unintentional, involuntary (lack of control), autonomous, and unaware. Behaviors may have some of the horsemen at work and not others.

Most social behavior, therefore, often does not have all four of these horsemen at work. It is clear that most social and cognitive behaviors are complex and do not represent all-or-none phenomena, even though they may seem automatic (have some of the horsemen active) in some aspects.[11,12] To the extent that complex mental processes can become unmonitored or unaware through practice, the scope of preconscious processing may be expandable to some degree. Thus if one allows complex judgments to become routine, these may be performed even on subliminal stimuli being presented, especially if they are presented at the subjective rather than the objective threshold. Yet, this does not necessarily make them unintentional or uncontrollable. Bargh explains that although initial research on preconscious information processing has shown that social behaviors can be brought about without apparent effort, that same research indicates that experiment subjects needed specific instructions to make a judgment or form an impression.[11] As such, they could not be unintentional. Bargh adds that other preconscious information processing experiments have shown measured behavior to be unintentional, but dependent on effort of attention.

As a further example, consider driving. One is aware that one is driving, and one intends to drive. What makes this still seem "automatic" is that while the qualities of unintentional and unawareness are lacking, are the other horsemen of

there is autonomy of the action (once set in motion we do not have to be aware of how to keep it in motion), and there is a low level of attentive effort required (autonomous). Hence, as per the popular statement of an individual's elemental abilities: "He can at least walk and chew gum at the same time." This form of "automaticity" (in one sense of the word) has been referred to by Bargh[11(p24)] as "intended goal-dependent automaticity."

So if one is to consider automaticity, one must further qualify which of the horsemen of automaticity is operative: unintentional, involuntary (lack of control), autonomy, and unaware.

Goal-Dependent Automaticity

The goal we have been considering here is adoption and maintenance of the sick role. It seems paradoxical to have an "intentional form of automaticity," but this simply refers to the fact that one may set a goal, and the process does not need to be controlled once it has started—it is autonomous. As Bargh points out, however, studies indicate that more attentional control and conscious decision making are needed when the situation has novel characteristics or nonroutine events arise.[11] The fact that such processes immediately demand and attract conscious attention at these nonroutine junctures indicates how closely controlled the processes are despite their otherwise autonomous nature. We suggest that over the lengthy process of adoption and maintenance of the sick role, such illness behavior entails encountering many novel situations and nonroutine events.

Illness brings events that entail losses that must be weighed each time they arrive, even though the loss may be expected only for a limited time. Alternatively, there may be events that challenge the legitimacy of the sick role in some way, and those nonroutine events must be dealt with to maintain the intended goal-oriented automaticity.

The proximal stimulus of a consideration of gains that ultimately recognizes an economy favoring adoption of the sick role may very well be processed preconsciously. But control is necessary for the remainder of the behavior to be maintained over time.

Preconscious processing categorizes, evaluates, and imputes the meaning of social input, and this input is available for conscious and controlled judgment and behavioral decisions; however, those judgments and decisions are not mandatory and uncontrollable, given the proximal stimulus event alone.[11]

It is true that automaticity can be seen in some social behaviors in the experimental setting in response to immediate stimuli, but this occurs only when the individual already associates a given situation with the behavioral representation being activated.[13] The question is thus not how often such automatic behavioral events occur but whether and how often they can be controlled or overridden by some conscious intention and purpose. We are all aware of the receipt of secondary gain as an expected consequence of illness, but the social behavior of adoption of the sick role is not simply enacted by that awareness or even the existence of motivations for such behavior alone. Fiske and Devine have suggested, for example, that the preconscious processing of prejudicial motivations such as racial discrimination requires conscious input to be enacted.[14,15] Although one may be able to affect people's behavior by making some motivations more salient than others, one cannot give people a motivation that they do not already have and make them do something for which they have no motive base.

CONCLUSION

The sick role exists in most societies as a social contract between those who are ill and those who are empowered to grant relief from one's normal societal role during the illness. The contract may be broken when the ill individual is motivated to not "get well." Such motivations may arise for many reasons, but most generally arise within the economy of secondary gain. Certain individuals are at risk for having an economy that favors maintenance of the sick role because the secondary gains afforded by the sick role outweigh the secondary losses from the illness.

The thought processing (cognition) underlying this behavior can best be appreciated by the more complete model of states of consciousness comprising the preconscious state (processing to focus attention on thoughts related to the goal-oriented motivations) and the conscious state (the thoughts that maintain and bind the process toward fulfillment of the goal-oriented motivations). To an extent, much of the thought processing in illness behavior may be preconscious and have some of the defining features of automaticity, but the overall behavior, being goal-oriented toward adoption of the sick role, yet requires elements of nonautomatic, and therefore controllable, behavior.

The long-held field theory of social behavior remains supported.[16] The field theory holds that individuals must at some time (or many times) decide their motivations, determine the value of those motivations, and weigh the consequences of those motivations should they be enacted. Otherwise, the goal-oriented behavior cannot be maintained. For preconscious processing to affect enactment of a motivation, it is necessary that relevant goal structures be activated. Thus, preconscious motivation to adopt the sick role would not be enough to achieve the illness behavior that would ensure others grant the sick role. Even if people were to engage in the consideration of the economy of secondary gain at a preconscious level (outside one's awareness), the illness behavior to adopt the sick role would not be chosen unless individuals decide they want the gains and intend to pursue those gains.[13] Conscious awareness of motivations is necessary at some point in the evaluation process and in ultimately enacting the illness behavior of adoption of the sick role. Further, it is the strength of motivations and conscious appreciation of negative and positive consequences that determine the extent to which behaviors are enacted.[11]

Thus, most complex social behaviors have some but not all features of automaticity. This is what has lead to confusion about whether an act or behavior is controllable. When an act is said to be outside of awareness, that does not mean on its own that it is automatic, as it still may be intentional and motivated. Yet many have held the misconception that because a thought process does not entail awareness, it is "automatic" and thus uncontrollable. Bargh points out that the view that there is a truly "automatic" nature to social behaviors is falsely held because of the belief that automatic social behaviors are an all-or-none phenomenon.[13] Complex social behaviors may seem to be automatic but are not, and the phenomenology of apparent automaticity suggests strongly that while many of the underlying processes are automatic, the behavior is not. Automatic reactions can be modulated by attention and intention, be suppressed, and be goal oriented.

Complex social behaviors where one has goal-oriented motivations (adoption of the sick role obviously being within this realm) necessarily require conscious control even though there are aspects of automaticity apparent. Preconscious processing does not remove control but allows for the convenience and efficiency of some aspects of automaticity. This misconception, as well as the difference between our common usage of "automatic" and the known phenomenology of automaticity (appreciated from experimental evidence), may have arisen because we have come to use an inappropriate contrasting scheme of definitions. When we contrast "automatic" with "controlled," we assume that automatic processes cannot be controlled. Alternatively, when we contrast "automatic" with "conscious," we mistakenly believe that automatic behaviors belong to our "unconscious minds." Experimental evidence suggests that for most behaviors "automatic" should not be contrasted with any of these, but rather with adjectives such as "attentive." Then "automaticity" in some cases comes to mean simply "nonattentiveness."[3] Control remains.

Understanding the states of consciousness and thought process interaction helps clinicians to understand that pain behaviors may indeed be nonmalingered and yet be under one's control in the grander appreciation of the illness behavior. This interaction between conscious and preconscious information processing allows for the enactment of one's motivations to adopt the sick role, which may further explain the efficacy of cognitive therapy in chronic pain and other disability syndromes. There seems to be little doubt that belief systems, for example, influence the behavior of chronic pain patients.[17] These belief systems may be processed on both a preconscious (unattended) and conscious (attended) level. Cognitive therapy allows conscious efforts to alter the response to and perhaps the very basis of these belief systems through insight, further evidence of the capacity of conscious thought processes to reach and thereby control the effect of preconscious information processing on enactment of motivations.

This same understanding allows for appropriate appreciation of the role secondary gain plays in illness behaviors when it is "not conscious." We see that "not conscious" does not mean unconscious. "Not conscious" does not necessarily mean "nonvolitional" or "automatic" either. The full appreciation of "nonconscious" processes that are perhaps yet intentional and subject to volition arises only through an appreciation of the role of preconscious thought processing in illness behavior—both its capabilities for aspects of automaticity and its limitations in leading to motivation enactment and complex social behaviors.

Indeed, understanding the interaction of automaticity, volition, and illness behavior likely has numerous clinical, social, and legal applications.

REFERENCES

1. Jang D, Coles EM. The evolution and definition of the concept of 'automatism' in Canadian Case Law. *Medicine and the Law.* 1995;14:221–238.

2. Civin M, Lombardi KL. The preconscious and potential space. *Psychoanalytic Review.* 1990;77(4):573–585.

3. Tzelgov J. Specifying the relations between automaticity and consciousness: a theoretical note. *Consciousness and Cognition.* 1997;6:441–451.

4. Velmans M. Is human information processing conscious? *Behavioral and Brain Sciences.* 1991;14:651–726.

5. Dorpat TL. The cognitive arrest hypothesis of denial. *International Journal of Psychoanalysis.* 1983;64:47–58.

6. Kihlstrom JF. The psychological unconscious and the self. Experimental and theoretical studies of consciousness. In: *Ciba Foundation Symposium 174.* Chichester, England: Wiley; 1993:147–167.

7. Ferrari R, Kwan O. Comment on study by Aaron et al. Perceived physical and emotional trauma as precipitating events in fibromyalgia [letter]. *Arthritis and Rheumatism.* 1998. In press.

8. Parsons T. *Social Structure and Personality.* London: Collier-MacMillan; 1964.

9. Pribram KH. Brain models of mind. In: Kaplan HR, Sadock BJ, ed. *Comprehensive Textbook of Psychiatry.* 6th ed. Baltimore: Williams & Wilkins; 1995:331.

10. Fleminger S. Seeing is believing: the role of 'preconscious' perceptual processing in delusional misidentification. *British Journal of Psychiatry.* 1992;160:293–303.

11. Bargh JA. Conditional automaticity: varieties of automatic influence in social perception and cognition. In: Uleman JS, Bargh JA, eds. *Unintended Thought.* New York: Guilford Press; 1989:3–52.

12. Bargh JA. The ecology of automaticity: Toward establishing the conditions needed to produce automatic processing effects. *American Journal of Psychology.* 1992; 105(2):181–199.

13. Bargh JA, Chen M, Burrows L. Automaticity of social behavior: direct effects of trait construct and stereotype activation on action. *Journal of Personality and Social Psychology.* 1996;71(2):230–244.

14. Fiske ST. Examining the Role of Intent: Toward Understanding Its Role in Stereotyping and Prejudice. In: Uleman JS, Bargh JA, eds. *Unintended Thought.* New York: Guilford Press; 1989:253–283.

15. Devine PG. Stereotypes and prejudice: their automatic and controlled components. *Journal of Personality and Social Psychology.* 1989;56:680–690.

16. Lewin K. Defining the "field at a given time." *Psychology Review.* 1943;50:292–310.

17. Kilhstrom JF. The cognitive unconscious. *Science.* 1987;237:1445–1452.

CHAPTER 24

Tertiary Gain

The following is part of a work in progress I have undertaken with Dr. Oliver Kwan and Dr. Jon Friel regarding the development of a conceptual framework for future research on the phenomenon of tertiary gain. Tertiary gain is also briefly dealt with in Chapter 10.

INTRODUCTION

Gain has long been a subject of debate in the health care and legal communities, particularly as an element operating within the context of illness behavior in disability syndromes. The focus has largely been on primary and secondary gain, despite the recognition decades ago of a need to appreciate the concept of tertiary gain (D. A. Dansak 1973). There has been no research on tertiary gain, and indeed few have attempted to establish a framework upon which to pursue research on this subject. In this regard, we suggest that a pragmatic approach is necessary. The first step in such an approach is phraseologic. The second step is an exploration of the quintessential elements from which tertiary gains arise and how the gains may be pursued. An understanding of how tertiary gain is achieved will lay the foundation for future discussion and research.

Because tertiary gain occurs in the setting of illness behavior, and because illness behavior is equally entwined with secondary and primary gain, to understand tertiary gain, one must fully understand primary and secondary gain. Primary and secondary gain have been discussed elsewhere in this book (see Chapters 10 and 11).

TERTIARY GAIN

Tertiary gain was first proposed by Dansak (1973) as an important modulating and motivating factor in illness behavior. He defined tertiary gains simply as

499

gains sought or attained from a patient's illness by someone other than the patient. In his discussion, he further implies that tertiary gain is the result of some self-serving intent. Although the term "secondary gain" also carries a negative connotation, it is actually a neutral phenomenon, available and received by virtually all of those who are ill. The malignancy is not the gain itself but rather the desire for gain as the motivation underlying and dictating one's behavior. We thus suggest that tertiary gain is a neutral phenomenon as well. Some, however, are motivated by the desire for tertiary gain.

Tertiary gain arises out of the social construct of the caregiver role. That is, society values the caregiver role to the extent that personal advantages are immediately conferred to the caregiver (monetary payment for services, special status and recognition in the community as a caregiver, excuse from one's responsibilities to some extent while dealing with the ill person, and other advantages that will be discussed later). These advantages are tertiary gains and are very often merely a valued, normal, and natural consequence of the caregiver role. That is, while these gains can be pursued, they also are attained automatically from the caregiver role, and their existence does not necessarily imply a motivation to receive gain or that the gain is dictating behavior.

The caregiver role must be broadly defined to appreciate the full extent of tertiary gains available. Health care workers are not the only caregivers. Legal professionals (eg, personal injury lawyers caring for the rights of injured or ill individuals), social workers, religious community members, and family members or friends may also be caregivers. Each can become entwined in or affected by the person's illness and thus play a caregiving role. Caregivers, in carrying out their role, can receive tertiary gains without any specific motivation other than to care for another. People apparently value this exchange. Yet people do not expect that caregivers be motivated to care chiefly because they expect and wish to receive tertiary gain. When tertiary gains are deliberately sought through the caregiver role, it breaches a contract caregivers have with society: they are expected to care for caring's sake and not for the sake of tertiary gain.

Of course, along with secondary gains, illness brings secondary losses (suffering, loss of income, reduced ability to carry out normal social roles, etc). It is the secondary losses that the ill person experiences that make illness undesirable. Just as there are tertiary gains, there are tertiary losses. Tertiary loss may be defined as the limitation or loss (linked to the patient's illness) experienced by an individual other than the patient. Obvious examples of tertiary loss include emotional distress over a family member's illness, loss of income, and increased responsibility upon "well" members of the family to accommodate the ill individual's incapacity to fulfill his or her normal role. Tertiary losses operate in an economy, balanced against tertiary gains. They influence behavior as much as tertiary gains do.

ECONOMY OF TERTIARY GAIN

As noted above, tertiary gains and losses operate in an economy, just as secondary gains and losses do. For most people, secondary losses so outweigh secondary gains that not only is illness undesirable but the ill individual is motivated to recover as soon as possible. This satisfies the social contract of the sick role. There is a small percentage of people, however, who may actually have an economy of secondary gain such that the gains dramatically outweigh the losses. In such cases, the individual is not motivated to relinquish the sick role but to continue to receive secondary gains. This is adoption of the sick role—pursuit of secondary gain—and is not simply malingering.

It is also possible to be motivated to pursue tertiary gain. In most cases, the caregiver need not "adopt the caregiver role," as that role is usually established in advance by social structures. Health care, legal, religious, and other professionals are already in that role, and indeed family members are usually automatically expected to fulfill that role when a family member is ill. While in that caregiver role, however, individuals may be motivated to care not simply for caring's sake but to pursue the recognized opportunity for tertiary gain. This pursuit of tertiary gain motivates them.

Yet tertiary gains must be balanced against tertiary losses. If a person's illness brings tertiary losses, is it ever desirable to receive tertiary gains in the face of those losses? It may be in some cases where the gains outweigh the losses. For most professional caregivers, the tertiary losses are low. It is likely that only true professionalism and sense of honor and duty preclude most caregivers from actively pursuing tertiary gain. They receive tertiary gain as part of their normal caregiver role, but that is not their primary motivation for caring. Yet it would be easy to function in the normal and honorable caregiver role but actually be motivated by tertiary gain.

For the family member caregiver, there are usually more tertiary losses expected, and so these people do not usually wish the individual's illness to continue. There may be circumstances, however, in which the tertiary gains for the family member outweigh the tertiary losses. Dansak offers an example where declaring a family member insane (and placing that family member in an asylum) results in more living space for the rest of the family—a definite gain.

The following section examines the tertiary gains and losses for family member caregivers and professional caregivers.

PURSUIT OF TERTIARY GAIN

The following tertiary gains are available to the professional caregiver:

- gratifying altruistic needs
- gratifying need (or sense of righteousness) to level the playing field against the "big corporation"

- obtaining fame and fortune after years of struggling and dutiful attention to responsibilities
- gaining admiration and respect from patients or their support groups
- withdrawing from or simply avoiding unpleasant or potentially litigious situations that may result from confronting the patient with a diagnosis or treatment the patient and his or her community might reject (giving a patient the diagnosis and treatment the patient clearly wants frees a physician from rebuke)
- gaining financial rewards from an increased client pool
- establishing one's position in one's field as a compassionate patient advocate—part of the popular "victimology"
- excusing oneself from the greater demands of intellectual honesty
- attacking professional detractors
- gratifying preexisting unresolved vengeful feelings wherein one's hostility toward the world is expressed thorough rebelling against established scientific facts
- validating one's own illness of the same type

The following tertiary losses are available to the professional caregiver:

- being viewed by some colleagues or others as dishonorable, feeling that the caregiver is disabling the patient
- feeling that one is ignoring one's duty to society by not directing patients to more appropriate diagnosis and treatment

The following tertiary gains are available to the family member caregiver:

- gratifying altruistic needs
- gaining financially
- making the ill individual develop a dependency on the caregiver, thus elevating the role of that caregiver in the relationship

The following tertiary losses are available to the family member caregiver:

- having increased responsibilities (perhaps having to work in place of the ill individual to maintain the family income and having more work to do at home)
- experiencing the suffering of a loved one
- suffering financially
- facing disturbance or discord (emotional and physical) within the relationship with the ill person
- facing guilt created by the ill individual that obligates the caregiver to remain in an already undesirable relationship
- facing stigmatization because the caregiver is associated with the ill individual

It is the economy of tertiary gain, the weighing and assigning of value to these gains and losses, that will determine how desirable is the pursuit of tertiary gain. Depending on the caregiver's previous relationship with the ill individual, the caregiver's own emotional and social state, the caregiver's own perceived needs, and so forth, the net balance may be quite varied. It seems that for the professional caregiver, the gains would most often substantially outweigh the losses, and yet one would like to believe the pursuit of tertiary gain is a key motivation in only a few professional caregivers. In most caregivers, it is assumed that honor and ethics outweigh the temptation of tertiary gain. Only when the behavior is blatant would one suspect a caregiver of pursuing tertiary gain.

Though there has been research into the risk factors for adoption of the sick role and pursuit of secondary gain, there is no research into the risk factors for pursuit of tertiary gain. The gains themselves may, in retrospect, implicate the risk factors. But clearly, more research is needed. Knowing the risk factors may enable identification of individuals who may be motivated by tertiary gain and enable intervention.

INTERACTION OF SECONDARY AND TERTIARY GAIN PURSUIT

It seems apparent that an individual adopting the sick role (pursuing secondary gain) and a caregiver pursuing tertiary gain will eventually meet. Do they meet because they seek each other out, or do they meet many individuals and finally remain with each other because, even without a formal declaration, they serve each other's needs and form a symbiotic relationship?

A person who is "looking" for a dependency relationship, who has the desire to adopt the sick role, may have many partners and have personally "unsatisfying" relationships with them. This person may then meet another person who desires the role of caregiver and is actually prepared to engage in a long-term relationship with a person who is reporting disability. For this new partner, the situation may satisfy some deep need, and the tertiary gains may outweigh the losses.

The partner's action and role (motivated by tertiary gain) will then reinforce the ill person's sick role behaviors and further satisfy the ill person's purpose (to pursue secondary gains offered when occupying the sick role). Yet there is no open conspiracy between these two people. One induces the other's behavior and reinforces it. We suggest this may be referred to as "gain induction," a principle analogous to one well known in electromagnetic theory. In electromagnetic theory, a coil of wire carrying an electric current from a power source will generate a magnetic field. If another coil of wire without a direct link to a power source is placed in that generated magnetic field, this second coil will produce its own current. The effect of the first coil upon the other is known as "electromagnetic induction."

Gain induction is an analogous concept. When one individual is motivated to pursue gain, he or she generates a "gain field" that another individual may enter.

The behavior of the second individual may be altered (induced) as a result. The nature and strength of the gain field is determined by the pattern of behavior (in the case of the one adopting the sick role, abnormal illness behavior), to which others respond.

The response may be different for different individuals. We believe that when the respondent is also motivated to seek gain, induction is more likely to occur. The respondent will behave in ways that satisfy this motivation to pursue gain as well. Beyond induction, the two individuals may reinforce each other's gain behaviors. As has been described in other sections of this book, an individual cannot adopt the sick role without an enabling gatekeeper, usually a physician. That gatekeeper may be motivated to pursue tertiary gain, and almost automatically the two will entwine their behaviors to satisfy each other's motivations. Hence, one induces and reinforces behavior in the other. There may thus be co-induction.

The co-induction may be psychodynamically complex. For some patients, "getting better" may actually be a guilt-producing procedure that in turn does not allow one to get better. What is the basis of that guilt? We suggest it is in some cases the caregiver's tertiary gain behavior. Through the negative behavior created by the pursuit of tertiary gain, the patient may be influenced to feel guilty or anxious when "getting better." The caregiver may send out negative messages to the patient who tries to become better, more independent, and so forth, as this directly threatens the tertiary gain of the caregiver. The caregiver is, although not necessarily consciously, responding in ways that provoke guilt in the recovering patient. That guilt then prevents recovery, and the tertiary gains continue. Thus, when patients encounter caregivers who are pursuing tertiary gain, patients may feel they should not get better because others would be angry with them or not love them anymore.

And yet these processes are not openly spoken about or planned. Various preconscious and conscious thought processes are operating. Some aspects of the behavior are clearly involuntary. Ultimately, however, a person is making a choice and controlling the process.

CONCLUSION

Dansak was hopeful that the concept of tertiary gain might have a therapeutic application—encouraging caregivers to realize that they may hamper recovery if they do not appreciate how their own behavior modulates patients' behavior. The most important reason to understand tertiary gain may be that individuals seeking to adopt the sick role (pursue secondary gain) depend on others' motivations for tertiary gain. In fact, researchers may be focusing too much on the motivations of patients adopting the sick role and too little on the fact that a caregiver's pursuit of tertiary gain is essential to a patient's adopting the sick role.

The therapeutic community has sometimes had a negative influence in controversial syndromes such as the late whiplash syndrome, fibromyalgia, and chronic fatigue syndrome. This effect may be partly the result of the pursuit of tertiary gain.

The clinical utility of the concept of tertiary gain remains to be seen. Researchers must first appreciate the structure of tertiary gain before it can be more effectively considered through clinical research and further discourse.

Glossary

One can understand many of this text's concepts without being able to define most medical terms. But to work successfully with whiplash-related cases, one must use medical language correctly. Hence, this glossary. Many of the most important terms are defined within the text itself as well; less important terms are dealt with only here.

accommodation—A process the eye undergoes to adjust vision for various distances.

adhesion—A fibrous tissue that will often adhere to other normal tissues.

Adson's maneuver (test)—The examiner places the patient in a seated position and with the patient's head tilted back (hyperextended) and to one side. The patient takes a deep breath. The examiner checks if the radial (wrist) pulse on that side becomes much weaker. If it does, then that is a positive Adson's test. Positive results are often found in normal subjects.

aetiology—See **etiology.**

annulus fibrosus—This is a fibrous ring around the intervertebral disk through which the gel-like center of the disk may bulge if the disc ruptures.

anterior—The position in front of or in the forward position.

anteroposterior—Moving in a direction from anterior to posterior (from front to back).

articular—Having to do with a joint.

articular cartilage—A thin layer of cartilage covering the surface of each of two bones that meet to form a joint.

articulation—The movement of the bones of a joint where they meet to form the joint.

asymptomatic—Having no symptoms.

avulsion—A tissue or part of the body being torn away.

benign—Not serious or malignant and usually having a good outcome.

blinded study—The method of conducting a study so that the researchers and the participants do not know whether they are receiving the active component of a trial (eg, the real drug) or the inactive component (eg, a placebo).

canal stenosis—A narrowing of the canal through which the spinal cord runs.

capsular—Relating to the capsule of the joint.

capsule—The lining or envelope that surrounds a joint. It attaches to the end of each bone forming the joint.

cardiac—Having to do with the heart.

cervical—Having to do with the neck.

cervical lordosis—The anterior curve of the cervical spine as viewed from the side on an X-ray.

cervical migraine—A migraine headache that derives from some abnormality in the neck.

cervical radiculitis—Inflammation of a cervical nerve.

cervical spine—That part of the spinal column lying within the neck and composed of 7 vertebrae.

cervical spondylosis—Another term for *disc degeneration*, producing changes to the vertebrae, discs, and nearby ligaments. Other terms for this include *cervical disc disease, degenerative disc disease of the cervical spine, degenerative disease of the cervical spine,* and *osteoarthritis of the cervical spine.*

cervicogenic—Of or arising from disorders of the cervical spine.

chronic—Persisting over a long period of time—in most cases, more than weeks or months.

cicatricial—Pertaining to or of the nature of a scar formed in the healing of a wound.

computed tomography—A type of scan using X-ray beams to form a cross-section image. Also called a *computer-assisted tomography (CAT) scan.*

condylar poles—The outermost or the peak of the surface of a condyle.

condyle—A rounded projection on a bone, often involved in forming a joint with another bone.

control population—A standard population that resembles, in all respects, the population being tested except for the absence of the one characteristic being evaluated.

convergence—The process in which the eyes move toward the middle of the field of view to help focus on a nearby point.

coronal suture—The line of junction between two types of skull bones, the frontal and the parietal bones.

cranial base—The bony support for the brain, separating the cranial from the facial region of the skull.

deep fascia—A layer of tissue that is fibrous and forms a sheath around muscles. Also called *aponeurotic fascia*.

diplopia—Seeing double. Also called *double vision*.

disc or disk—See **intervertebral disc**.

disc-condyle complex—The dynamic structure referring to the relationship of the condyle of the mandible (jaw) and the disc of cartilage articulating between it and the temporal bone of the skull. The temporomandibular joint contains these structures.

disc disease—Degeneration of the vertebral discs, with flattening, and a tendency to be associated with bony spurs near the edges of the vertebrae involved. Also called *degenerative disc disease*.

diskogenic (discogenic)—Of or deriving from any process affecting the intervertebral disc.

dorsal—The position toward the back or behind. It is similar to *posterior*.

edema—The collection of extra fluid in tissues, often causing swelling.

electroencephalogram—The result of recording electrical activity of nerve cells in the brain. Abbreviated *EEG*.

electroencephalographic patterns—Specific patterns of the recordings of an electroencephalogram that can be interpreted as normal or abnormal.

electromyography—The recording and study of the intrinsic electrical properties of skeletal muscle by recording its activity through electrodes and by inducing activity with electrical stimulation of its supplying nerve. Abbreviated *EMG*.

electronystagmography—The process of recording electrical potentials in the retina of the eye that come about with eye movements. Abbreviated *ENG*.

etiologic(al)—Having to do with the cause of a disease or illness.

etiology—The study of causes of diseases or illnesses.

extension—What occurs when a joint moves so that the parts are drawn away from each other. *Hyperextension* is an extreme or excessive degree of extension, that is, beyond what is considered the normal range.

extravasation—Leaking of blood into tissues.

fibrocartilage—A type of cartilage made up of typical cartilage cells, with parallel thick, compact bundles of collagen.

fibromyalgia—One of the chronic pain syndromes, a primarily nonorganic illness characterized by diffuse pain in the trunk and extremities, numbness and/or tingling in the extremities, headaches, jaw pain, fatigue, malaise, poor sleep, and poor concentration. Often associated with irregular bowel habits (irritable bowel syndrome) and benign chest pain.

fibrosis—The formation of abnormal tissue containing mainly collagen fibers.

fibrositis—See **fibromyalgia**. The term *fibrositis* was originally coined to suggest inflammation in the tissues such as muscle and fascia, but when none was discovered, the term was changed to *fibromyalgia*.

flexion—The movement by which two ends of any jointed part are drawn toward each other. *Hyperflexion* is an extreme or excessive degree of flexion, that is, beyond what is considered the normal range.

flushing—Sudden and usually brief redness of the face, neck, or other body parts.

foramen—An opening or passage, usually in a bone.

foramina—Plural of *foramen*.

frontal lobe—The anterior portion of the brain.

gluteal fold—The crease separating the buttock from the thigh, where the sun don't shine.

hemorrhage—Bleeding.

hyperextension—See **extension**.

hyperflexion—See **flexion**.

hypertrophic degenerative change—The enlargement or overgrowth of bone at the ends of the vertebrae, often seen in association with degenerative disc disease.

hypertrophy—The enlargement or overgrowth of an organ.

hypochondriasis—Being preoccupied with bodily symptoms in a maladaptive way.

hysteria—More specifically now replaced with the *Diagnostic and Statistical Manual of Mental Disorders,* 4th Edition, conversion disorder.

iatrogenic—The result of actions by physicians in causing symptoms or illness.

interarticular disc—The *fibrocartilage* tissue in some joints, covering the ends of the bones making up the joint and representing the contact point of the joint surface where movement occurs.

intervertebral disc—Fibrocartilage found between the adjacent vertebrae. Each one consists of a fibrous ring (*annulus fibrosus*) and a gel-like center (*nucleus pulposus*).

intervertebral disc space—The space between two vertebral bones that is occupied by the disc.

intrapsychic—Taking place in the mind only.

kinematics—The study of the mechanics of movement.

kyphosis—Abnormally increased curvature (more convex) of the thoracic spine as viewed from the side.

lateral—Pertaining to a position farther away from the middle or away from the midline of the body or structure.

ligament—Fibrous tissue that connects bones or cartilage to other tissues to give more strength.

ligamentous—Having to do with a ligament.

longus colli—Muscle that runs vertically along the posterior aspect of the neck and is attached to the vertebrae there.

magnetic resonance imaging—A form of imaging in which images may be produced through various planes of a body part of interest, using magnetic properties of the tissues to obtain the signal for the image. Abbreviated *MRI*.

malocclusion—Abnormal position and contact of the upper and lower teeth that interferes with the movements that occur during chewing.

mandible—The name of the bone normally called the jaw.

mastication—The act of chewing food.

medial—Pertaining to the middle, or closer to the midline of the body or a structure.

migraine—A form of headache sometimes referred to as a *vascular headache*, with periodic attacks, usually on one side of the head, sometimes associated with irritability, nausea, vomiting, aversion to light, and occasionally unusual visual phenomena prior to the headache onset.

muscular rheumatism—A vague term sometimes used synonymously with *fibromyalgia*. The reason Granny consumed spirits for medicinal purposes.

musculature—The muscles.

musculoskeletal—Having to do with the skeleton and the muscles.

myelogram—An X-ray of the spinal cord taken after a special dye is injected around the spinal cord.

myospasm—Muscle spasm.

nerve conduction studies—Studies that measure the velocity, amplitude, and character of electrical signals conducted along stimulated nerves.

neuralgia—Pain arising from some disorder of the nerves themselves.

neurasthenia—An older term for *chronic fatigue syndrome.*

neurologic(al)—Having to do with the nervous system.

neurology—The study of the nervous system.

neuromuscular tension—The condition of mild to moderate contraction of a muscle in response to stimulation of the nervous system.

neurons—The cells of the nervous system that conduct electrical impulses.

neurosis—Also called a *psychoneurosis,* it refers to a disorder arising from some intrapsychic conflict or disorder.

nociceptor—A nerve receptor for pain.

nonorganic—In the context of illness, *nonorganic* is used to indicate that the origin of the illness is chiefly psychosocial rather than physical (biological).

nucleus pulposus—The gel-like center of an intervertebral disc.

nystagmus—A rapid, involuntary movement of the eyeball. The movement may be of horizontal, vertical, rotatory, or mixed directions.

occipital region—The posterior part of the brain or skull.

ocular—Of or having to do with the eyes or vision.

ophthalmologic—Having to do with diseases and defects of the eye.

organic—Used to indicate that the origin of the illness is chiefly through physical rather than psychosocial factors.

osseous—Having to do with bone.

osteoarthritis—A degenerative joint disease resulting in degeneration of the articular cartilage and inflammation within the joint, often causing pain.

osteophyte—Abnormal bone outgrowth.

paresthesia—An abnormal sensation such as burning, prickling, or pins and needles.

pathogenesis—The development of disease or illness.

pathology—The study of the tissue changes underlying disease.

pathophysiological mechanisms—The mechanisms of disease or abnormal functioning of the body.

periosteum—A specialized tissue covering all bones of the body and possessing bone-forming potential.

PET (positron emission tomography)—A scan that uses a nuclear particle (a positron) to produce the image.

photophobia—Abnormal visual intolerance to light.

physiologic(al)—Having to do with the normal functioning of the body.

physiology—The study of the body, its parts, and the physical and chemical processes involved in normal function.

placebo—An inactive substance used in controlled studies to determine the true effect of a drug or other therapy.

positional nystagmus—Nystagmus that is brought on by certain head positions.

positron emission tomography—See **PET**.

posterior intervertebral joints—Joints between the bones along the posterior aspect of the spine.

posterior osteophytes—The formation of osteophytes along the posterior aspects of the vertebrae.

posteroanterior—Moving in a direction from posterior to anterior (from back to front).

prevertebral soft-tissue space—The space anterior to the vertebrae of the spine; in the neck, it contains the airways, esophagus, and major blood vessels.

psychical—Having to do with the psyche (mind).

psychologic(al)—Having to do with psychology.

psychology—The study of the mental processes underlying human behavior.

psychoneurosis—See **neurosis**.

psychoneurotic—Having to do with a psychoneurosis.

psychopathologic(al)—Pertaining to the pathology of mental disorders.

psychosomatic—Bodily symptoms arising from emotional or mental origin.

radial pulse—The pulse felt at the wrist and arising from the radial artery.

radicular neuralgia—A type of neuralgia ("nerve pain") where the pain follows the path or distribution of a specific nerve.

radiculitis—Inflammation of a spinal nerve.

radiologic(al)—Having to do with radiology.

radiology—The study of uses of radiant energy to diagnose disease.

radionuclide—A substance that contains a specific element that gives off radiation at a known rate.

radiopaque—The quality of a substance that does not allow X-rays to pass through readily and produces a white image (ie, the appearance of bone) on the X-ray.

roentgen—The measurement unit of X-ray radiation.

roentgenogram—An X-ray image.

roentgenographic—Having to do with X-ray images.

roentgenographic studies—See **roentgenogram**.

roentgenography—The production of an X-ray film. Also referred to as *radiography*.

sacral—Having to do with the sacrum.

sacrum—The triangular bone at the end of the last lumbar vertebrae and formed by 5 fused vertebrae.

scintigraphic—Having to do with scintigraphy.

scintigraphy—The use of radionuclides to produce an image.

sequelae—In medicine, any lesions or results upon the person following from an injury, illness, disease, or other such factor.

shoulder girdle—A group of bones that forms the major skeletal support for the muscles and soft tissues around the upper back and shoulders.

single photon emission computed tomography—See **SPECT**.

soft diet—A diet consisting mainly of semisolid foods requiring little or no chewing before swallowing.

soft tissues—A general term referring to such tissues as fat, muscle, ligaments, tendons, and nervous tissue, as opposed to bones.

soma—The body as distinguished from the mind.

somatic—Pertaining to or characteristic of the body or *soma*.

somatoform disorder—See **Chapter 10**.

SPECT (single photon emission computed tomography)—A scan formed by passing the energy of a particle of light (a photon) through tissues onto a detector.

spinal canal—The canal running through the center of the vertebrae and holding the spinal cord. Also called *vertebral canal*.

spinal meningeal branches—The blood vessel branches that supply the membranes lining the spinal cord.

spinous process—A slender, bony projection from the vertebrae. These are the only parts of the spine that can be felt through the skin.

spondylarthritis—Arthritis of the spine. Also called *spondyloarthritis*.

spondylochondrosis—See **spondylosis**.

spondylosis—A general term for degenerative changes of the spine.

spondylosis cervicalis—Spondylosis in the cervical spine. See **spondylosis**.

spontaneous extensor recoil—A nebulous term sometimes used to describe the reflex contraction of the posterior neck muscles in response to sudden neck flexion.

spur—In medicine, a sharp, bony projection.

sternocleidomastoid—One of the anterior neck muscles, largely responsible for turning the head left and right.

subclavian artery—The main artery underlying the clavicle (collarbone).

subluxation—Partial dislocation.

syndrome—A set of symptoms that when grouped identify a distinct illness pattern.

synovial—Pertaining to the synovium.

synovial joint—A specific type of joint where there is a joint capsule and an inner layer of synovium.

synovium—The innermost lining of certain joints; it produces the lubricating and nutrient joint fluid.

temporal bone—One of a pair of bones of the skull, lying in the region commonly referred to as the *temples*.

temporomandibular joint—The joint formed by the articulation of the temporal and mandibular bones, forming the active joint of the mouth as it opens and closes.

thermography—A technique wherein an infrared camera is used to portray the surface temperatures of the body photographically, based on the self-emanating infrared radiation.

thoracic spine—That part of the spine lying between the cervical and lumbar spine and having 12 vertebrae.

thoracic vertebra—One of the vertebrae in the thoracic spine.

thyroid cartilage—The cartilage making up the larynx, or "voice box," in the neck. "Adam's apple."

vascular—Having to do with blood vessels.

vertebral disc—See **intervertebral disc**.

vertigo—The sensation that one's environment is spinning (*objective vertigo*) or that one's body is spinning and the environment is remaining still (*subjective vertigo*).

vestibular—Having to do with a vestibule.

vestibule—A space or cavity to the entrance of a canal (eg, vestibular canals in the inner ear used for balance).

Index